PARASITOLOGY: A CONCEPTUAL APPROACH

Edited by
Patricia Marques

ArclerPress

Parasitology: A Conceptual Approach

Edited by Patricia Marques

Edition 2018

ArclerPress

Published by
Arcler Press LLC
708 3rd Avenue, 6th Floor
New York
NY 10017
United States of America
www.arclerpress.com

ISBN: 978-1-68094-531-7 (Hardback)

Printed in United States of America

Library of Congress Control Number: 2017933108

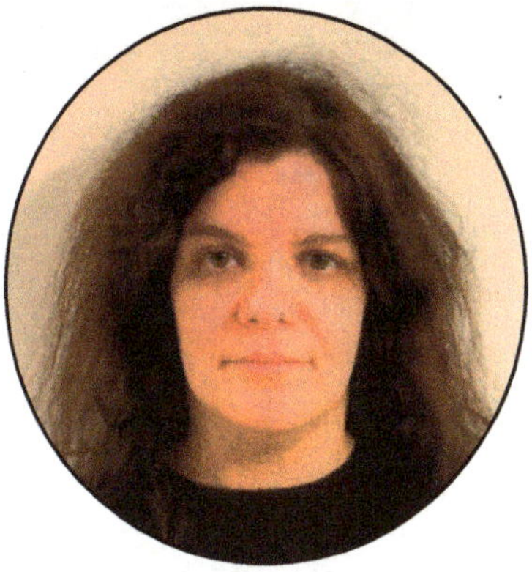

About the Editor

Patricia Marques

Patricia obtained her PhD form University College Dublin in 2010. Her interests are on Microbiology and Parasitology. She is currently working as a Postdoc at University of Maryland Baltimore, USA on Chlamydia infections.

Table of Contents

3 PROTOZOAN PARASITES

4 HELMINTHS

5 VETERINARY PARASITOLOGY

6 HUMAN PARASITOLOGY

7 NEGLECTED PARASITES

8 QUANTITATIVE PARASITOLOGY

9 BROOD PARASITES

List of Abbreviations

ALA	alpha-Linolenic acid
AI	Artificial insemination
BAC	blood alcohol concentration
CAMRA	Campaign for Real Ale
CDC	Centers for Disease Control
CMA	Cow's milk allergy
DRI	daily recommended intake
ESL	extended shelf life
FDA	Food and Drug Administration
HTST	high temperature short time
IGF-1	insulin-like growth factor-1
IBU	International Bitterness Units scale
LIBS	laser induced breakdown spectroscopy
MVH	Microwave volumetric heating
MESA	Multi-Ethnic Study of Atherosclerosis
PMO	Pasteurized Milk Ordinance
UHT	ultra-heat treatment
UV	Ultraviolet
VM	voluntary milking

Preface

Parasitology is the study of parasites, their hosts, and the relationship between them. As a biological discipline, the scope of parasitology is not determined by the organism or environment in question, but by their way of life. This means it forms a synthesis of other disciplines, and draws on techniques from fields such as cell biology, bioinformatics, biochemistry, molecular biology, immunology, genetics, evolution and ecology. Medical parasitology traditionally has included the study of three major groups of animals: parasitic protozoa, parasitic helminths (worms), and those arthropods that directly cause disease or act as vectors of various pathogens. A parasite is a pathogen that simultaneously injures and derives sustenance from its host. Some organisms called parasites are actually commensals, in that they neither benefit nor harm their host (for example, Entamoeba coli). Although parasitology had its origins in the zoologic sciences, it is today an interdisciplinary field, greatly influenced by microbiology, immunology, biochemistry, and other life sciences. Infections of humans caused by parasites number in the billions and range from relatively innocuous to fatal. The diseases caused by these parasites constitute major human health problems throughout the world. (For example, approximately 30 percent of the world's population is infected with the nematode Ascaris lumbricoides.) The incidence of many parasitic diseases (e.g., schistosomiasis, malaria) have increased rather than decreased in recent years. Other parasitic illnesses have increased in importance as a result of the AIDS epidemic (e.g., cryptosporidiosis, Pneumocystis carinii pneumonia, and strongyloidiasis). The migration of parasite-infected people, including refugees, from areas with high prevalence rates of parasitic infection also has added to the health problems of certain countries. In this book, several deal with the structure and classification of parasites and the mechanisms of parasitic diseases. The remaining chapters describe the specific human parasites and the diseases they cause. Emphasis is placed throughout on the basic biology of the pathogens and their host-parasite relationships. Thus, descriptions of the basic properties of the pathogens, the pathogenesis of the diseases they cause, host defenses, and epidemiology are highlighted.

Content Coverage

Chapter One presents the theory of parasitism is a non-mutual symbiotic relationship between species, where one species, the parasite, benefits at the expense of the other, the host.

Chapter Two presents an emphasis on history and life cycle of parasites.

Chapter Three focuses on the characteristics and classification of Protozoan parasites.

Chapter Four discusses about helminths, also commonly known as parasitic worms, are large multicellular organisms, which when mature can generally be seen with the naked eye. They are often referred to as intestinal worms even though not all helminths reside in the intestines; for example schistosomes are not intestinal worms, but rather reside in blood vessels.

Chapter Five presents the study of the genesis and development of parasitoses in animal hosts, as well as the taxonomy and systematics of parasites, including the morphology, life cycles, and living needs of parasites in the environment and in animal hosts.

Chapter Six presents the information of parasitic diseases caused by infestation (infection) with parasites such as protozoa (one-celled animals), worms, or insects.

Chapter Seven is about the neglected tropical diseases (NTDs) caused by neglected parasites, which are especially common in low-income populations in developing regions of Africa, Asia, and the Americas.

Chapter Eight discusses the quantitative study of parasitism in a host population that involves the use of statistics to draw meaningful conclusions from observations of the prevalence and intensity of parasitic infection.

Chapter Nine provides the knowledge of brood parasites that rely on others to raise their young. Brood parasitism relieves the parasitic parents from the investment of rearing young or building nests for the young, enabling them to spend more time on other activities such as foraging and producing further offspring.

Chapter Ten is about obligate parasites that is advantageous for the parasite to preserve the health of their host when this is compatible with their nutritional and reproductive requirements, except when the death of the host is necessary for transmission.

CHAPTER 1

Parasitism

Chapter Contents

Parasitism describes a relationship between two organisms where one benefits, and the other is harmed. The parasite is the organism that benefits from the relationship, while the host is harmed by the relationship. Parasites can be a number of things including plants, animals and even viruses and bacteria.

It is useful to know about parasitism because, technically, anything that is benefited while we are harmed is considered a parasite. Yes, that pesky mosquito that keeps biting you just gained an official title. While some of the parasites that affect humans can be a nuisance, such as lice or bedbugs, there are other parasites that can make us really sick, such as a bite from a tick, which can cause Lyme disease, or giardia, which we ingest by drinking contaminated water.

INTRODUCTION

In biology/ecology, parasitism is a non-mutual symbiotic relationship between species, where one species, the parasite, benefits at the expense of the other, the host. Traditionally parasite (in biological usage) referred primarily to organisms visible to the naked eye, or macroparasites (such as helminths). Parasites can be microparasites, which are typically smaller, such as protozoa, viruses, and bacteria. Examples of parasites include the plants mistletoe and cuscuta, and animals such as hookworms.

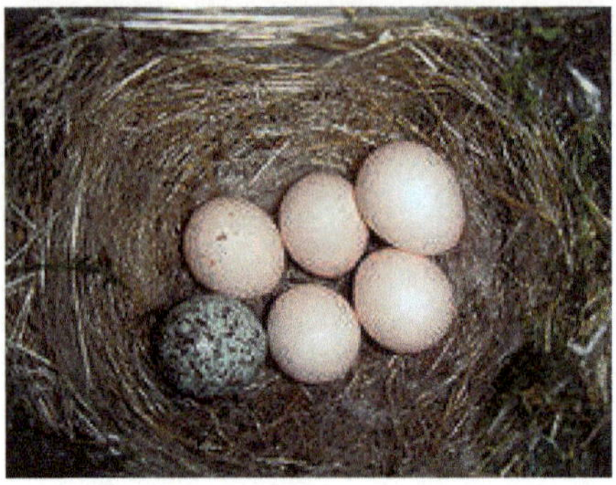

Brood parasitism is a form of parasitism.

A *Tetragnatha montana* spider parasitised by an *Acrodactyla quadrisculpta* larva

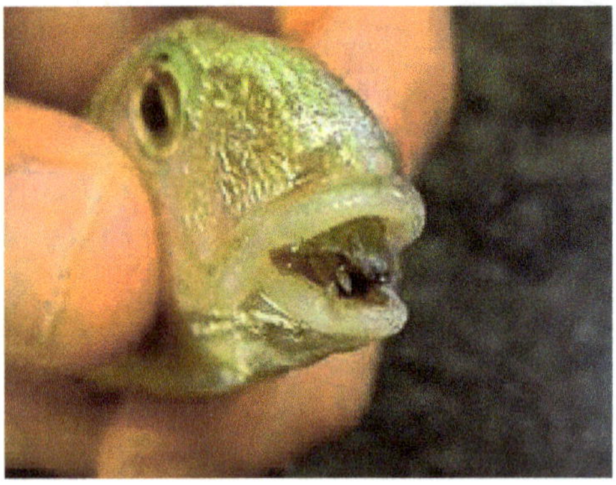

A *Lithognathus* fish parasitised by a *Cymothoa exigua* parasite

Unlike predators, parasites typically do not kill their host, are generally much smaller than their host, and will often live in or on their host for an extended period. Both are special cases of consumer-resource interactions. Parasites show a high degree of specialization, and reproduce at a faster rate than their hosts. Classic examples of parasitism include interactions between vertebrate hosts and tapeworms, flukes, the *Plasmodium* species, and fleas. Parasitism differs from the parasitoid relationship in that parasitoids generally kill their hosts.

Parasites reduce host biological fitness by general or specialized pathology, such as parasitic castration and impairment of secondary sex characteristics, to the modification of host behavior. Parasites increase their own fitness by exploiting hosts for resources necessary for their survival, e.g. food, water, heat, habitat, and transmission. Although parasitism applies unambiguously to many cases, it is part of a continuum of types of interactions between species, rather than an exclusive category. In many cases, it is difficult to demonstrate harm to the host. In others, there may be no apparent specialization on the part of the parasite, or the interaction between the organisms may remain short-lived.

ETYMOLOGY

First used in English 1539, the word *parasite* comes from the Medieval French *parasite*, from the Latin *parasitus*, the latinisation of the Greek ϖαράσιτος (*parasitos*), "one who eats at the table of another" and that from ϖαρά (*para*), "beside, by" + σῖτος (*sitos*), "wheat". Coined in English in 1611, the word *parasitism* comes from the Greek ϖαρά (*para*) + σιτισμός (*sitismos*) "feeding, fattening". In its original sense, it was not strictly pejorative in nature; being a *parasitos* was an accepted lifestyle, whereby a person could live off the hospitality of others, and in return provide "flattery, simple services, and a willingness to endure humiliation".

TYPES OF PARASITES

Parasites are classified based on their interactions with their hosts and on their life cycles. An obligate parasite is totally dependent on the host to complete its life cycle, while a facultative parasite is not. A direct parasite has only one host while an indirect parasite has multiple hosts. For indirect parasites, there will always be a definitive host and an intermediate host.

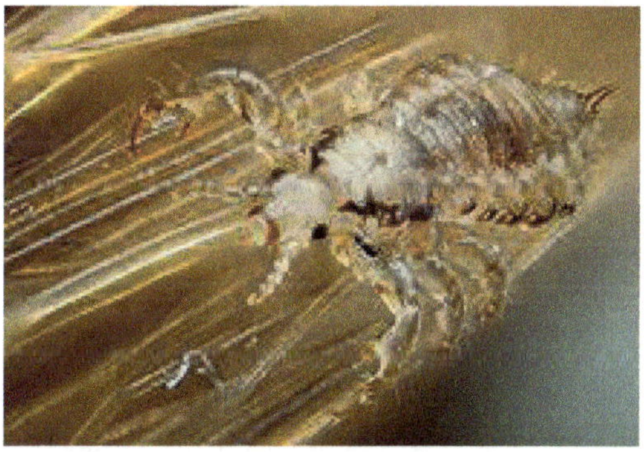

Human head lice (*Pediculus humanus capitis*) are ectoparasites.

Parasites that live on the outside of the host, either on the skin or the outgrowths of the skin, are called ectoparasites (e.g. lice, fleas, and some mites).

Those that live inside the host are called endoparasites (including all parasitic worms). Endoparasites can exist in one of two forms: intercellular parasites (inhabiting spaces in the host's body) or intracellular parasites (inhabiting cells in the host's body). Intracellular parasites, such as protozoa, bacteria or viruses, tend to rely on a third organism, which is generally known as the carrier or vector. The vector does the job of transmitting them to the host. An example of this interaction is the transmission of malaria, caused by a protozoan of the genus *Plasmodium*, to humans by the bite of an anopheline mosquito.

Those parasites living in an intermediate position, being half-ectoparasites and half-endoparasites, are called mesoparasites.

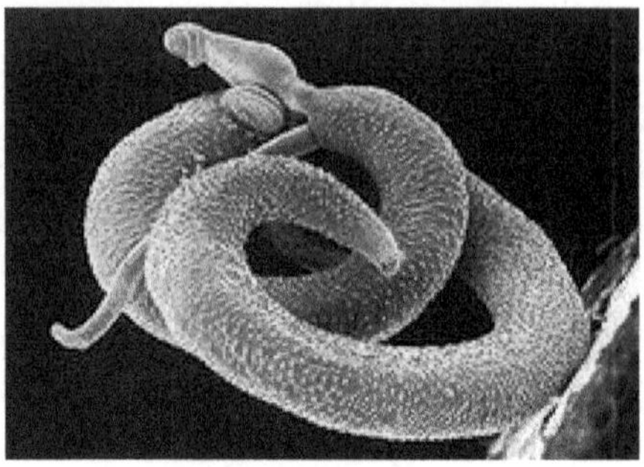

Schistosoma mansoni is an endoparasite that lives in human blood vessels.

An epiparasite is one that feeds on another parasite. This relationship is also sometimes referred to as *hyperparasitism,* exemplified by a protozoan (the hyperparasite) living in the digestive tract of a flea living on a dog.

Social parasites take advantage of interactions between members of social organisms such as ants, termites, and bumblebees. Examples include *Phengaris arion*, a butterfly whose larvae employ mimicry to parasitize certain species of ants, *Bombus bohemicus*, a bumblebee who invades the hives of other species of bee and takes over reproduction, their young raised by host workers, and *Melipona scutellaris,* a eusocial bee where virgin queens escape killer workers and invade another colony without a queen. An extreme example of social parasitism is the ant species of *Tetramorium inquilinum* of the Alps, which spend their whole lives on the back of *Tetramorium* host ants. With tiny and deprecated bodies they have evolved for one single task: holding on to their host. If they fall off, they most likely would not have the strength to climb back on top of another ant, and eventually they will die.

In kleptoparasitism (from the Greek κλέπτης (kleptes), thief), parasites appropriate food gathered by the host. An example is the brood parasitism practiced by cowbirds, whydahs, cuckoos, and black-headed ducks which do not build nests of their own and leave their eggs in nests of other species. The host behaves as a "babysitter" as they raise the young as their own. If the host removes the cuckoo's eggs, some cuckoos will return and attack the nest to compel host birds to remain subject to this parasitism.

Intraspecific social parasitism may also occur. One example of this is *parasitic nursing*, where some individuals take milk from unrelated females. In wedge-capped capuchins, higher ranking females sometimes take milk from low ranking females without any reciprocation. The high ranking females benefit at the expense of the low ranking females.

Parasitism can take the form of isolated *cheating* or *exploitation* among more generalized mutualistic interactions. For example, broad classes of plants and fungi exchange carbon and nutrients in common mutualistic mycorrhizal relationships; however, some plant species known as myco-heterotrophs "cheat" by taking carbon from a fungus rather than donating it.

An adelpho-parasite (from the Greek αδελφός (adelphos), brother) is a parasite in which the host species is closely related to the parasite, often being a member of the same family or genus. An example of this is the citrus blackfly parasitoid, *Encarsia perplexa*, unmated females of which may lay haploid eggs in the fully developed larvae of their own species. These result in the production of male offspring. The marine worm *Bonellia viridis* has a similar reproductive strategy, although the larvae are planktonic.

Autoinfection is the infection of a primary host with a parasite, particularly a helminth, in such a way that the complete life cycle of the parasite happens in a single organism, without the involvement of another host. Therefore, the primary host is at the same time the secondary host of the parasite. Some of the organisms where autoinfection occurs are *Strongyloides stercoralis*, *Enterobius vermicularis*, *Taenia solium*, and *Hymenolepis nana*. Strongyloidiasis for example involves premature transformation of noninfective larvae in infective larvae, which can then penetrate the intestinal mucosa (internal autoinfection) or the skin of the perineal area (external autoinfection). Infection can be maintained by repeated migratory cycles for the remainder of the person's life.

HOST DEFENSES

Animal defenses

Skin

The first line of defense against invading parasites is the skin. Skin is made up of layers of dead cells and acts as a physical barrier to invading organisms. These dead cells contain the protein keratin, which makes skin tough and waterproof. Most microorganisms needs a moist environment to survive. By keeping the skin dry, it prevents invading organisms from colonizing. Furthermore, human skin also secretes sebum, which is toxic to most microorganisms.

Mouth

The mouth contains saliva, which prevents foreign organisms from getting into the body orally. Furthermore, the mouth also contains lysozyme, an enzyme found in tears and the saliva. This enzyme breaks down cell walls of invading microorganisms.

Stomach

Should the organism pass the mouth, the stomach is the next line of defense. The stomach contains hydrochloric acid and gastric acids, which makes its pH level around 2. In this environment, the acidity of the stomach helps kill most microorganisms that try to invade the body through the gastric intestinal tract.

Eyes

Parasites can also invade the body through the eyes. The lashes on the eyelid prevents invading microorganisms from entering the eye in the first place. Even if the microorganism does get into the eye, tears contain the enzyme lysozyme, which will kill most invading microorganisms.

Immune System

Should the parasite enter the body, the immune system is a vertebrate's major defense against parasitic invasion. The immune system is made up of different families of molecules. These include serum proteins and pattern recognition receptors (PRRs). PRRs are intracellular and cellular receptors that activate dendritic cells, which in turn activate the adaptive immune system's lymphocytes. Lymphocytes such as the T cells and antibody producing B cells with variable receptors that recognize parasites.

Insect Defenses

Insects often adapt their nests to aid in parasite defense. For example, one of the key reasons the *Polistes canadensis* nests across multiple combs rather than building a single comb like much of the rest of its genus is as a defense mechanism against the infestation of tineid moths. The tineid moth lays its eggs within the wasps' nests and then these eggs hatch into larvae that can burrow from cell to cell and prey on wasp pupae. Adult wasps attempt to remove and kill moth eggs and larvae by chewing down the edges of cells, coating the cells with an oral secretion that gives the nest a dark brownish appearance.

Plant Defenses

In response to parasitic attack, plants undergo a series of metabolic and biochemical reaction pathways that will enact defensive responses. For example, parasitic invasion causes an increase in the jasmonic acid-insensitivel (JA) and NahG (SA) pathway. These pathways produce chemicals that induce defensive responses, such as the production of chemicals or defensive molecules to fight off the attack. Different biochemical pathways are activated by different parasites. In general, there are two types of responses that can be activated by the pathways. Plants can either initiate a specific or non-specific response. Specific responses involve gene-gene recognition of the plant and parasite. This can be mediated by the ability of the plant's cell receptors recognizing and binding molecules that are located on the cell surface of parasites. Once the plant's receptors recognizes the parasite, the plant localizes the defensive compounds to that area creating a hypersensitive response. This form of defense mechanism localizes the area of attack and keeps the parasite from spreading. Furthermore, a specific response against parasitic attack prevents the plants from wasting its energy by increasing defenses where it's not need. However, specific defensive responses only target specific parasites. If the plant lacks the ability to recognize a parasite, specific defense responses won't be activated. Nonspecific defensive responses work against all parasites. These responses are active over time and are systematic, meaning that the responses are not confined to an area of the plant, but rather spread throughout the entirety of the organism. However, nonspecific responses are energy costly, since the plant has to ensure that the genes producing the nonspecific responses are always expressed.

EVOLUTIONARY ASPECTS

Parasitism has arisen independently many times. Depending on the definition used, as many as half of all animals have at least one parasitic phase in their life cycles, and is frequent in plants and fungi. Almost all free-living animals are host to one or more parasitic taxa.

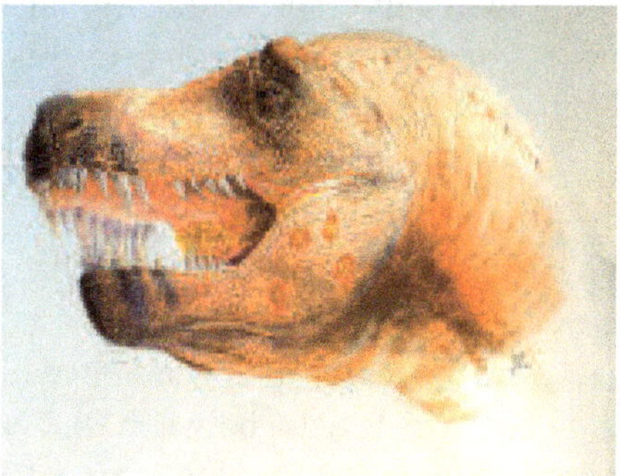

Restoration of a *Tyrannosaurus* with parasite infections. A 2009 study showed that holes in the skulls of several specimens might have been caused by *Trichomonas*-like parasites

Parasites evolve in response to their hosts' defences, sometimes in a manner specific to a particular host taxon and specializing to the point where they infect only a single species. Such narrow host specificity can be costly over evolutionary time, however, if the host species becomes extinct. Therefore, many parasites can infect a variety of more or less closely related host species, with different success rates.

In turn, host defenses coevolve in response to attacks by parasites. Theoretically, parasites may have an advantage in this evolutionary arms race because their generation time commonly is shorter. Hosts reproduce less quickly than parasites, and therefore have fewer chances to adapt than their parasites do over a given span of time.

Long-term coevolution sometimes leads to a relatively stable relationship tending to commensalism or mutualism, as, all else being equal, it is in the evolutionary interest of the parasite that its host thrives. A parasite may evolve to become less harmful for its host or a host may evolve to cope with the unavoidable presence of a parasite—to the point that the parasite's absence causes the host harm. For example, although animals infected with parasitic worms are often clearly harmed, and therefore parasitized, such infections may also reduce the prevalence and effects of autoimmune disorders in animal hosts, including humans. In a more extreme example, some nematode worms cannot reproduce, or even survive, without infection by Wolbachia bacteria.

Competition between parasites tends to favor faster reproducing and therefore more virulent parasites. Parasites whose life cycle involves the death of the host, to exit the present host and sometimes to enter the next, evolve to be more virulent or even alter the behavior or other properties of the host to make it more vulnerable to predators. Parasites that reproduce largely to the offspring of the previous host tend to become less virulent or mutualist, so that its hosts reproduce more effectively.

The presumption of a shared evolutionary history between parasites and hosts can sometimes elucidate how host taxa are related. For instance, there has been dispute about whether flamingos are more closely related to the storks and their relatives, or to ducks, geese and their relatives. The fact that flamingos share parasites with ducks and geese is evidence these groups may be more closely related to each other than either is to storks.

Parasitism is part of one explanation for the evolution of secondary sex characteristics seen in breeding males throughout the animal world, such as the plumage of male peacocks and manes of male lions. According to this theory, female hosts select males for breeding based on such characteristics because they indicate resistance to parasites and other disease.

Co-speciation

In rare cases, a parasite may even undergo co-speciation with its host. One particularly remarkable example of co-speciation exists between the simian foamy virus (SFV) and its primate hosts. In one study, the phylogenies of SFV polymerase and the mitochondrial cytochrome oxidase subunit II from African and Asian primates were compared. Surprisingly, the phylogenetic trees were very congruent in branching order and divergence times. Thus, the simian foamy viruses may have co-speciated with Old World primates for at least 30 million years.

Evolutionary events like host switch, host shift, the duplication or extinction of parasite species (without similar events on the host phylogeny) often erode topographical similarities between host and parasite phylogenies.

ECOLOGY

Quantitative Ecology

A single parasite species usually has an aggregated distribution across host individuals, which means that most hosts harbor few parasites, while a few hosts carry the vast majority of parasite individuals. This poses considerable problems for students of parasite ecology: the use of parametric statistics should be avoided. Log-transformation of data before the application of parametric test, or the use of non-parametric statistics is recommended by several authors. However, this can give rise to further problems. Therefore, modern day quantitative parasitology is based on more advanced biostatistical methods.

Diversity ecology

Hosts represent discrete habitat patches that can be occupied by parasites. A hierarchical set of terminology has come into use to describe parasite assemblages at different host scales.

The diversity ecology of parasites differs markedly from that of free-living organisms. For free-living organisms, diversity ecology features many strong conceptual frameworks including Robert MacArthur and E. O. Wilson's theory of island biogeography, Jared Diamond's assembly rules and, more recently, null models such as Stephen Hubbell's unified neutral theory of biodiversity and biogeography. Frameworks are not so well-developed for parasites and in many ways they do not fit the free-living models. For example, island biogeography is predicated on fixed spatial relationships between habitat patches ("sinks"), usually with reference to a mainland ("source"). Parasites inhabit hosts, which represent mobile habitat patches with dynamic spatial relationships. There is no true "mainland" other than the sum of hosts (host population), so parasite component communities in host populations are metacommunities.

Nonetheless, different types of parasite assemblages have been recognized in host individuals and populations, and many of the patterns observed for free-living organisms are also pervasive among parasite assemblages. The most prominent of these is the interactive-isolationist continuum. This proposes that parasite assemblages occur along a cline from interactive communities, where niches are saturated and interspecific competition is high, to isolationist communities, where there are many vacant niches and interspecific interaction is not as important as stochastic factors in providing structure to the community. Whether this is so, or whether community patterns simply reflect the sum of underlying species distributions (no real "structure" to the community), has not yet been established.

ADAPTATION

Parasites infect hosts that exist within their same geographical area (sympatric) more effectively. This phenomenon supports the "Red Queen hypothesis—which states that interactions between species (such as host and parasites) lead to constant natural selection for adaptation and counter adaptation." The parasites track the locally common host phenotypes, therefore the parasites are less infective to allopatric (from different geographical region) hosts.

Experiments published in 2000 discuss the analysis of two different snail populations from two different sources—Lake Ianthe and Lake Poerua in New Zealand. The populations were exposed to two pure parasites (digenetic trematode) taken from the same lakes. In the experiment, the snails were infected by their sympatric parasites, allopatric parasites and mixed sources of parasites. The results suggest that the parasites were more highly effective in infecting their sympatric snails than their allopatric snails. Though the allopatric snails were still infected by the parasites, the infectivity was much less when compared to the sympatric snails. Hence, the parasites were found to have adapted to infecting local populations of snails.

Transmission

Parasites have a variety of methods to infect hosts. For example, the *Acanthamoeba* enters the body when the environment is not hostile, and *Strongyloides stercoralis* enters the body when a host steps on infected ground while barefoot. Many parasites enter the food of their hosts and wait to be eaten. *Plasmodium malariae* uses a mosquito host to transmit malaria, and *Loa loa* parasites use deer flies to enter hosts.

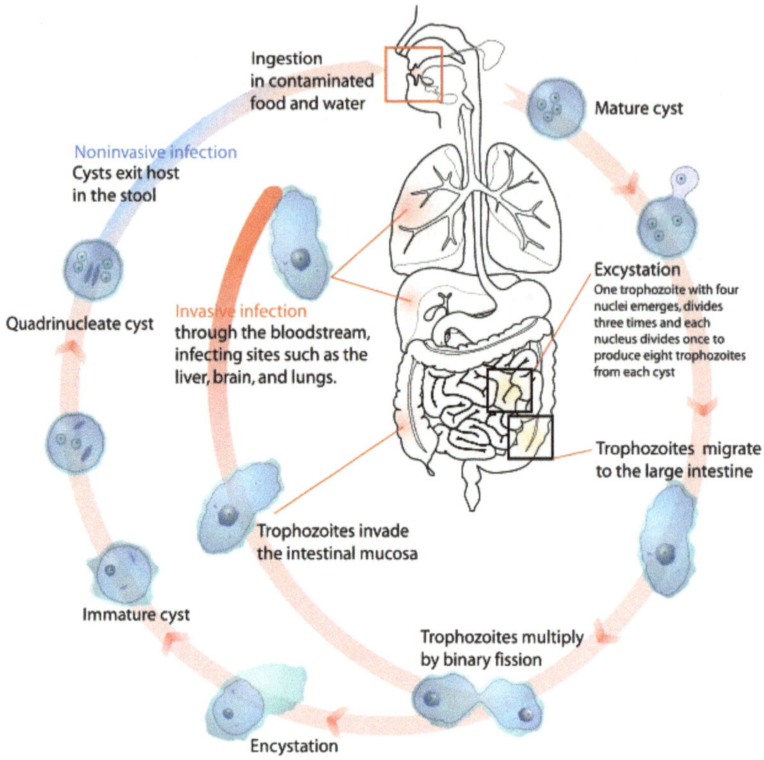

Life cycle of *Entamoeba histolytica*, an anaerobic parasitic protozoan.

Parasites inhabit living organisms and therefore face problems that free-living organisms do not. Hosts, the only habitats in which parasites can survive, actively try to avoid, repel, and destroy parasites. Parasites employ numerous strategies for getting from one host to another, a process sometimes referred to as parasite *transmission* or *colonization*.

Some endoparasites infect their host by penetrating its external surface, while others must be ingested. Once inside the host, adult endoparasites need to shed offspring into the external environment to infect other hosts. Many adult endoparasites reside in the host's gastrointestinal tract, where offspring can be shed along with host excreta. Adult stages of tapeworms, thorny-headed worms and most flukes use this method.

Among protozoan endoparasites, such as the malarial parasites and trypanosomes, infective stages in the host's blood are transported to new hosts by biting-insects, or vectors.

Larval stages of endoparasites often infect sites in the host other than the blood or gastrointestinal tract. In many such cases, larval endoparasites require their host to be consumed by the next host in the parasite's life cycle in order to survive and reproduce. Alternatively, larval endoparasites may shed free-living transmission stages that migrate through the host's tissue into the external environment, where they actively search for or await ingestion by other hosts. The foregoing strategies are used, variously, by larval stages of tapeworms, thorny-headed worms, flukes and parasitic roundworms.

Some ectoparasites, such as monogenean worms, rely on direct contact between hosts. Ectoparasitic arthropods may rely on host-host contact (e.g. many lice), shed eggs that survive off the host (e.g. fleas), or wait in the external environment for an encounter with a host (e.g. ticks). Some aquatic leeches locate hosts by sensing movement and only attach when certain temperature and chemical cues are present.

Some parasites modify host behavior in order to increase the transmission between hosts, often in relation to predator and prey (parasite increased trophic transmission). For example, in California salt marshes, the fluke *Euhaplorchis californiensis* reduces the ability of its killifish host to avoid predators. This parasite matures in egrets, which are more likely to feed on infected killifish than on uninfected fish. Another example is the protozoan *Toxoplasma gondii*, a parasite that matures in cats but can be carried by many other mammals. Uninfected rats avoid cat odors, but rats infected with *T. gondii* are drawn to this scent, which may increase transmission to feline hosts.

Roles in Ecosystems

Modifying the behavior of infected hosts, to make transmission to other hosts more likely to occur, is one way parasites can affect the structure of ecosystems. For example, in the case of *Euhaplorchis californiensis* (discussed above) it is plausible that the local predator and prey species might be different if this parasite were absent from the system.

Although parasites are often omitted in depictions of food webs, they usually occupy the top position. Parasites can function like keystone species, reducing the dominance of superior competitors and allowing competing species to co-exist. Many parasites require multiple hosts of the different species to complete their life cycles and rely on predator-prey or other stable ecological interactions to get from one host to another. In this sense, the parasites in an ecosystem reflect the health of that system.

Although parasites are generally considered to be harmful, the eradication of all parasites would not necessarily be beneficial. Parasites account for as much as or more than half of life's diversity; they perform an important ecological role (by weakening prey) that ecosystems would take some time to adapt to; and without parasites organisms may eventually tend to asexual reproduction, diminishing the diversity of sexually dimorphic traits. Parasites provide an opportunity for the transfer of genetic material between species. On rare, but significant, occasions this may facilitate evolutionary changes that would not otherwise occur, or that would otherwise take even longer.

PHYLUM

In biology, a **phylum** is a taxonomic rank below kingdom and above class. Traditionally, in botany the term division was used instead of "phylum", although from 1993 the International Code of Nomenclature for algae, fungi, and plants accepted the designation "phylum". The kingdom Animalia contains approximately 35 phyla, Plantae contains 12, and Fungi contains 7. Current research in phylogenetics is uncovering the relationships between phyla, which are contained in larger clades, like Ecdysozoa and Embryophyta.

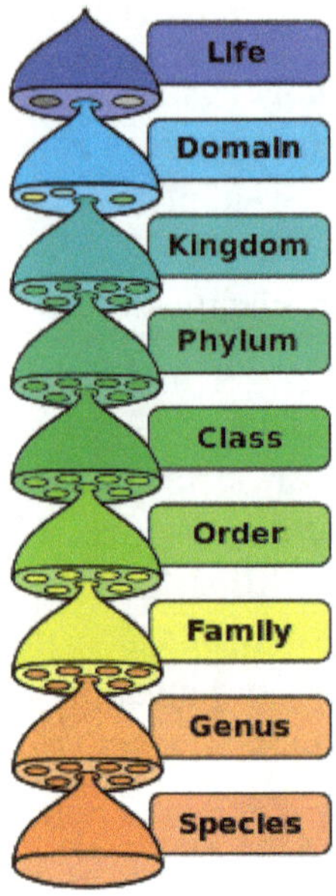

The hierarchy of biological classification's eight major taxonomic ranks. A kingdom contains one or more phyla. Intermediate minor rankings are not shown.

General Description and Familiar Examples

The definitions of zoological phyla have changed importantly from their origins in the six Linnaean classes and the four "embranchements" of Georges Cuvier. Haeckel introduced the term *phylum*, based on the Greek word *phylon* ('tribe' or 'stock'). In plant taxonomy, Eichler (1883) classified plants into five groups, named divisions.

Informally, phyla can be thought of as grouping organisms based on general specialization of body plan. At its most basic, a phylum can be defined in two ways: as a group of organisms with a certain degree of morphological or developmental similarity (the phenetic definition), or a group of organisms with a certain degree of evolutionary relatedness (the phylogenetic definition). Attempting to define a level of the Linnean hierarchy without referring to (evolutionary) relatedness is unsatisfactory, but a phenetic definition is useful when addressing questions of a morphological nature—such as how successful different body plans were.

Definition

The most important objective measure in the above definitions is the "certain degree"—how unrelated do organisms need to be to be members of different phyla? The minimal requirement is that all organisms in a phylum should be clearly more closely related to one another than to any other group. Even this is problematic because the requirement depends on knowledge of organisms' relationships: as more data become available, particularly from molecular studies, we are better able to judge the relationships between groups. So phyla can be merged or split if it becomes apparent that they are related to one another or not. For example, the bearded worms were described as a new phylum (the Pogonophora) in the middle of the 20th century, but molecular work almost half a century later found them to be a group of annelids, so the phyla were merged (the bearded worms are now an annelid family). On the other hand, the highly parasitic phylum Mesozoa was divided into two phyla, Orthonectida and Rhombozoa, when it was discovered the Orthonectida are probably deuterostomes and the Rhombozoa protostomes.

This changeability of phyla has led some biologists to call for the concept of a phylum to be abandoned in favour of cladistics, a method in which groups are placed on a "family tree" without any formal ranking of group size.

Definition based on Body Plan

A definition of a phylum based on body plan has been proposed by paleontologists Graham Budd and Sören Jensen (as Haeckel had done a century earlier). The definition was posited because extinct organisms are hardest to classify: they can be offshoots that diverged from a phylum's line before the characters that define the modern phylum were all acquired. By Budd and Jensen's definition, a phylum is defined by a set of characters shared by all its living representatives.

This approach brings some small problems—for instance, ancestral characters common to most members of a phylum may have been lost by some members. Also, this definition is based on an arbitrary point of time: the present. However, as it is character based, it is easy to apply to the fossil record. A greater problem is that it relies on a subjective decision about which groups of organisms should be considered as phyla.

The approach is useful because it makes it easy to classify extinct organisms as "stem groups" to the phyla with which they bear the most resemblance, based only on the taxonomically important similarities. However, proving that a fossil belongs to the crown group of a phylum is difficult, as it must display a character unique to a sub-set of the crown group.Furthermore, organisms in the stem group of a phylum can possess the "body plan" of the phylum without all the characteristics necessary to fall within it.This weakens the idea that each of the phyla represents a distinct body plan.

A classification using this definition may be strongly affected by the chance survival of rare groups, which can make a phylum much more diverse than it would be otherwise. Representatives of many modern phyla did not appear until long *after* the Cambrian.

REFERENCES

1. Leong, K. L. H.; M. A. Yoshimura; H. K. Kaya; H. Williams (1997). "Instar Susceptibility of the Monarch Butterfly (Danaus plexippus) to the Neogregarine Parasite, Ophryocystis elektroscirrha". Journal of Invertebrate Pathology. 69 (1): 79–83. doi:10.1006/jipa.1996.4634. PMID 9028932.
2. Bartel, Rebecca; Oberhauser, Karen; De Roode, Jacob; Atizer, Sonya (February 2011). "Monarch butterfly migration and parasite transmission in eastern North America". Ecology. 92 (2): 342–351. doi:10.1890/10-0489.1. PMID 21618914.
3. Getz WM (2011). "Biomass transformation webs provide a unified approach to consumer-resource modelling". Ecol. Lett. 14 (2): 113–24. doi:10.1111/j.1461-0248.2010.01566.x. PMC 3032891. PMID 21199247.
4. Godfray HC (2004). "Parasitoids". Current Biology Magazine. 14 (12): R456. doi:10.1016/j.cub.2004.06.004. PMID 15203011.

5. H.Charles J Godfray (22 June 2004). "Parasitoids". Current Biology. Vol. 14 no. 2. p. R456. doi:10.1016/j.cub.2004.06.004.
6. Henry George Liddell, Robert Scott, A Greek-English Lexicon, on Perseus Digital Library
7. Toussaint-Samat, M. (2009) A History of Food. Wiley-Blackwell Publishers.
8. Donahue, J.F. (2014) Food and Drink in Antiquity: A Sourcebook: Readings from the Graeco-Roman World. Bloomsbury Publishers.
9. Garcia LS (1999). "Classification of Human Parasites, Vectors, and Similar Organisms" . Clin Infect Dis. 29 (4): 734–6. doi:10.1086/520425. PMID 10589879.
10. C.E. Hopla; L.A. Durden; J.E. Keirans. "Ectoparasites and classification" (PDF). Rev. sci. tech. Off. int. Epiz. 13 (4): 985–1017.
11. "Pathogenic Parasitic Infections". PEOI. Retrieved 2013-07-18.
12. Thomas JA, Schönrogge K, Bonelli S, Barbero F, Balletto E (2010). "Corruption of ant acoustical signals by mimetic social parasites: Maculinea butterflies achieve elevated status in host societies by mimicking the acoustics of queen ants". Commun Integr Biol. 3 (2): 169–71. doi:10.4161/cib.3.2.10603. PMC 2889977Freely accessible. PMID 20585513.
13. Van Oystaeyen, Annette; Araujo Alves, Denise; Caliari Oliveira, Ricardo; Lima do Nascimento, Daniela; Santos do Nascimento, Fábio; Billen, Johan; Wenseleers, Tom (2013-09-01). "Sneaky queens in Melipona bees selectively detect and infiltrate queenless colonies". Animal Behaviour. 86 (3): 603–609. doi:10.1016/j.anbehav.2013.07.001.
14. "Social Parasites in the Ant Colony". Antkeepers. Retrieved 4 April 2016.
15. "Bullies of the Bird World". National Wildlife Magazine. Aug/Sep 1997, Vol. 35 No. 5
16. O'Brien, Timothy G. (1988). "Parasitic nursing behavior in the wedge-capped capuchin monkey (Cebus olivaceus)". American Journal of Primatology. 16 (4): 341–344. doi:10.1002/ajp.1350160406.
17. Featured Creatures
18. Larry Gonick and Mark Wheelis, The Cartoon Guide to Genetics. HarperCollins, 1991.
19. "Host-Parasite Interactions Innate Defenses of the Host" (PDF). University of Colorado website.
20. Maizels RM (2009). "Parasite immunomodulation and polymorphisms of the immune system". J. Biol. 8 (7): 62. doi:10.1186/jbiol166. PMC 2736671. PMID 19664200.
21. Jeanne, Robert L. "Construction and Utilization of Multiple Combs in Polistes canadensis in Relation to the Biology of a Predaceous Moth." Behavioral Ecology and Sociobiology 4.3 (1979): 293-310.
22. Runyon JB, Mescher MC, De Moraes CM (2010). "Plant defenses against parasitic plants show similarities to those induced by herbivores and pathogens". Plant

Signal Behav. 5 (8): 929–31. doi:10.4161/psb.5.8.11772. PMC 3115164Freely accessible. PMID 20495380.

23. .Hatcher, J. M. & Dunn, M. A. (2011). Parasites in Ecological Communities. Cambridge, UK: Cambridge University Press.
24. Frank SA (2000). "Specific and non-specific defense against parasitic attack". J. Theor. Biol. 202 (4): 283–304. doi:10.1006/jtbi.1999.1054. PMID 10666361.
25. Price, P.W. 1980. Evolutionary Biology of Parasites. Princeton University Press, Princeton
26. Wolff, Ewan D. S.; Steven W. Salisbury; John R. Horner; David J. Varricchio (2009). Hansen, Dennis Marinus, ed. "Common Avian Infection Plagued the Tyrant Dinosaurs". PLoS ONE. 4 (9): e7288. doi:10.1371/journal.pone.0007288. PMC 2748709Freely accessible. PMID 19789646. .
27. Rook GA (2007). "The hygiene hypothesis and the increasing prevalence of chronic inflammatory disorders". Transactions of the Royal Society of Tropical Medicine and Hygiene. 101 (11): 1072–4. doi:10.1016/j.trstmh.2007.05.014. PMID 17619029.
28. Werren, John H. (February 2003). "Invasion of the Gender Benders: by manipulating sex and reproduction in their hosts, many parasites improve their own odds of survival and may shape the evolution of sex itself" (Reprint). Natural History. 112 (1): 58. ISSN 0028-0712. OCLC 1759475. Retrieved 15 November 2008.
29. Switzer WM, Salemi M, Shanmugam V, Gao F, Cong ME, Kuiken C, Bhullar V, Beer BE, Vallet D, Gautier-Hion A, Tooze Z, Villinger F, Holmes EC, Heneine W (2005). "Ancient co-speciation of simian foamy viruses and primates". Nature. 434 (7031): 376–80. doi:10.1038/nature03341. PMID 15772660.
30. Rózsa L, Reiczigel J, Majoros G (2000). "Quantifying parasites in samples of hosts". J. Parasitol. 86 (2): 228–32. doi:10.1645/0022-3395(2000)086[0228:QPISOH]2.0.CO;2. PMID 10780537.
31. Lively CM, Dybdahl MF (2000). "Parasite adaptation to locally common host genotypes". Nature. 405 (6787): 679–81. doi:10.1038/35015069. PMID 10864323.
32. Lafferty KD, Morris AK (1996). "Altered behavior of parasitized killifish increases susceptibility to predation by bird final hosts". Ecology. 77: 1390. doi:10.2307/2265536.
33. Berdoy M, Webster JP, Macdonald DW (2000). "Fatal attraction in rats infected with Toxoplasma gondii". Proc. Biol. Sci. 267 (1452): 1591–4. doi:10.1098/rspb.2000.1182. PMC 1690701Freely accessible. PMID 11007336.
34. Holt RD (2010). "IJEE Soapbox". Israel Journal of Ecology and Evolution. 56 (3): 239–250. doi:10.1560/IJEE.56.3-4.239.

CHAPTER 2

History and Life Cycle

Chapter Contents

- **Introduction**
- **History**
- **Most Common Parasites**
- **Endoparasites**
- **Taxonomy**

Parasites live in or on another organism called the host organism. They use the half-digested food that is found in their host's intestines as their own food supply. Parasites use host organisms for their nutrients and thrive in environments where they have a ready supply of food.

Parasites cause damage and destroy the tissues of their hosts as well as producing their own toxic waste products that can cause a whole range of unwanted and often debilitating health problems. Hosts suffer from discomforts, infections and disease as a result of parasitic infection.

INTRODUCTION

Human parasites include various protozoa and worms which may infect humans that cause parasitic diseases.

Human parasites are divided into endoparasites, which cause infection inside the body, and ectoparasites, which cause infection superficially within the skin.

The cysts and eggs of endoparasites may be found in feces which aids in the detection of the parasite in the human host while also providing the means for the parasitic species to exit the current host and enter other hosts.- Although there are number of ways in which humans can contract parasitic infections, observing basic hygiene and cleanliness tips can reduce its probability. The most accurate diagnosis is by qPcr DNA antigen assay, not generally available by primary care physicians in the USA: most labs offer research only service.

HISTORY

Archaeological Evidence

It was assumed that early human ancestors generally had parasites, but until recently there was no evidence to support this claim. Generally, the discovery of parasites in ancient humans relies on the study of feces and other fossilized material. The earliest known parasite in a human was eggs of the lung fluke found in fossilized feces in northern Chile and is estimated to be from around 5900BC. There are also claims of hookworm eggs from around 5000BC in Brazil and large roundworm eggs from around 2330BC in Peru. Tapeworm eggs have also been found present in Egyptian mummies dating from around 2000BC, 1250BC, and 1000BC along with a well preserved and calcified female worm inside of a mummy.

Written Evidence

The first written records of parasites date from 3000 to 400BC in Egyptian papyrus records. They identify parasites such as roundworms, Guinea worms, threadworms, and some tapeworms of unknown varieties. In ancient Greece, Hippocrates and Aristotle documented several parasites in his collection of works Corpus Hippocraticus. In this book, they documented the presence of worms and other parasites inside of fish, domesticated animals, and humans. The bladder worm is well documented in its presence in pigs along with the larval stages of a tapeworm (Taenia Solium). These tapeworms were mentioned in a play by Aristophanes as “hailstones” with Aristotle in the section about pig diseases in his book History of Animals. The cysts of the Echinococcus granulosus tapeworm were also well known in ancient cultures mainly because of their presence in slaughtered and sacrificed animals. The major parasitic disease which has been documented in early records is dracunculiasis. This disease is caused by the Guinea worm and is characterized by the female worm emerging from the leg. This symptom is so specific to the disease that it is mentioned in many texts and plays which predate 1000AD.

Greece and Rome

In Greece, Hippocrates and Aristotle created considerable medical documentation about parasites in the Corpus Hippocraticus. In this work, they documented the presence of parasitic worms in many animals ranging from fish to domesticated animals and humans. Among the most extensively documented was the Bladder Worm (Taenia solium). This condition was called “measly pork” when present in pigs and was characterized by the presence of the larval stages of the Bladder Worm in muscle tissue. This disease was also mentioned by the playwright Aristophanes when he referred to "hailstones" in one of his plays. This naming convention is also reflected by Aristotle when he refers to "bladders that are like hailstones." Another worm which was commonly written about in ancient Greek texts was the tapeworm Echinococccus granulosus. This worm was distinguished by the presence of "massive cysts" in the liver of animals. This condition was documented so well mainly because of its presence in slaughtered and sacrificed animals. It was documented by several different cultures of the time other than the Greeks including the Arabs, Romans, and Babylonians. Not many parasitic diseases were identified in ancient Greek and Roman texts mainly because the symptoms for parasitic diseases are shared with many other illnesses such as the flu, the common cold, and dysentery. However, several diseases such as Dracunculiasis (Guinea worm disease), Hookworm, Elephantiasis, Schistosomiasis, Malaria, and Amebiasis cause unique and specific symptoms and are well documented because of this. The most documented by far was Guinea worm disease mainly because the grown female worm emerges from the skin which causes considerable irritation and which cannot really be ignored. This particular disease is widely accepted to also be the "fiery serpents" written about in the Old Testament of the Bible. This disease was mentioned by Hippocrates in Greece along with Pliny the Elder, Galen, Aetius of Amida, and Paulus Aegineta of Alexandria in Rome. Strangely, this disease was never present in Greece even though it was documented.

Northern Africa, The Middle East, and Mesopotamia

The medieval Persian doctor Avicenna records the presence of several parasites in animals and in his patients including Guinea worm, threadworms, tapeworms, and the Ascaris worm. This followed a tradition of Arab medical writings spanning over 1000 years in the area near the Red Sea. However, the Arabs never made the connection between parasites and the diseases they caused. As with Greek and Roman texts, the Guinea worm is very well documented in Middle Eastern medical texts. Several Assyrian documents in the library of King Ashurbanipal refer to an affliction which has been interpreted as Guinea worm disease. In Egypt, the Ebers Papyrus contains one of the few references to hookworm disease in ancient texts. This disease does not have very specific symptoms and was vaguely mentioned. However vague the reference, it is one of the few that connect the disease to the hookworm parasite. Another documented disease is elephantiasis. Symptoms of this disease are highly visible, since it causes extreme swelling in the limbs, breasts, and genitals. A number of surviving statues indicate that Pharaoh Mentuhotep II is likely to have suffered from elephantiasis. This disease was well known to Arab physicians and Avicenna, who noted specific differences between elephantiasis and leprosy. That the disease schistosomiasis was extremely common in Ancient Egyptis suggested by mummified evidence, but it is not specifically documented in surviving texts. Other names for this disease include bilharzia, Katayama disease, Red Water fever, snail fever, and big belly. The only really defining symptom is bloody urine, but this can easily be overlooked as several other diseases exhibit the same symptom. However, the main reason it was not documented is probably because it was simply so common. In the same way, the Greeks and Romans did not acknowledge the existence of colds and coughs because of how common they were.

China

The Chinese mostly documented diseases rather than the parasites associated with them. Chinese texts contain one of the few references to Hookworm disease found in ancient records, but no connection to hookworm is made.[:174] The Emperor Huang Ti recorded the earliest mentioning (2700BC) of malaria in his text Nei Ching. He lists chills, headaches, and fevers as the main symptoms and distinguished between the different kinds of fevers.

India

In India, the Charaka Samhita and Sushruta Samhita document Malaria. These documents list the main symptoms as fever and enlarged spleens The Bhrigu Samhita from 1000 BCE makes the earliest reference to Amebiasis. The symptoms were given as bloody and mucosal diarrhea.

MOST COMMON PARASITES

As of 2013, the parasites causing the most deaths globally were as follows:

Parasitic Disease	**Global Deaths in 2013**
Malaria	854,600
Leishmaniasis (Kala-azar)	62,500
Cryptosporidiosis	41,900
Amoebiasis	11,300
Chagas disease	10,600
African Trypanosomiasis	6,900
Schistosomiasis	5,500
Ascariasis	4,500
Cystic Echinococcosis	2,200
Cysticercosis	700
Total Deaths from Parasitic Infections	**1,000,700**

ENDOPARASITES

Protozoa

Plasmodium ***spp. - causes Malaria***

Plasmodium is a genus of parasitic protozoa, many of which cause malaria in their hosts. The parasite always has two hosts in its life cycle: a Dipteran insect host and a vertebrate host. Sexual reproduction always occurs in the insect, making it the definitive host.

The life-cycles of *Plasmodium* species involve several different stages both in the insect and the vertebrate host. These stages include sporozoites, which are injected by the insect vector into the vertebrate host's blood. Sporozoites infect the host liver, giving rise to merozoites and (in some species) hypnozoites. These move into the blood where they infect red blood cells. In the red blood cells, the parasites can either form more merozoites to infect more red blood cells, or produce gametocytes which are taken up by insects which feed on the vertebrate host. In the insect host, gametocytes merge to sexually reproduce. After sexual reproduction, parasites grow into new sporozoites, which move to the insect's salivary glands, from which they can infect a vertebrate host bitten by the insect.

The genus *Plasmodium* was first described in 1885. It now contains about 200 species, which are spread across the world where both the insect and vertebrate hosts are present. Five species regularly infect humans, while many others infect birds, reptiles, rodents, and various primates.

Life cycle

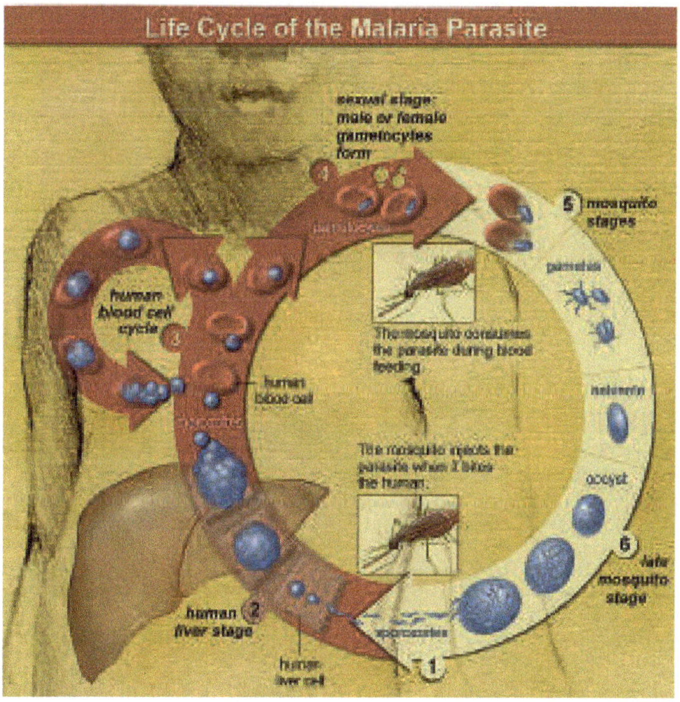

The life cycle of malaria parasites. Parasites enter the vertebrate host through a mosquito bite. Sporozoites enter the skin and travel through the bloodstream to the liver, where they multiply into merozoites, which return to the bloodstream. Merozoites infect red blood cells, where they develop through several stages to produce either more merozoites, or gametocytes. Gametocytes are taken up by a mosquito and infect the insect, continuing the life cycle.

The life cycle of *Plasmodium* involves several distinct stages in the insect and vertebrate hosts. In infected mosquitoes, parasites in the salivary gland are called sporozoites. When the mosquito bites a vertebrate host, sporozoites are injected into the host with the saliva. From there, the sporozoites enter the bloodstream and are transported to the liver, where they invade and replicate within hepatocytes. At this point, some species of *Plasmodium* can form a long-lived dormant stage called a hypnozoite which can remain in the liver for many years. The parasites that emerge from infected hepatocytes are called merozoites, and these return to the blood to infect red blood cells.

Within the red blood cells, the merozoites grow first to a ring-shaped form and then to a larger form called a trophozoite. Trophozoites then mature to schizonts which divide several times to produce new merozoites. The infected red blood cell eventually bursts, allowing the new merozoites to travel within the bloodstream to infect new red blood cells. Most merozoites continue this replicative cycle, however some merozoites differentiate into male or female sexual forms called gametocytes. These gametocytes circulate in the blood until they are taken up when a mosquito feeds on the infected vertebrate host, taking up blood which includes the gametocytes.

In the mosquito, the gametocytes move along with the blood meal to the mosquito's midgut. Here the gametocytes develop into male and female gametes which fertilize each other, forming a zygote. Zygotes then develop into a motile form called an ookinete, which penetrates the wall of the midgut. Upon traversing the midgut wall, the ookinete embeds into the gut's exterior membrane and develops into an oocyst. Oocysts divide many times to produce large numbers of small elongated sporozoites. These sporozoites migrate to the salivary glands of the mosquito where they can be injected into the blood of the next host the mosquito bites, repeating the cycle.

Genome

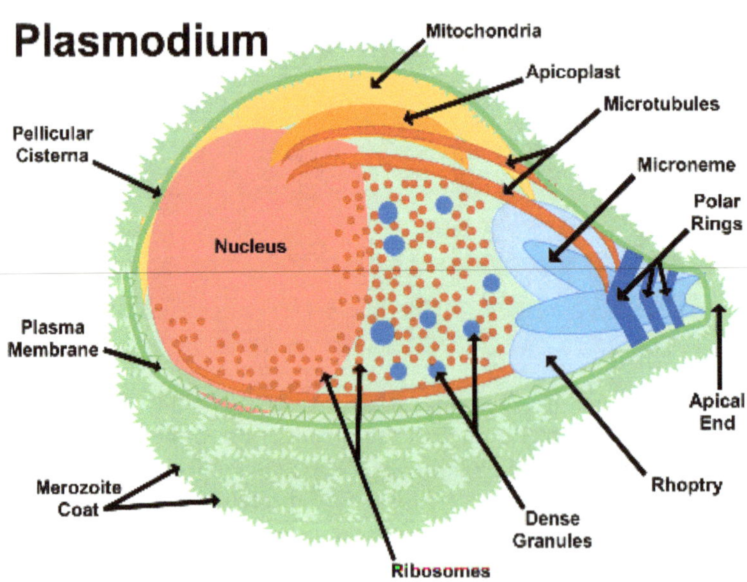

Plasmodium is a Eukaryote but with unusual features

Plasmodium species each have 14 chromosomes in the nucleus, as well as genetic material in the mitochondrion and in the apicoplast. The chromosomes vary from 500 kilobases to 3.5 megabases in length. The apicoplast is involved in isoprenoid metabolism, Fe-S cluster synthesis, fatty acid synthesis, and phospholipid biosynthesis.

On a molecular level, the parasite damages red blood cells using plasmepsin enzymes — aspartic acid proteases which degrade hemoglobin.

Taxonomt and Evolution

Plasmodium is a member of the family Plasmodiidae, order Haemosporidia and phylum Apicomplexa which, along with dinoflagellates and ciliates, make up the taxonomic group Alveolata.

Plasmodium species were originally classified into subgenera based on their morphology, location, and host specificity. However, more recent studies of *Plasmodium* species using molecular methods have occasionally given results which conflict with the original taxonomic system.

Evolutionary relationships of species within the genus *Plasmodium* have been controversial. *Plasmodium* species were originally divided by morphology, life-cycle characteristics, and host species. However, modern molecular approaches for determining evolutionary relationships have given results which conflict with older classification methods. Many attempts to clarify *Plasmodium* taxonomy with molecular methods have also run into technical challenges. Ribosomal RNA sequencing, which is often used in other organisms to determine evolutionary relationships, is challenging to interpret from *Plasmodium* species as *Plasmodia* maintain several different copies of ribosomal RNA which are expressed at different stages of the life cycle and which may be able to recombine with one another. Another commonly used marker for evolutionary studies has been the circumsporozoite protein (CSP) which is present in all *Plasmodium* species. However, analyses of CSP sequences are complicated by the fact that the sequence of CSP, which is present on the surface of the parasite during infection, is under heavy selective pressure from the host immune system. This could potentially obscure relevant changes.

Environmental factors play a considerable role in the evolution of *Plasmodium* and the transmission of malaria. The genetic information of *Plasmodium falciparum* has signaled a recent expansion that coincides with the agricultural revolution. It is likely that the development of extensive agriculture increased mosquito population densities by giving rise to more breeding sites, which may have triggered the evolution and expansion of *Plasmodium falciparum*.

There are over one hundred species of mosquito-transmitted *Plasmodium*. The phylogeny of these malarial parasites suggests that the *Plasmodium* of mammalian hosts forms a well-defined clade strongly associated with the specialization to the *Anopheles* mosquito vector. This was a major evolutionary transition that allowed Plasmodium to exploit humans and other mammals.

P. falciparum, the most lethal malaria parasite of humans, evolved from a "nearly identical" parasite of western gorillas.

The high mortality and morbidity caused by malaria—especially that caused by *P. falciparum*—has placed the greatest selective pressure on the human genome in recent history. Several genetic factors provide some resistance to *Plasmodium* infection, including sickle cell trait, thalassaemia traits, glucose-6-phosphate dehydrogenase deficiency, and the absence of Duffy antigens on red blood cells.

Although there are therapeutic medications to treat malaria, *Plasmodium* has accumulated increasing drug resistance over time. A recent examination has shown that even artemisinin, one of the most powerful anti-malarial drugs, has been experiencing decreased efficacy due to the development of resistance.

Plasmodium species have been subdivided into subgenera, which group species of similar morphology and with similar hosts.

- Subgenus *Asiamoeba* (lizards)
- Subgenus *Bennettinia* (birds)
- Subgenus *Carinamoeba* (reptiles)
- Subgenus *Giovannolaia* (birds)
- Subgenus *Haemamoeba* (birds)
- Subgenus *Huffia* (birds)
- Subgenus *Lacertamoeba* (reptiles)
- Subgenus *Laverania* (higher primates)
- Subgenus *Novyella* (birds)
- Subgenus *Paraplasmodium* (lizards)
- Subgenus *Plasmodium* (monkeys, higher primates)
- Subgenus *Sauramoeba* (reptiles)
- Subgenus *Vinckeia* (non-primate mammals)

Species infecting monkeys and apes (the higher primates) with the exceptions of *P. falciparum* and *P. reichenowi* (which together make up the subgenus *Laverania*) are classified in the subgenus *Plasmodium*. Parasites infecting other mammals including lower primates (lemurs and others) are classified in the subgenus *Vinckeia*. The distinction between *P. falciparum* and *P. reichenowi* and the other species infecting higher primates was based on morphological findings but have since been confirmed by DNA analysis.

The four subgenera *Giovannolaia*, *Haemamoeba*, *Huffia* and *Novyella* were created by Corradetti et al. for the known avian malarial species. A fifth — *Bennettinia* — was created in 1997 by Valkiunas. The relationships between the subgenera are a matter of current investigation.

P. juxtanucleare is the only member of the subgenus *Bennettinia*.

Unlike the mammalian and bird malarias those affecting reptiles have been more difficult to classify. In 1966 Garnham classified those with large schizonts as *Sauramoeba*, those with small schizonts as *Carinamoeba* and the single then-known species infecting snakes (*Plasmodium wenyoni*) as *Ophidiella*. In 1988, Telford used this scheme as the basis for the current system.

Hosts

All Plasmodia are parasitic and require both a vertebrate host and an insect host to reproduce. Known vertebrate hosts include various primates (including humans), birds, rodents, bats, porcupines and squirrels. Mosquitoes of the genera *Culex*, *Anopheles*, *Culiseta*, *Mansonia* and *Aedes* often serve as insect hosts for various *Plasmodium* species.

Non-human Primates

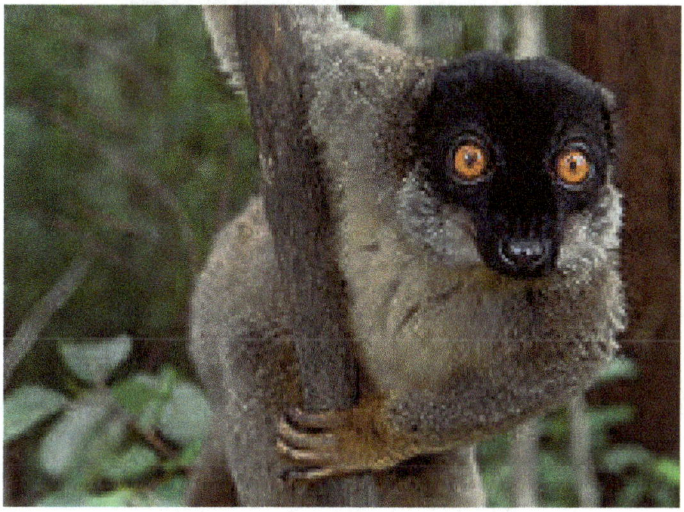

Species of *Plasmodium* infect many primates across the world, such as the brown lemur, *Eulemur fulvus*, of Madagascar.

The species that infect primates other than humans include: *P. bouillize*, *P. brasilianum*, *P. bucki*, *P. cercopitheci*,*P. coatneyi*, *P. coulangesi*, *P. cynomolgi*, *P. eylesi*, *P. fieldi*, *P. foleyi*, *P. fragile*, *P. girardi*, *P. georgesi*, *P. gonderi*, *P. hylobati*, *P. inui*, *P. jefferyi*, *P. joyeuxi*, *P. knowlesi*, *P. lemuris*, *P. percygarnhami*, *P. petersi*, *P. reichenowi*, *P. rodhaini*, *P. sandoshami*, *P. semnopitheci*, *P. silvaticum*, *P. simiovale*, *P. simium*, *P. uilenbergi*, *P. vivax* and *P. youngei*.

Many *Plasmodium* species infect more than one primate host species. Primates which have been found to be infected with *Plasmodium* include species of the genera *Alouatta* (also known as howler monkeys), *Ateles* (spider monkeys), *Brachyteles* (muriqui or wooly spider monkeys), *Callicebus* (titi monkeys), *Chiropotes* (bearded sakis), *Lagothrix* (woolly monkeys), *Lemur* (lemurs), *Macaca* (macaques), *Pan* (chimpanzees), *Pongo* (orangutans), and *Saimiri* (squirrel monkeys).

The insect hosts of the *Plasmodium* species which infect primates are various species of Anopheles mosquitoes. Different species of *Plasmdodium* generally infect different species of mosquito, although some mosquito species can carry several *Plasmodium* species.

Non-primate Mammals

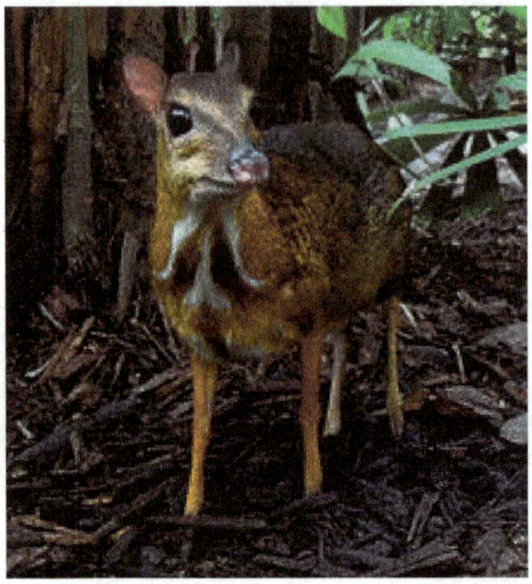

Many non-primate mammals, such as mouse-deer (*Tragulus kanchil*) can carry malaria parasites.

The subgenus *Vinckeia* was created by Cyril Garnham to accommodate the mammalian parasites other than those infecting primates. Species infecting lemurs have also been included in this subgenus. *Plasmodium* species can infect a wide variety of mammals including rodents, ungulates, and bats. Several of the species which infect rodents have been shown to also infect the mosquito *Anopheles stephensi.*

P. aegyptensis, *P. bergei*, *P. chabaudi*, *P. inopinatum*, *P. yoelli* and *P. vinckei* infect rodents. *P. bergei*, *P. chabaudi*, *P. yoelli* and *P. vinckei* have been used to study malarial infections in the laboratory. Other members of this subgenus infect other mammalian hosts.

Birds

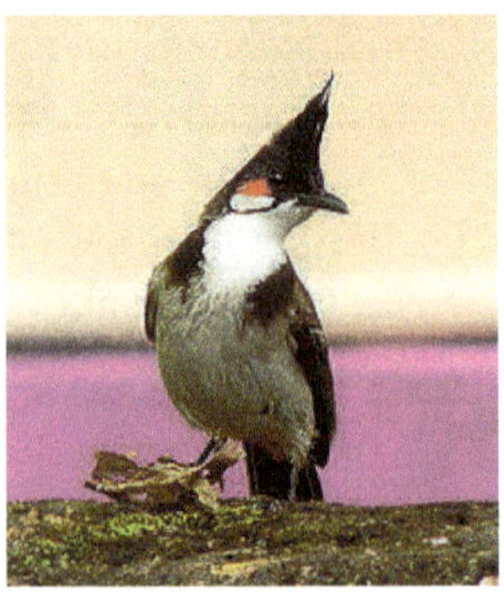

Many bird species, from raptors to passerines like the red-whiskered bulbul (*Pycnonotus jocosus*), can carry malaria.

Species in five *Plasmodium* subgenera infect birds — *Bennettinia*, *Giovannolaia*, *Haemamoeba*, *Huffia* and *Novyella*. *Giovannolaia* appears to be a polyphyletic group and may be sudivided in the future. Species that infect birds include *P. accipiteris*, *P. alloelongatum*, *P. anasum*, *P. ashfordi*, *P. bambusicolai*, *P. bigueti*, *P. biziurae*, *P. buteonis*, *P. cathemerium*, *P. circumflexum*, *P. coggeshalli*, *P. corradettii*, *P. coturnix*, *P. dissanaikei*, *P. durae*, *P. elongatum*, *P. fallax*, *P forresteri*, *P. gallinacium*, *P. garnhami*, *P. giovannolai*, *P. griffithsi*, *P. gundersi*, *P. guangdong*, *P. hegneri*, *P. hermani*, *P. hexamerium*, *P. huffi*, *P. jiangi*, *P. juxtanucleare*, *P. kempi*, *P. lophurae*, *P.lutzi*, *P. matutinum*, *P. nucleophilum*, *P. papernai*, *P. paranucleophilum*, *P. parvulum*, *P. pediocetti*, *P. paddae*, *P. pinotti*, *P. polare*, *P. relictum*, *P. rouxi*, *P. tenue*, *P. tejerai*, *P. tumbayaensis* and *P. vaughani*.

These infect a variety of bird species. In general each species of *Plasmodium* infects one to a few species of birds. Each species is also generally transmitted by a single insect species. Insect hosts include *Aedes aegypti*, *Mansionia crassipes*, and various *Culex* species.

Reptiles

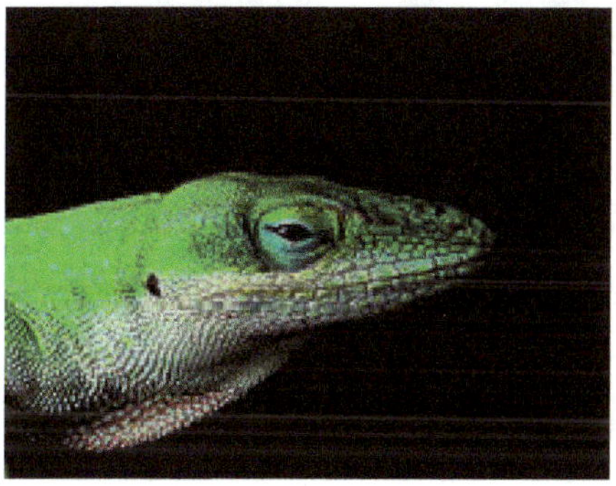

Over 3000 species of lizard, including the Carolina anole (*Anolis carolinensis*), carry some 90 kinds of malaria.

Species in the subgenera *Asiamoeba*, *Carinamoeba*, *Lacertaemoba*, *Paraplasmodium* and *Sauramoeba* infect reptiles. These species of *Plasmodium* include: *P. achiotense*, *P. aeuminatum*, *P. agamae*, *P. arachniformis*, *P. attenuatum*,*P. aurulentum*, *P. australis*, *P. azurophilum*, *P. balli*, *P. basilisci*, *P. beebei*, *P. beltrani* , *P. brumpti*, *P. brygooi*, *P. chiricahuae*, *P. circularis*, *P. cnemaspi*, *P. cnemidophori*, *P. colombiense*, *P. cordyli*, *P. diminutivum*, *P. diploglossi*, *P. egerniae*, *P. fairchildi*, *P. floridense*, *P. gabaldoni*, *P. giganteum*, *P. gologoense*, *P. gracilis*, *P. guyannense*, *P. heischi*, *P. holaspi*, *P. icipeensis*, *P. iguanae*, *P. josephinae*, *P. kentropyxi*, *P. lacertiliae*, *P. lainsoni*, *P. lepidoptiformis*, *P. lionatum*, *P. loveridgei*, *P. lygosomae*, *P. mabuiae*, *P. mackerrasae*, *P. maculilabre*, *P. marginatum*, *P. mexicanum*, *P. michikoa*, *P. minasense*, *P. pelaezi*, *P. pessoai*, *P. pifanoi*, *P. pitmani*, *P. rhadinurum*, *P. sasai*,*P. saurocaudatum*, *P. scorzai*, *P. siamense*, *P. robinsoni*, *P. sasai*, *P. scorzai*, *P. tanzaniae*, *P. tomodoni*, *P. torrealbai*, *P. tribolonoti*, *P. tropiduri*, *P. uluguruense*, *P. uzungwiense*, *P. vacuolatum*, *P. vastator*, *P. volans*, *P. wenyoni* and *P. zonuriae*.

Plasmodium species have been reported from over 3200 species of lizard and 29 species of snake. Only three species — *P. pessoai*, *P. tomodoni* and *P. wenyoni* — infect snakes. Species infecting lizards have been reported in relatively few insect hosts, including *Lutzomyia* and *Culicoides* species, *Culex fatigans* and *Aedes aegypti*.

Insects

Mosquitoes of the genera *Culex*, *Anopheles*, *Culiseta*, *Mansonia* and *Aedes* may act as insect hosts for various *Plasmodia* species. The best studies of these have been the *Anopheles* mosquitoes which host *Plasmodia* which cause human malaria, as well as *Culex* mosquitoes which host the *Plasmodia* that cause malaria in birds. In all cases, only female mosquitoes can be infected with *Plasmodia* species, since only the females feed on the blood of vertebrate hosts.

The survivorship and relative fitness of mosquitoes are not adversely affected by *Plasmodium* infection, which indicates the importance of vector fitness in shaping the evolution of *Plasmodium*. *Plasmodium* has evolved the capability to manipulate mosquito feeding behavior. Mosquitoes harboring *Plasmodium* have a higher propensity to bite than uninfected mosquitoes. This tendency has facilitated the spread of *Plasmodium* to the various hosts.

Species reclassified into other genera

Further information: Hepatocystis and Garnia (protist)

Several species of *Plasmodium* have been reclassified, mostly to *Hepatocystis*. These include:

- *Plasmodium epomophori* to *Hepatocystis epomophori*
- *Plasmodium kochi* to *Hepatocystis kochi*
- *Plasmodium limnotragi* to *Hepatocystis limnotragi* (Van Denberghe 1937)
- *Plasmodium pteropi* to *Hepatocystis pteropi* (Breinl 1911)
- *Plasmodium ratufae* to *Hepatocystis ratufae* (Donavan 1920)
- *Plasmodium vassali* to *Hepatocystis vassali* (Laveran 1905)
- *Plasmodium gonatodi* to *Garnia gonatodi*

Link to Ebola virus

In August 2016, the National Institute Of Allergy and Infectious Diseases (NIAID) came out with a study that showed that people with the Ebola virus were 20 percent more likely to survive it if they were infected with the Plasmodium parasite. The study was published in *Clinical Infectious Diseases*. Researchers did their work at an ebola treatment unit in Monrovia, Liberia. Researchers also found that the greater the number of Plasmodium parasites in the body, the greater the rate of Ebola survival. NIAID is part of the National Institutes of Health.

Species

Several species are found in humans and animals. *Entamoeba histolytica* is the pathogen responsible for invasive 'amoebiasis' (which includes amoebic dysentery and amoebic liver abscesses). Others such as *Entamoeba coli* (not to be confused with *Escherichia coli*) and *Entamoeba dispar* are harmless. With the exception of *Entamoeba gingivalis*, which lives in the mouth, and *E. moshkovskii*, which is frequently isolated from river and lake sediments, all *Entamoeba* species are found in the intestines of the animals they infect. *Entamoeba invadens* is a species that can cause a disease similar to *E. histolytica* but in reptiles. In contrast to other species, *E. invadens* forms cysts in vitro in the absence of bacteria and is used as a model system to study this aspect of the life cycle. Many other species of *Entamoeba* have been described and it is likely that many others remain to be found.

Structure

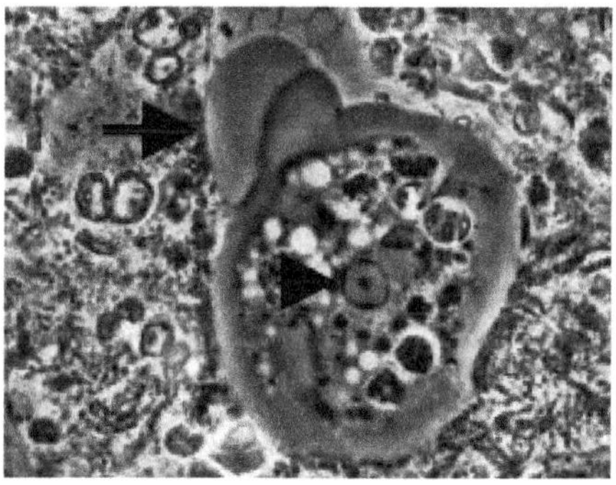

Entamoeba gingivalis

Entamoeba cells are small, with a single nucleus and typically a single lobose pseudopod taking the form of a clear anterior bulge. They have a simple life cycle. The trophozoite (feeding-dividing form) is approximately 10-20 µm in diameter and feeds primarily on bacteria. It divides by simple binary fission to form two smaller daughter cells. Almost all species form cysts, the stage involved in transmission (the exception is *Entamoeba gingivalis*). Depending on the species, these can have one, four or eight nuclei and are variable in size; these characteristics help in species identification.

Entamoeba belongs to the Archamoebae, which like many other anaerobic eukaryotes lack mitochondria. This group also includes *Endolimax* and *Iodamoeba*, which also live in animal intestines and are similar in appearance to *Entamoeba*, although this may partly be due to convergence. Also in this group are the free-living amoebo-flagellates of the genus *Mastigamoeba* and related genera. Certain other genera of symbiotic amoebae, such as *Endamoeba*, might prove to be synonyms of *Entamoeba* but this is still unclear.

Reproduction

Asexual Reproduction: Fission

Studying *Entamoeba invadens*, David Biron of the Weizmann Institute of Science and coworkers found that about one third of the cells are unable to separate unaided and recruit a neighboring amoeba (dubbed the "midwife") to complete the fission.He writes:

When an amoeba divides, the two daughter cells stay attached by a tubular tether which remains intact unless mechanically severed. If called upon, the neighbouring amoeba midwife travels up to 200 μm towards the dividing amoeba, usually advancing in a straight trajectory with an average velocity of about 0.5 μm/s. The midwife then proceeds to rupture the connection, after which all three amoebae move on.

They also reported a similar behavior in *Dictyostelium*.

Since *E. histolytica* does not form cysts in the absence of bacteria, *E. invadens* has become used as a model for encystation studies as it will form cysts under axenic growth conditions, which simplifies analysis. After inducing encystation in *E. invadens*, DNA replication increases initially and then slows down. On completion of encystation, predominantly tetra-nucleate cysts are formed along with some uni-, bi- and tri-nucleate cysts.

Differentiation and cell biology

Uni-nucleated trophozoites convert into cysts in a process called encystation. The number of nuclei in the cyst varies from 1 to 8 among species and is one of the characteristics used to tell species apart. Of the species already mentioned, *Entamoeba coli* forms cysts with 8 nuclei while the others form tetra-nucleated cysts. Since *E. histolytica* does not form cysts *in vitro* in the absence of bacteria, it is not possible to study the differentiation process in detail in that species. Instead the differentiation process is studied using *E. invadens*, a reptilian parasite that causes a very simiilar disease to *E. histolytica* and which can be induced to encyst *in vitro*. Until recently there was no genetic transfection vector available for this organism and detailed study at the cellular level was not possible. However, recently a transfection vector was developed and the transfection conditions for *E. invadens* were optimised which should enhance the research possibilities at the molecular level of the differentiation process.

Sexual Reproduction

In sexually reproducing eukaryotes, homologous recombination (HR) ordinarily occurs during meiosis. The meiosis-specific recombinase, Dmc1, is required for efficient meiotic HR, and Dmc1 is expressed in *E. histolytica*. The purified Dmc1 from *E. histolytica* forms presynaptic filaments and catalyzes ATP-dependent homologous DNA pairing and DNA strand exchange over at least several thousand base pairs. The DNA pairing and strand exchange reactions are enhanced by the eukaryotic meiosis-specific recombination accessory factor (heterodimer) Hop2-Mnd1. These processes are central to meiotic recombination, suggesting that *E. histolytica* undergoes meiosis.

Studies of *E. invadens* found that, during the conversion from the tetraploid uninucleate trophozoite to the tetranucleate cyst, homologous recombination is enhanced. Expression of genes with functions related to the major steps of meiotic recombination also increased during encystations. These findings in *E. invadens*, combined with evidence from studies of *E. histolytica* indicate the presence of meiosis in the *Entamoeba*.

Structure

Like other diplomonads, *Giardia* have two nuclei, each with four associated flagella, and were thought to lack both mitochondria and a Golgi apparatus. However they are now known to possess a complex endomembrane system as well as mitochondrial remnants, called mitosomes, through mitochondrial reduction. The mitosomes are not used in ATP synthesis the way mitochondria are, but are involved in the maturation of iron-sulfur proteins. The synapomorphies of genus *Giardia* include cells with duplicate organelles, absence of cytostomes, and ventral adhesive disc.

Infection and Prevention

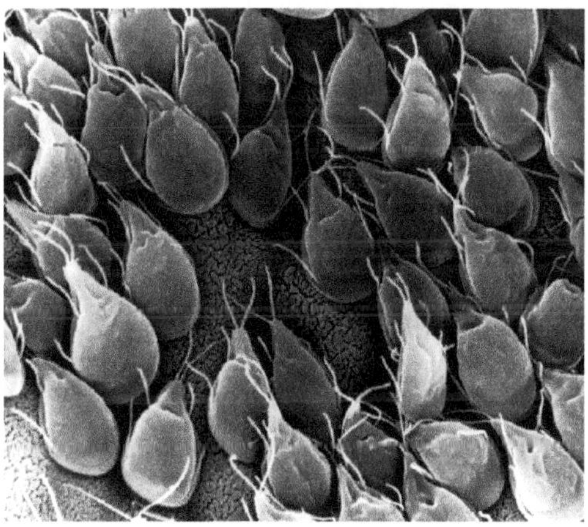

An SEM micrograph of the small intestine of a gerbil infested with *Giardia* reveals a mucosa surface almost entirely obscured by attached trophozoites

Giardia lives in the intestines of infected humans or other animals, individuals of which become infected by ingesting or coming into contact with contaminated foods, soil, or water tainted by the feces of an infected carrier.

The symptoms of *Giardia*, which may begin to appear 2 days after infection, include violent diarrhea, excess gas, stomach or abdominal cramps, upset stomach, and nausea. Resulting dehydration and nutritional loss may need immediate treatment. A typical infection can be slight, resolve without treatment, and last between 2–6 weeks, although it can sometimes last longer and/or be more severe. Coexistence with the parasite is possible (symptoms fade), but an infected individual can remain a carrier and transmit it to others. Medication containing tinidazole or metronidazole decreases symptoms and time to resolution. Albendazole is also used, and has an anti-helmintic (anti-worm) property as well, ideal for certain compounded issues when a general vermicidal agent is preferred. *Giardia* causes a disease called Giardiasis, which causes the villi of the small intestine to atrophy and flatten, resulting in malabsorption in the intestine. Lactose intolerance can persist after the eradication of *Giardia* from the digestive tract.

Person-to-person transmission accounts for the majority of *Giardia* infections and is usually associated with poor hygiene and sanitation. *Giardia* is found on the surface of the ground, in the soil, in undercooked foods, and water along with improper cleaning of fecal material from the hands after handling infected feces. Water-borne transmission is associated with the ingestion of contaminated water. In the U.S., outbreaks typically occur in small water systems using inadequately treated surface water. Venereal transmission happens through fecal-oral contamination. Additionally, diaper changing and inadequate hand washing are risk factors for transmission from infected children. Lastly, food-borne epidemics of *Giardia* have developed through the contamination of food by infected food-handlers.

The CDC recommends hand-washing and avoiding potentially contaminated food and untreated water.

Boiling suspect water for one minute is the surest method to make water safe to drink and kill disease-causing microorganisms such as *Giardia lamblia* if in doubt about whether water is infected. Chemical disinfectants or filters may be used.

According to a review of the literature from 2000, there is little evidence linking the drinking of water in the N. American wilderness and Giardia. The researcher notes that treatment of drinking water for *Giardia* may not be as important as recommended hand-washing in wilderness regions in North America. CDC surveillance data (for 2005 and 2006) reports one outbreak (6 cases) of waterborne giardiasis contracted from drinking wilderness river water in Colorado. However, less than 1% of reported giardiasis cases are associated with outbreaks.

Taxonomy

About 40 species have been described from different animals, but many of them are probably synonyms. Currently, five to six morphologically distinct species are recognised. *Giardia lamblia* (=*G. intestinalis*, =*G. duodenalis*) infect humans and other mammals, *G. muris* is found from other mammals, *G. ardeae* and *G. psittaci* from birds, *G. agilis* from amphibians and *G. microti* from voles. Other described, (but not certainly valid) species include: Many different species of *Giardia* exist and to discriminate between species very specific PCR (Polymerase Chain Reactions) have been developed to detect specific *Giardia* spp. Gene probe-based detection is also used to differentiate between species of *Giardia*. A more common and less time consuming means of identifying different species of *Giardia* includes microscopy and immunofluorescence techniques.

- *Giardia beckeri*
- *Giardia beltrani*
- *Giardia botauri*

- *Giardia bovis*
- *Giardia bradypi*
- *Giardia canis*
- *Giardia caprae*
- *Giardia cati*
- *Giardia caviae*
- *Giardia chinchillae*
- *Giardia dasi*
- *Giardia equii*
- *Giardia floridae*
- *Giardia hegneri*
- *Giardia herodiadis*
- *Giardia hyderabadensis*
- *Giardia irarae*
- *Giardia marginalis*
- *Giardia melospizae*
- *Giardia nycticori*
- *Giardia ondatrae*
- *Giardia otomyis*
- *Giardia pitymysi*
- *Giardia pseudoardeae*
- *Giardia recurvirostrae*
- *Giardia sanguinis*
- *Giardia serpentis*
- *Giardia simoni*
- *Giardia sturnellae*
- *Giardia suricatae*
- *Giardia tucani*
- *Giardia varani*
- *Giardia viscaciae*
- *Giardia wenyoni*

Genetic and biochemical studies have revealed the heterogeneity of *Giardia lamblia*, which contains probably at least eight lineages or cryptic species.

Genome

A *Giardia* isolate (WB) was the first diplomonad to have its genome sequenced. Its

11.7 million basepair genome is compact in structure and content with simplified basic cellular machineries and metabolism. Currently the genomes of several other *Giardia* isolates and diplomonads (the fish pathogens *Spironucleus vortens* and *S. salmonicida*) are being sequenced.

A second isolate (the B assemblage) from humans has been sequenced along with a species from a pig (the E assemblage). There are ~5000 genes in the genome. The E assemblage is more closely related to the A assemblage than is the B. A number of chromosomal rearrangements are present.

Species

T. brucei comprises a species complex that includes:

- *T. brucei gambiense* — Causes slow onset chronic trypanosomiasis in humans. Most common in central and western Africa, where humans are thought to be the primary reservoir.
- *T. brucei rhodesiense* — Causes fast onset acute trypanosomiasis in humans. Most common in southern and eastern Africa, where game animals and livestock are thought to be the primary reservoir.
- *T. brucei brucei* — Causes animal African trypanosomiasis, along with several other species of trypanosoma. *T. b. brucei* is not infective to humans due to its susceptibility to lysis by trypanosome lytic factor-1 (TLF-1). However, it is closely related to, and shares fundamental features with the human infective subspecies.

Structure

T. brucei is a typical unicellular eukaryotic cell, and measures 8 to 50 μm in length. It has an elongated body having a streamlined and tapered shape. Its cell membrane (called pellicle) encloses the cell organelles, including the nucleus, mitochondria, endoplasmic reticulum, Golgi apparatus, and ribosomes. In addition, there is an unusual organelle called the kinetoplast, which is made up of numerous circular DNA (mitochondrial DNA) and functions as a single large mitochondrion. The kinetoplast lies near the basal body with which it is indistinguishable under microscope. From the basal body arises a single flagellum that run towards the anterior end. Along the body surface, the flagellum is attached to the cell membrane forming an undulating membrane. Only the tip of the flagellum is free at the anterior end. The cell surface of the bloodstream form features a dense coat of variant surface glycoproteins (VSGs) which is replaced by an equally dense coat of procyclins when the parasite differentiates into the procylic in the tsetse fly midgut.

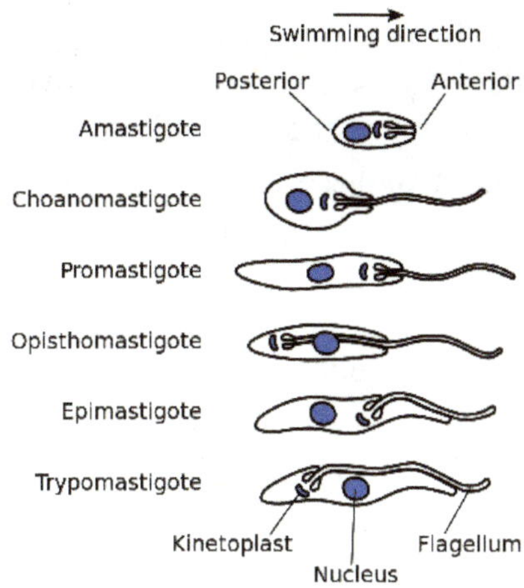

The six main morphologies of trypanosomatids. The different life cycle stages of *Trypanosoma brucei* fall into the trypomastigote and epimastigote morphological categories.

Trypanosomatids show several different classes of cellular organisation of which two are adopted by *Trypanosoma brucei* at different stages of the life cycle:

- Epimastigote, which is found in tsetse fly. Its kinetoplast and basal body lie anterior to the nucleus, with a long flagellum attached along the cell body. The flagellum starts from the centre of the body.
- Trypomastigote, which is found in mammalian hosts. The kinetoplast and basal body are posterior of nucleus. The flagellum arises from the posterior end of the body.

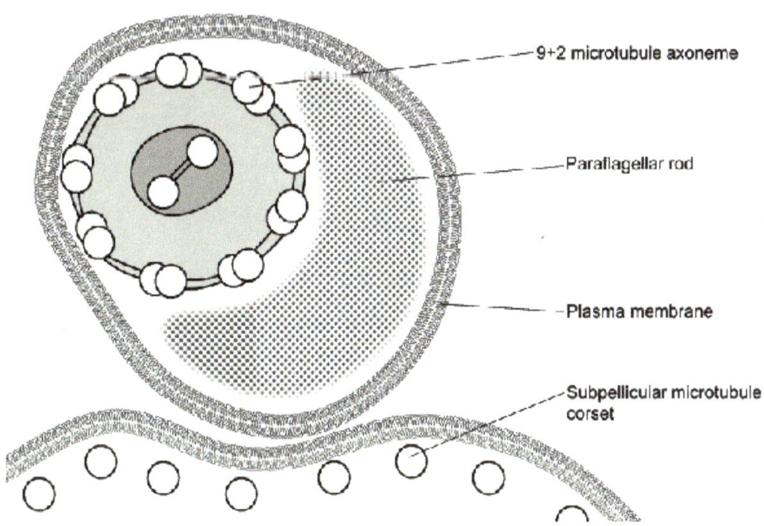

Trypanosoma Brucei flagellar structure.

These names are derived from the Greek *mastig-* meaning whip, referring to the trypanosome's whip-like flagellum. The trypanosome flagellum has two main structures. It is made up of a typical flagellar axoneme which lies parallel to the paraflagellar rod, a lattice structure of proteins unique to the kinetoplastida, euglenoids and dinoflagellates.

The microtubules of the flagellar axoneme lie in the normal 9+2 arrangement, orientated with the + at the anterior end and the - in the basal body. The a cytoskeletal structure extends from the basal body to the kinetoplast. The flagellum is bound to the cytoskeleton of the main cell body by four specialised microtubules, which run parallel and in the same direction to the flagellar tubulin.

The flagellar function is twofold — locomotion via oscillations along the attached flagellum and cell body, and attachment to the fly gut during the procyclic phase.

Life cycle

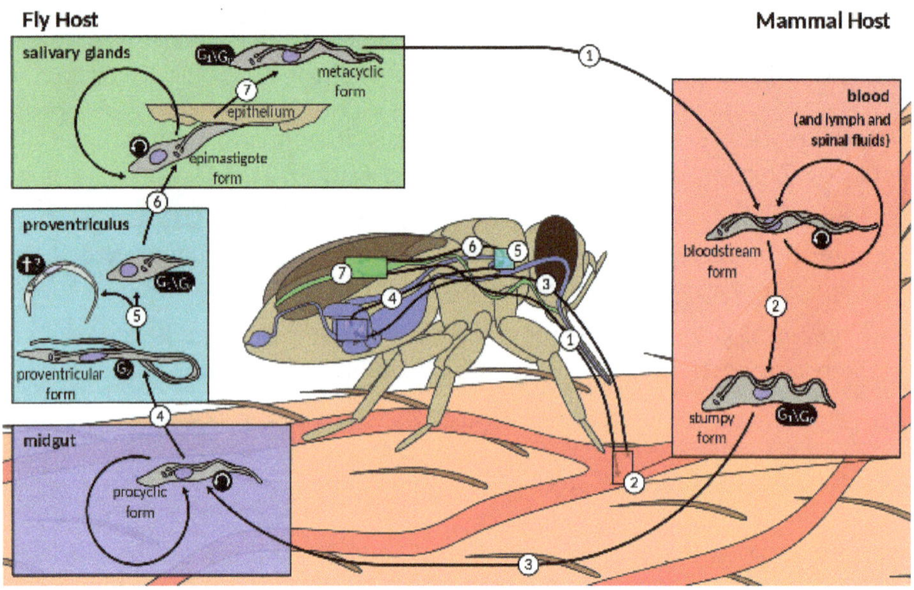

Life cycle of the *Trypanosoma brucei*

T. brucei completes its life cycle between tsetsefly (of the genus *Glossina*) and mammalian hosts, including humans, cattle, horses, and wild animals.

Hosts: Mammalian Tsetse fly

Infection occurs when a vector tsetse fly bites a mammalian host. The fly injects the metacyclic trypomastigotes into the skin tissue. The trypomastigotes enter the lymphatic system and into the bloodstream. The initial trypomastigotes are short and stumpy. Once inside the bloodstream, they grow into long and slender forms. Then, they multiply by binary fission. The daughter cells then become short and stumpy again. The long slender forms are able to penetrate the blood vessel endothelium and invade extravascular tissues, including the central nervous system (CNS).

Sometimes, wild animals can be infected by the tsetsefly and they act as reservoirs. In these animals, they do not produce the disease, but the live parasite can be transmitted back to the normal hosts.

The short and stumpy trypomastigotes are taken up by tsetse fly during blood meal. The trypomastigotes enter the midgut of the fly where they become procyclic trypomastigotes. These rapidly divide to become epimastigotes. The epimastigotes migrate from the gut via the proventriculus to the salivary glands where they get attached to the salivary gland epithelium. In the salivary glands, some parasites detach and undergo transformation into short and stumpy trypomastigotes. These become the infective metacyclic trypomastigotes. They are injected into the mammalian host along with the saliva on biting. Complete development in the fly takes about 20 days.

Reproduction

Asexual Reproduction: Binary fission

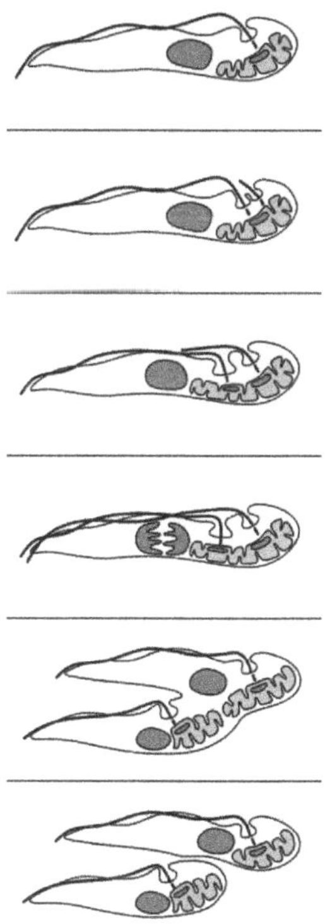

Trypanosome cell cycle (procyclic form).

The reproduction of *T. brucei* is unusual compared to most eukaryotes. The nuclear membrane remains intact and the chromosomes do not condense during mitosis. The basal body, unlike the centrosome of most eukaryotic cells, does not play a role in the organisation of the spindle and instead is involved in division of the kinetoplast. The events of reproduction are:

- The basal body duplicates and both remain associated with the kinetoplast. Each basal body forms a separate flagellum.
- Kinetoplast DNA undergoes synthesis then the kinetoplast divides coupled with separation of the two basal bodies.
- Nuclear DNA undergoes synthesis while a new flagellum extends from the younger, more posterior, basal body.
- The nucleus undergoes mitosis.
- Cytokinesis progresses from the anterior to posterior.
- Division completes with abscission.

Sexual Reproduction

In the 1980s, DNA analyses of the developmental staged of *T. brucei* started to indicate the trypomastigote in tsetse fly undergo meiosis, i.e. sexual reproduction stage. But it is not always necessary for a complete life cycle. The existence of meiosis-specific proteins was reported in 2011. The haploid gametes (daughter cells produced after meiosis) were discovered in 2014. The haploid trypomastigote-like gametes can interact with each other via their flagella and undergo cell fusion (the process called syngamy). Thus, in addition to binary fission, *T. brucei* can multiply by sexual reproduction. Trypanosomes belong to the supergroup Excavata and are one of the earliest diverging lineages among eukaryotes. The discovery of sexual reporduction in *T. brucei* supports the hypothesis that meiosis and sexual reproduction are ancestral and ubiquitous features of eukaryotes.

Infection and Pathogenicity

The insect vector for *T. brucei* is the tsetse fly (genus *Glossina*). In later stages of a *T. brucei* infection of a mammalian host the parasite may migrate from the bloodstream to also infect the lymph and cerebrospinal fluids. It is under this tissue invasion that the parasites produce the sleeping sickness.

In addition to the major form of transmission via the tsetse fly *T. brucei* may be transferred between mammals via bodily fluid exchange, such as by blood transfusion or sexual contact, although this is thought to be rare.

Distribution, Evolution ans Genetic

T. brucei is found where the tsetse fly vectors are prevalent. It is present in tropical and subtropical areas of Africa north of the equator, covering East, Central and West Africa. Hence, the equatorial region of Africa is called the "sleeping sickness" belt. However, the specific type of the trypanosome differs according to geography. *T. b. rhodesiense* is found primarily in East Africa (Botswana, Ethiopia, Kenya, Malawi, Tanzania, Uganda, Zaire, and Zimbabwe), while *T. b. gambiense* is found in Central and West Africa.

Trypanosoma brucei gambiense evolved from a single progenitor ~10,000 years ago. It is evolving asexually and its genome shows the Meselson effect.

There are two subpopulations of *T. b. gambiense* that possesses two distinct groups that differ in genotype and phenotype. Group 2 is more akin to *T. b. brucei* than group 1 *T. b. gambiense*.

All *T. b. gambiense* are resistant to killing by a serum component — trypanosome lytic factor (TLF) of which there are two types: TLF-1 and TLF-2. Group 1 *T. b. gambiense* parasites avoid uptake of the TLF particles while those of group 2 are able to either neutralize or compensate for the effects of TLF.

In contrast *T. b. rhodesiense* is dependent upon the expression of a serum resistance associated (SRA) gene. This gene is not found in *T. b. gambiense*.

Genome

The genome of *T. brucei* is made up of:

- 11 pairs of large chromosomes of 1 to 6 megabase pairs.
- 3–5 intermediate chromosomes of 200 to 500 kilobase pairs.
- Around 100 minichromosomes of around 50 to 100 kilobase pairs. These may be present in multiple copies per haploid genome.

Most genes are held on the large chromosomes, with the minichromosomes carrying only *VSG* genes. The genome has been sequenced and is available online .

The mitochondrial genome is found condensed into the kinetoplast, an unusual feature unique to the kinetoplastea class. The kinetoplast and the basal body of the flagellum are strongly associated via a cytoskeletal structure.

In 1993, a new base, beta-d-glucopyranosyloxymethyluracil (base J), was identified in the nuclear DNA of Trypanosoma brucei

VSG Coat

The surface of the trypanosome is covered by a dense coat of ~5 x 10^6 molecules of variant surface glycoprotein (VSG).This coat enables an infecting *T. brucei* population to persistently evade the host's immune system, allowing chronic infection. VSG is highly immunogenic, and an immune response raised against a specific VSG coat rapidly kills trypanosomes expressing this variant. Antibody-mediated trypanosome killing can also be observed in vitro by a complement-mediated lysisassay. However, with each cell division there is a possibility that one or both of the progeny will switch expression to change the VSG that is being expressed. The frequency of VSG switching has been measured to be approximately 0.1% per division. As *T. brucei* populations can peak at a size of 10^{11} within a host this rapid rate of switching ensures that the parasite population is typically highly diverse. Because host immunity against a specific VSG does not develop immediately, some parasites will have switched to an antigenically-distinct VSG variant, and can go on to multiply and continue the infection. The clinical effect of this cycle is successive 'waves' of parasitaemia (trypanosomes in the blood).

Expression of *VSG* genes occurs through a number of mechanisms yet to be fully understood. The expressed VSG can be switched either by activating a different expression site (and thus changing to express the *VSG* in that site), or by changing the *VSG* gene in the active site to a different variant. The genome contains many hundreds if not thousands of *VSG* genes, both on minichromosomes and in repeated sections ('arrays') in the interior of the chromosomes. These are transcriptionally silent, typically with omitted sections or premature stop codons, but are important in the evolution of new VSG genes. It is estimated up to 10% of the *T. brucei* genome may be made up of VSG genes or pseudogenes. It is thought that any of these genes can be moved into the active site by recombination for expression.

Trypanosoma brucei brucei (as well as related species *T. equiperdum* and *T. evansi*) is not human infective because it is susceptible to innate immune system 'trypanolytic' factors present in the serum of some primates, including humans. These trypanolytic factors have been identified as two serum complexes designated trypanolytic factors (TLF-1 and -2) both of which contain haptoglobin related protein (HPR) and apolipoprotein LI (ApoL1). TLF-1 is a member of the high density lipoprotein family of particles while TLF-2 is a related high molecular weight serum protein binding complex. The protein components of TLF-1 are haptoglobin related protein (HPR), apolipoprotein L-1 (apoL-1) and apolipoprotein A-1 (apoA-1). These three proteins are colocalized within spherical particles containing phospholipids and cholesterol. The protein components of TLF-2 include IgM and apolipoprotein A-I.

Trypanolytic factors are found only in a few species including humans, gorillas, mandrills, baboons and sooty mangabeys.This appears to be because haptoglobin related protein and apolipoprotein L-1 are unique to primates. This suggests these gene appeared in the primate genome 25 million years ago-35 million years ago.

Human infective subspecies *T. b. gambiense* and *T. b. rhodesiense* have evolved mechanisms of resisting the trypanolytic factors, described below.

ApoL1 is a member of a six gene family, ApoL1-6, that have arisen by tandem duplication. These proteins are normally involved in host apoptosis or autophagic death and possess a Bcl-2 homology domain 3. ApoL1 has been identified as the toxic component involved in trypanolysis. ApoLs have been subject to recent selective evolution possibly related to resistance to pathogens

The gene encoding ApoL1 is found on the long arm of chromosome 22 (22q12.3). Variants of this gene, termed G1 and G2, provide protection against *T. b. rhodesiense*. These benefits are not without their downside as a specific ApoL1 glomeropathy has been identified. This glomeropathy may help to explain the greater prevalence of hypertension in African populations.

The gene encodes a protein of 383 residues, including a typical signal peptide of 12 amino acids. The plasma protein is a single chain polypeptide with an apparent molecular mass of 42 kiloDaltons. ApoL1 has a membrane pore forming domain functionally similar to that of bacterial colicins. This domain is flanked by the membrane addressing domain and both these domains are required for parasite killing.

Within the kidney, ApoL1 is found in the podocytes in the glomeruli, the proximal tubular epithelium and the arteriolar endothelium. It has a high affinity for phosphatidic acid and cardiolipin and can be induced by interferon gamma and tumor necrosis factor alpha.

Hpr is 91% identical to haptoglobin (Hp), an abundant acute phase serum protein, which possesses a high affinity for haemoglobin (Hb). When Hb is released from erythrocytes undergoing intravascular hemolysis Hp forms a complex with the Hb and these are removed from the circulation by the CD163 scavenger receptor. In contrast to Hp–Hb, the Hpr–Hb complex does not bind CD163 and the Hpr serum concentration appears to be unaffected by haemolysis.

The association HPR with haemoglobin allows TLF-1 binding and uptake via the trypanosome haptoglobin-hemoglobin receptor (TbHpHbR). TLF-2 enters trypanosomes independently of TbHpHbR. TLF-1 uptake is enhanced in the low levels of haptoglobin which competes with haptoglobin related protein to bind free haemoglobin in the serum. However the complete absence of haptoglobin is associated with a decreased killing rate by serum. The trypanosome haptoglobin-hemoglobin receptor is an elongated three a-helical bundle with a small membrane distal head. This protein extends above the variant surface glycoprotein layer that surrounds the parasite.

The first step in the killing mechanism is the binding of TLF to high affinity receptors—the haptoglobin-hemoglobin receptors—that are located in the flagellar pocket of the parasite. The bound TLF is endocytosed via coated vesicles and then trafficked to the parasite lysosomes. ApoL1 is the main lethal factor in the TLFs and kills trypanosomes after insertion into endosomal / lysosomal membranes. After ingestion by the parasite, the TLF-1 particle is trafficked to the lysosome wherein Apo1 is activated by a pH mediated conformational change. After fusion with the lysosome the pH drops from ~7 to ~5. This induces a conformational change in the ApoL1 membrane addressing domain which in turn causes a salt bridge linked hinge to open. This releases ApoL1 from the HDL particle to insert in the lysosomal membrane. The ApoL1 protein then creates anionic pores in the membrane which leads to depolarization of the membrane, a continuous influx of chloride and subsequent osmotic swelling of the lysosome. This influx in its turn leads to rupture of the lysosome and the subsequent death of the parasite.

Resistance Mechanisms: *T. b. Gambiense*

Trypanosoma brucei gambiense causes 97% of human cases of sleeping sickness. Resistance to ApoL1 is principally mediated by the hydrophobic ß-sheet of the *T. b. gambiense* specific glycoprotein. Other factors involved in resistance appear to be a change in the cysteine protease activity and TbHpHbR inactivation due to a leucine to serine substitution (L210S) at codon 210. This is due to a thymidine to cytosine mutation at the second codon position. These mutations may have evolved due to the coexistence of malaria where this parasite is found. Haptoglobin levels are low in malaria because of the haemolysis that occurs with the release of the merozoites into the blood. The rupture of the erythrocytes results in the release of free haem into the blood where it is bound by haptoglobin. The haem is then removed along with the bound haptoglobin from the blood by the reticuloendothelial system.

Resistance Mechanisms: T. b. Rhodesiense

Trypanosoma brucei rhodesiense relies on a different mechanism of resistance: the serum resistance associated protein (SRA). The SRA gene is a truncated version of the major and variable surface antigen of the parasite, the variant surface glycoprotein. It has a low sequence homology with the VSGc (<25%). SRA is an expression site associated gene in *T. b. rhodesiense* and is located upstream of the VSGs in the active telomeric expression site. The protein is largely localized to small cytoplasmic vesicles between the flagellar pocket and the nucleus. In *T. b. rhodesiense* the TLF is directed to SRA containing endosomes while some dispute remain on its presence in the lysosome. SRA binds to ApoL1 using a coiled–coiled interaction at the ApoL1 SRA interacting domain while within the trypanosome lysosome. This interaction prevents the release of the ApoL1 protein and the subsequent lysis of the lysosome and death of the parasite.

Baboons are known to be resistant to *Trypanosoma brucei rhodesiense*. The baboon version of the ApoL1 gene differs from the human gene in a number of respects including two critical lysines near the C terminus that are necessary and sufficient to prevent baboon ApoL1 binding to SRA. Experimental mutations allowing ApoL1 to be protected from neutralization by SRA have been shown capable of conferring trypanolytic activity on *T. b. rhodesiense*. These mutations resemble those found in baboons, but also resemble natural mutations conferring protection of humans against *T. b. rhodesiense* which are linked to kidney disease .

Lifecycle

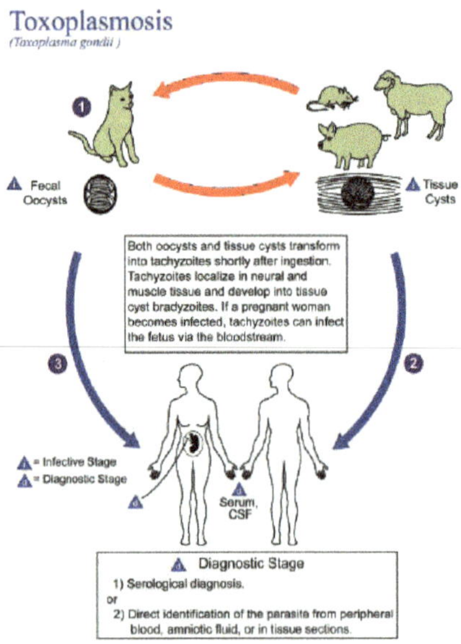

Lifecycle of *Toxoplasma gondii*

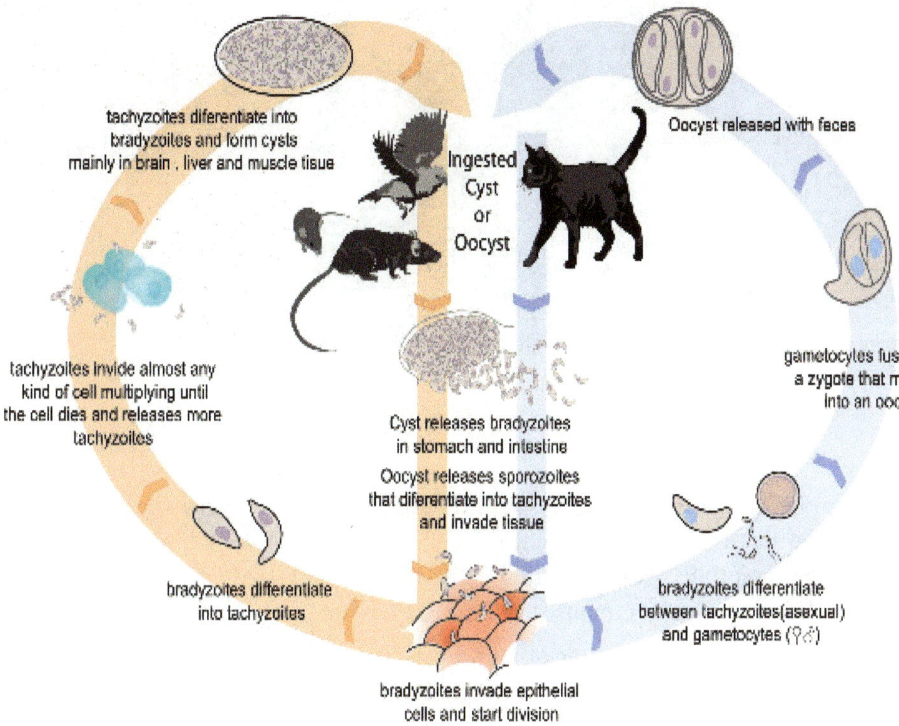

Lifecycle of *T. gondii*

The lifecycle of *T. gondii* can be broadly summarized into two components: a sexual component that occurs only within cats (felids, wild or domestic), and an asexual component that can occur within virtually all warm-blooded animals, including humans, cats, and birds. Because *T. gondii* can sexually reproduce only within cats, they are defined as the definitive host of *T. gondii*. All other hosts – hosts in which only asexual reproduction can occur – are defined as intermediate hosts.

Reproduction: Sexual Reproduction Asexual Reproduction

When a member of the cat family is infected with *T. gondii* (e.g. by consuming an infected mouse laden with the parasite's tissue cysts), the parasite survives passage through the stomach, eventually infecting epithelial cells of the cat's small intestine.Inside these intestinal cells, the parasites undergo sexual development and reproduction, producing millions of thick-walled, zygote-containing cysts known as oocysts.

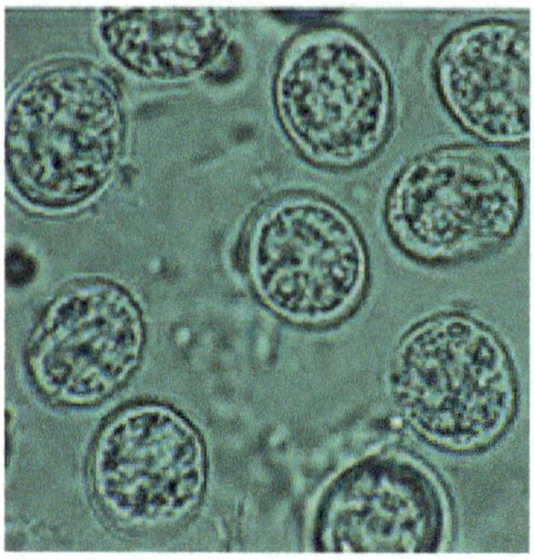

T. gondii oocysts in a fecal flotation

Infected epithelial cells eventually rupture and release oocysts into the intestinal lumen, whereupon they are shed in the cat's feces. Oocysts can then spread to soil, water, food, or anything potentially contaminated with the feces. Highly resilient, oocysts can survive and remain infective for many months in cold and dry climates.

Ingestion of oocysts by humans or other warm-blooded animals is one of the common routes of infection. Humans can be exposed to oocysts by, for example, consuming unwashed vegetables or contaminated water, or by handling the feces (litter) of an infected cat. Although cats can also be infected by ingesting oocysts, they are much less sensitive to oocyst infection than are intermediate hosts.

Asexual Reproduction in the Intermediate Host

Inside host cells, the tachyzoites replicate inside specialized vacuoles (called the parasitophorous vacuoles) created during parasitic entry into the cell. Tachyzoites multiply inside this vacuole until the host cell dies and ruptures, releasing and spreading the tachyzoites via the bloodstream to all organs and tissues of the body, including the brain.

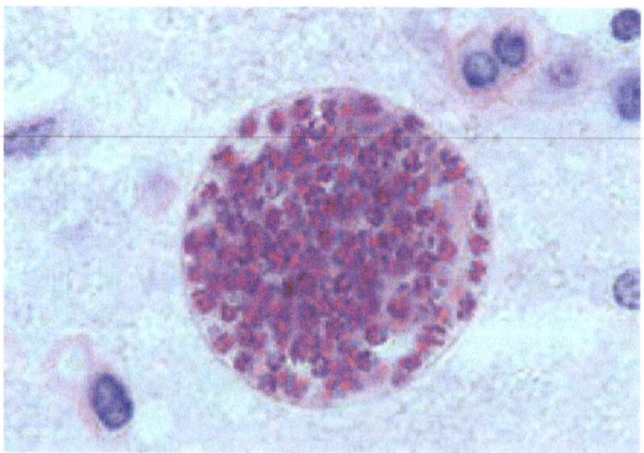

T. gondii tissue cyst in a mouse brain, individual bradyzoites can be seen within

Initial Infection of the Intermediate Host

T. gondii is considered to have three stages of infection; the tachyzoite stage of rapid division, the bradyzoite stage of slow division within tissue cysts, and the oocyst environmental stage. When an oocyst or tissue cyst is ingested by a human or other warm-blooded animal, the resilient cyst wall is dissolved by proteolytic enzymes in the stomach and small intestine, freeing sporozoites from within the oocyst. The parasites first invade cells in and surrounding the intestinal epithelium, and inside these cells, the parasites differentiate into tachyzoites, the motile and quickly multiplying cellular stage of *T. gondii*. Tissue cysts in tissues such as brain and muscle tissue, form approximately 7–10 days after initial infection.

Formation of Tissue Cysts

Following the initial period of infection characterized by tachyzoite proliferation throughout the body, pressure from the host's immune system causes *T. gondii* tachyzoites to convert into bradyzoites, the semidormant, slowly dividing cellular stage of the parasite. Inside host cells, clusters of these bradyzoites are known as tissue cysts. The cyst wall is formed by the parasitophorous vacuole membrane. Although bradyzoite-containing tissue cysts can form in virtually any organ, tissue cysts predominantly form and persist in the brain, the eyes, and striated muscle (including the heart). However, specific tissue tropisms can vary between species; in pigs, the majority of tissue cysts are found in muscle tissue, whereas in mice, the majority of cysts are found in the brain.

Cysts usually range in size between five and 50 µm in diameter, (with 50 µm being about two-thirds the width of the average human hair).

Consumption of tissue cysts in meat is one of the primary means of *T. gondii* infection, both for humans and for meat-eating, warm-blooded animals. Humans consume tissue cysts when eating raw or undercooked meat (particularly pork and lamb). Tissue cyst consumption is also the primary means by which cats are infected.

Chronic Infection

Tissue cysts can be maintained in host tissue for the lifetime of the animal. However, the perpetual presence of cysts appears to be due to a periodic process of cyst rupturing and re-encysting, rather than a perpetual lifespan of individual cysts or bradyzoites. At any given time in a chronically infected host, a very small percentage of cysts are rupturing, although the exact cause of this tissue cysts rupture is, as of 2010, not yet known.

Theoretically, *T. gondii* can be passed between intermediate hosts indefinitely via a cycle of consumption of tissue cysts in meat. However, the parasite's lifecycle begins and completes only when the parasite is passed to a feline host, the only host within which the parasite can again undergo sexual development and reproduction.

Population Structure in the Wild

Khan et al. reviewed evidence that despite the occurrence of a sexual phase in its life cycle, *T. gondii* has an unusual population structure dominated by three clonal lineages (Types I, II and III) that occur in North America and Europe. They estimated that a common ancestor founded these clonal lineages about 10,000 years ago. In a further and larger study (with 196 isolates from diverse sources including *T. gondii* found in the bald eagle, gray wolves, Arctic foxes and sea otters), Dubey et al. also found that *T. gondii* strains infecting North American wildlife have limited genetic diversity with the occurrence of only a few major clonal types. They found that 85% of strains in North America were of one of three widespread genotypes (Types II, III and Type 12). Thus *T. gondii* has retained the capability for sex in North America over many generations, producing largely clonal populations, and matings have generated little genetic diversity.

Immune Response and Behaviour Alterations

Initially, a *T. gondii* infection stimulates production of IL-2 and IFN-γ by the innate immune system. Continuous IFN-c production is necessary for control of both acute and chronic *T. gondii* infection. These two cytokines elicit a CD4+ and CD8+ T-cell mediated immune response. IL-12 is also produced during *T. gondii* infection to activate natural killer (NK) cells. Tryptophan is an essential amino acid for *T. gondii,* which it scavenges from host cells. IFN-γ induces the activation of indole-amine-2,3-dioxygenase (IDO) and tryptophan-2,3-dioxygenase (TDO), two enzymes that are responsible for the degradation of tryptophan. Immune pressure eventually leads the parasite to form cysts that normally are deposited in the muscles and in the brain of the hosts.

The IFN-γ-mediated activation of IDO and TDO is an evolutionary mechanism that serves to starve the parasite, but it can result in depletion of tryptophan in the brain of the host. IDO and TDO degrade tryptophan to N-formylkynurenine and administration of L-kynurenine is capable of inducing depressive-like behaviour in mice. *T. gondii* infection has been demonstrated to increase the levels of kynurenic acid (KYNA) in the brains of infected mice and KYNA has also been demonstrated to be increased in the brain of schizophrenic persons. Low levels of tryptophan and serotonin in the brain were already associated to depression.

Cellular Stages

During different periods of its life cycle, individual parasites convert into various cellular stages, with each stage characterized by a distinct cellular morphology, biochemistry, and behavior. These stages include the tachyzoites, merozoites, bradyzoites (found in tissue cysts), and sporozoites (found in oocysts).

Tachyzoites

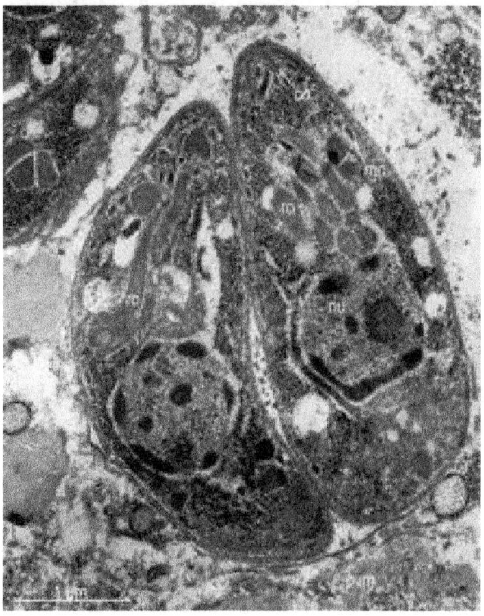

Two tachyzoites, transmission electron microscopy

Motile, and quickly multiplying, tachyzoites are responsible for expanding the population of the parasite in the host. When a host consumes a tissue cyst (containing bradyzoites) or an oocyst (containing sporozoites), the bradyzoites or sporozoites stage-convert into tachyzoites upon infecting the intestinal epithelium of the host. During the initial, acute period of infection, tachyzoites spread throughout the body via the blood stream. During the later, latent (chronic) stages of infection, tachyzoites stage-convert to bradyzoites to form tissue cysts.

Merozoites

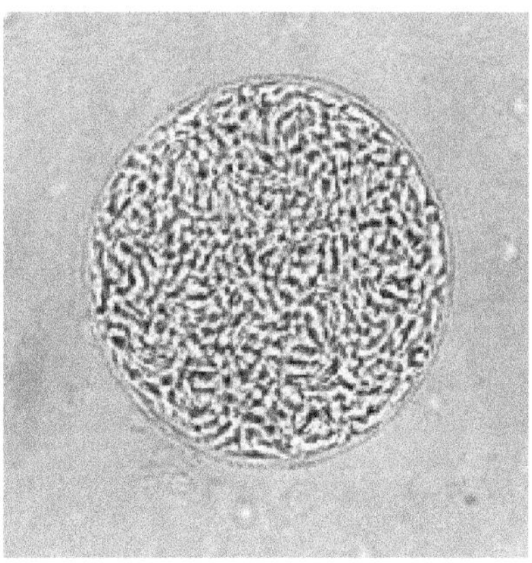

An unstained *T. gondii* tissue cyst, bradyzoites can be seen within

Like tachyzoites, merozoites divide quickly, and are responsible for expanding the population of the parasite inside the cat intestine prior to sexual reproduction.When a feline definitive host consumes a tissue cyst (containing bradyzoites), bradyzoites convert into merozoites inside intestinal epithelial cells. Following a brief period of rapid population growth in the intestinal epithelium, merozoites convert into the noninfectious sexual stages of the parasite to undergo sexual reproduction, eventually resulting in the formation of zygote-containing oocysts.

Bradyzoites

Bradyzoites are the slowly dividing stage of the parasite that make up tissue cysts. When an uninfected host consumes a tissue cyst, bradyzoites released from the cyst infect intestinal epithelial cells before converting to the proliferative tachyzoite stage.Following the initial period of proliferation throughout the host body, tachyzoites then convert back to bradyzoites, which reproduce inside host cells to form tissue cysts in the new host.

Sporozoites

Sporozoites are the stage of the parasite residing within oocysts. When a human or other warm-blooded host consumes an oocyst, sporozoites are released from it, infecting epithelial cells before converting to the proliferative tachyzoite stage.

Risk factors for Human Infection

The following have been identified as being risk factors for *T. gondii* infection:

Infection in humans and other warm-blooded animals can occur:

- by consuming raw or undercooked meat containing *T. gondii* tissue cysts. The most common threat to citizens in the United States is from eating raw or undercooked lamb or pork. It is possible, though unlikely, to ingest the parasite through other products:
- by ingesting water, soil, vegetables, or anything contaminated with oocysts shed in the feces of an infected animal.Cat fecal matter is particularly dangerous: Just one cyst consumed by a cat can result in thousands of oocysts. This is why physicians recommend pregnant or ill persons do not clean the cat's litter box at home. These oocysts are resilient to harsh environmental conditions and can survive over a year in contaminated soil.
- from a blood transfusion or organ transplant
- from transplacental transmission from mother to fetus, particularly when *T. gondii* is contracted during pregnancy
- from drinking unpasteurized goat milk
- by contact with soil
- from eating unwashed raw vegetables or fruits

Cleaning cat litter boxes is a potential route of infection; however, numerous studies have shown living in a household with a cat is not a significant risk factor for *T. gondii* infection, though living with several kittens has some significance.

In warm-blooded animals, such as brown rats, sheep, and dogs, *T. gondii* has also been shown to be sexually transmitted, and it is hypothesized that it may be sexually transmitted in humans, although not yet proven.Although *T. gondii* can infect, be transmitted by, and asexually reproduce within humans and virtually all other warm-blooded animals, the parasite can sexually reproduce only within the intestines of members of the cat family (felids). Felids are therefore defined as the definitive hosts of *T. gondii*, with all other hosts defined as intermediate hosts like human or other mammals.

Sewage has been identified as a carriage medium for the organism.

Preventing Infection

The following precautions are recommended to prevent or greatly reduce the chances of becoming infected with *T. gondii*. This information has been adapted from the websites of United States Centers for Disease Control and Prevention and the Mayo Clinic.

From Food

Basic food handling safety practices can prevent or reduce the chances of becoming infected with *T. gondii*, such as washing unwashed fruits and vegetable and avoiding raw or undercooked meat, poultry, and seafood. Other unsafe practices such as drinking unpasteurized milk or untreated water can increase odds of infection. Because *T. gondii* is typically transmitted through cysts that reside in the tissues of infected animals, meat that is not properly prepared can present an increased risk of infection. Freezing meat for several days at subzero temperatures (0 °F or −18 °C) before cooking eliminates tissue cysts, which can rarely survive these temperatures. During cooking, whole cuts of red meat should be cooked to an internal temperature of 145 °F (63 °C). Medium rare meat is generally cooked between 130 and 140 °F (55 and 60 °C), so cooking whole cuts of meat to medium is recommended. After cooking, a rest period of 3 min should be allowed before consumption. However, ground meat should be cooked to an internal temperature of at least 160 °F (71 °C) with no rest period. All poultry should be cooked to an internal temperature of at least 165 °F (74 °C). After cooking, a rest period of 3 min should be allowed before consumption.

From Environment

Oocysts in cat feces take at least a day to sporulate and become infectious after they are shed, so disposing of cat litter daily greatly reduces the chances of infectious oocysts being present in litter. As infectious oocysts from cat feces can spread and survive in the environment for months, humans should wear gloves when gardening or working with soil, and should wash their hands promptly after disposing of cat litter. The same precautions apply to outdoor sandboxes, which should be covered when not in use.

Furthermore, pregnant or immunocompromised people are at higher risk of becoming infected or transmitting the parasite to their fetus. Because of this, they should not change or handle cat litter boxes. Ideally, cats should be kept indoors and only fed food that has low to no risk of carrying oocysts, such as commercial cat food or well-cooked table food.

Vaccination

As of 2016, no approved human vaccine exists against *Toxoplasma gondii*. Research on human vaccines is ongoing.

For sheep there is an approved live vaccine available called Toxovax (MSD Animal Health) which provides lifetime protection.

Behavioral Differences of Infected Hosts

Once healthy humans are infected with *Toxoplasma gondii*, it may lead to altered behavioral differences like psychomotor performance and neurological disorders like depression and/or suicide and even schizophrenia. There are many instances where behavioural changes were reported in rodents with *T. gondii*. The changes seen were a reduction in their innate dislike of cats, which made it easier for cats to prey on the rodents. In an experiment conducted by Berdoy and colleagues the infected rats showed preference for the cat odour area versus the area with the rabbit scent, therefore making it easier for the parasite to take its final step in its definitive feline host. This is an example of the extended phenotype concept, that is, the idea that the behaviour of the infected animal changes in order to maximize survival of the genes that increase predation of the intermediate rodent host.

Differences in behaviour observed in infected hosts compared to non-infected individuals have been shown to be sex dependent. Looking at humans, studies using the Cattell's 16 Personality Factor questionnaire, found that infected men scored lower on Factor G (superego strength/rule consciousness) and higher on Factor L (vigilance) while the opposite pattern was observed for infected women. This means that men were more likely to disregard rule and were more expedient, suspicious and jealous. On the other hand, women were more warm hearted, outgoing, conscientious and moralistic. However, human studies have not been able to show causation as they have all been observational studies. Mice infected with *T. gondii* have a worse motor performance than non-infected mice. Thus, a computerized simple reaction test was given to both infected and non-infected adults. It was found that the infected adults performed much more poorly and lost their concentration more quickly than the control group. But, the effect of the infection only explains less than 10% of the variability in performance. (i.e., there could be other confounding factors) Correlation has also been observed between seroprevalence of *T. gondii* in humans and increased risk of traffic accidents. Infected subjects have a 2.65 times higher risk of getting into a traffic accident. A similar study done in Turkey showed that there is a higher incidence of *Toxoplasma gondii* antibodies among drivers who have been involved in traffic accidents. Furthermore, this parasite has been associated with many neurological disorders such as schizophrenia. In a meta-analysis, 23 studies met inclusion criteria. The results demonstrate that the seroprevalence of antibodies to *T.gondii* in people with schizophrenia is significantly higher than in control populations (OR=2.73, P<0.000001). In more recent studies, it was found that suicide attempters has significantly higher IgG antibody levels to *T. gondii* as compared with patients without a suicide attempt. Infection was also shown to be associated with suicide in women over the age of 60. ($P<0.005$) As mentioned before, these results of increased proportions of people seropositive for the parasite in cases of these neurological disorders does not indicate a causal relationship between the infection and disorder. It is important to mention that in 2016 a population-representative birth cohort study which was done, to test a hypothesis that toxoplasmosis is related to impairment in brain and behaviour measured by a range of phenotypes including neuropsychiatric disorders, poor impulse control, personality and neurocognitive deficits. Unfortunately, the results do not support any previously mentioned study. None of the P-values showed significance for any outcome measure. Therefore, they concluded that *T. gondii* antibodies does not result in increase susceptibility to any of the phenotypes. This team did not observe any significant association between *T. gondii* serpositivity and schizophrenia. The team reports that the null findings may be a false negative due to low statistical power because of small sample sizes.

Distribution

Acanthamoeba spp. are among the most prevalent protozoa found in the environment. They are distributed worldwide, and have been isolated from soil, air, sewage, seawater, chlorinated swimming pools, domestic tap water, bottled water, dental treatment units, hospitals, air-conditioning units, and contact lens cases. Additionally, *Acanthamoeba* have been isolated from human skin, nasal cavities, throats, and intestines, as well as plants and other mammals.

Role in disease

Diseases caused by *Acanthamoeba* include keratitis and granulomatous amoebic encephalitis (GAE). The latter is often but not always seen in immunosuppressed patients. GAE is caused by the amoeba entering the body through an open wound then spreading to the brain. The combination of host immune response and amoebal proteases causes massive brain swelling resulting in death in ~95% of those infected.

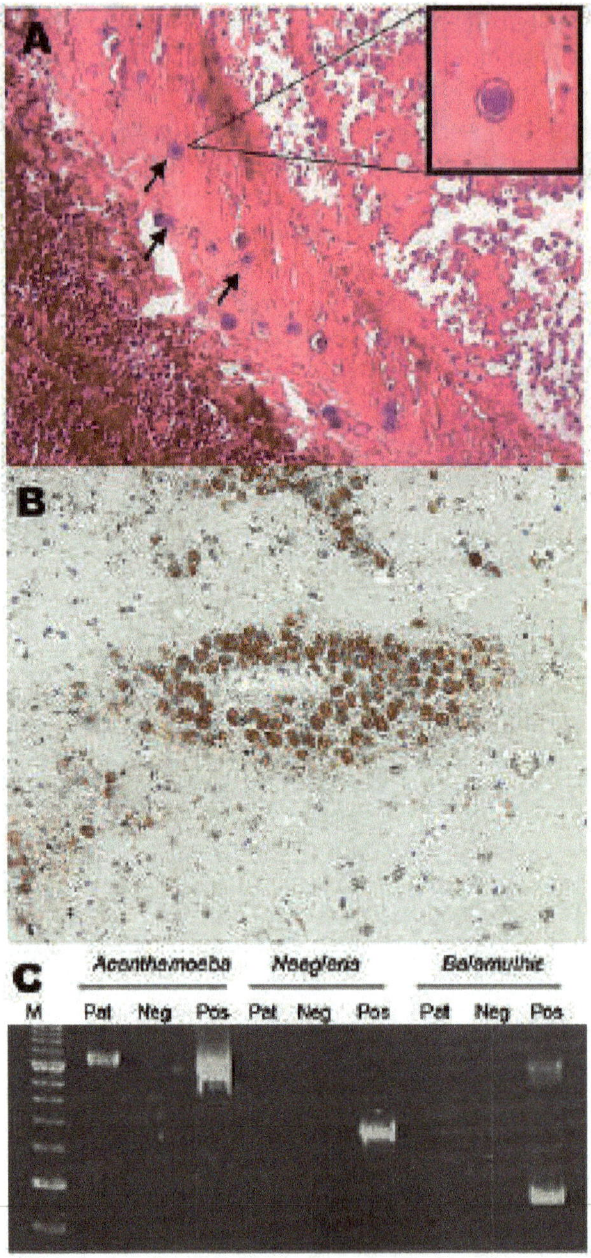

Acanthamoeba encephalitis. Scale bar: 10 µm

Granulomatous Amoebic Encephalitis

Granulomatous amoebic encephalitis is caused by amoeba infection of the central nervous system. It is characterized by neurological symptoms including headache, seizures, and mental status abnormalities. These worsen progressively over weeks to months, leading to death in most patients. Infection is generally associated with underlying conditions such as immunodeficiency, diabetes, malignancies, malnutrition, systemic lupus erythematosus, and alcoholism. The parasite enters the body through cuts in the skin or by being inhaled into the upper respiratory tract. The parasite then spreads through the blood into the central nervous system. *Acanthamoeba* crosses the blood–brain barrier by means that are not yet understood. Subsequent invasion of the connective tissue and induction of pro-inflammatory responses leads to neuronal damage that can be fatal within days. Pure granulomatous lesions are rare in patients with AIDS and other related immunodeficiency states as the patients do not have adequate numbers of CD+ve T-cells to mount a granulomatous response to Acanthamoeba infection in CNS and other organ and tissues. A perivascular cuffing with amoebae in necrotic tissue is usual finding in the AIDS and related T-cell immunodeficiency conditions. A *post mortem* biopsy reveals severe oedema and hemorrhagic necrosis. A patient who has contracted this illness usually displays subacute symptoms, including altered mental status, headaches, fever, neck stiffness, seizures, focal neurological signs (such as cranial nerve palsies and coma), all leading to death within one week to several months. Due to the rarity of this parasite and a lack of knowledge, there are currently no good diagnoses or treatments for *Acanthamoeba* infection. *Acanthamoeba* keratitis cases in the past, when were managed by atropine given as an adjuvant therapy without anti-parasitic drugs added to the regime, had been reported to halt the vision loss. Recent publications debate these successes related to an action of Atropine on muscarinic receptors on *Acanthamoeba* spp.

Infection usually mimics that of bacterial leptomeningitis, tuberculous meningitis, or viral encephalitis. The misdiagnosis often leads to erroneous, ineffective treatment. In the case that the *Acanthamoeba* is diagnosed correctly, the current treatments, such as amphotericin B, rifampicin, trimethoprim-sulfamethoxazole, ketoconazole, fluconazole, sulfadiazine, or albendazole, are only tentatively successful. Correct and timely diagnosis, as well as improved treatment methods and an understanding of the parasite are important factors in improving the outcome of infection by *Acanthamoeba*. A recent paper published in 2013 has shown substantial effects of some FDA approved drugs with a kill rate above 90%. These results were *in-vitro* effects, but as the drugs are already approved, human infections can be targeted after dose calculations in clinical trials with them.

Acanthamoebic Keratitis

When present in the eye, *Acanthamoeba* strains can cause acanthamoebic keratitis, which may lead to corneal ulcers or even blindness. This condition occurs most often among contact lens wearers who do not properly disinfect their lenses, exacerbated by a failure to wash hands prior to handling the lenses. Multipurpose contact lens solutions are largely ineffective against *Acanthamoeba*, whereas hydrogen peroxide-based solutions have good disinfection characteristics.

In May 2007, Advanced Medical Optics, manufacturer of Complete Moisture Plus Contact Lens Solution products, issued a voluntary recall of their Complete Moisture Plus solutions. The fear was that contact lens wearers who used their solution were at higher risk of acanthamoebic keratitis than contact lens wearers who used other solutions. The manufacturer recalled the product after the Centers for Disease Control in the United

States found that 21 individuals had possibly received an *Acanthamoeba* infection after using Complete Moisture Plus in the month prior to diagnosis.

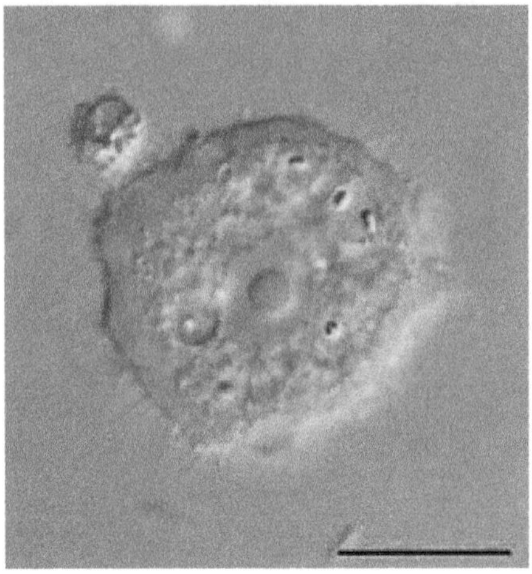

Acanthamoeba Causing Keratitis

Bacterial Infection

Several species of bacteria which can cause human disease are also able to infect and replicate within *Acanthamoeba* species. These include *Legionella pneumophila*, *Pseudomonas aeruginosa*, and some strains of *Escherichia coli* and *Staphylococcus aureus*. For some of these bacteria, replication inside *Acanthamoeba* has been associated with enhanced growth in macrophages, and increased resistance to some antibiotics. Furthermore, due to the high prevalence of *Acanthamoeba* in the environment, it has been proposed that these amoeba could serve as an environmental reservoir for some human pathogens.

Ecology

A. castellanii can be found at high densities in various soil ecosystems. It preys on bacteria, but also fungi and other protozoa.

This species is able to lyse bacteria and produce a wide range of enzymes, such as cellulases or chitinases, and probably contributes to the breakdown of organic matter in soil, contributing to the microbial loop.

Physiology

Role as a Model Organism

Because *Acanthamoeba* does not differ greatly at the ultrastructural-level from a mammalian cell, it is an attractive model for cell biology studies. *Acanthamoeba* is important in cellular microbiology, environmental biology, physiology, cellular interactions, molecular biology, biochemistry, and evolutionary studies, due to the organisms' versatile roles in the ecosystem and ability to capture prey by phagocytosis, act as vectors and reservoirs for microbial pathogens, and to produce serious human infections. In addition, *Acanthamoeba* has been used extensively to understand the molecular biology of cell motilityand cancer cell dormancy by in-depth exploration of the process of encystation

The recently available *Acanthamoeba* genome sequence revealed several orthologs of genes employed in meiosis of sexual eukaryotes. These genes included *Spo11, Mre11, Rad50, Rad51, Rad52, Mnd1, Dmc1, Msh* and *Mlh*. This finding suggests that *Acanthamoeba* is capable of some form of meiosis and may be able to undergo sexual reproduction. Furthermore, since *Acanthamoeba* diverged early from the eukaryotic family tree, these results suggest that meiosis was present early in eukaryotic evolution.

Owing to its ease and economy of cultivation, the Neff strain of *A. castellanii* discovered in a pond in Golden Gate Park in the 1960s, has been effectively used as a classic model organism in the field of cell biology. From just 30 liters of simple medium inoculated with *A. castellanii*, approximately one kilogram of cells can be obtained after several days of aerated culture at room temperature. Pioneered in the laboratory of Edward D. Korn at the National Institutes of Health (NIH), many important biological molecules have been discovered and their pathways elucidated using the *Acanthamoeba* model. Thomas Dean Pollard applied this model at the NIH, Harvard Medical School, Johns Hopkins University School of Medicine, and the Salk Institute for Biological Studies to discover and characterize many proteins that are essential for cell motility, not only in amoebas, but also in many other eukaryotic cells, especially those of the human nervous and immune systems, the developing embryo, and cancer cells. Acanthamoeba also has served as a model to study the evolution of certain G-Proteins. This unicellular eukaryote expresses few GPCRs over its cell membrane that serve vital role for the microorganism, structural homology bioinformatics tools have been used to show the presence of a homolog of human M1-Muscarinic receptor in Acanthamoeba castellanii. Blocking these muscarinic receptors in past studies has proven to be amoebicidal in Acanthamoeba spp.

Endosymbionts of *Acanthamoeba*

Acanthamoeba spp. contain diverse bacterial endosymbionts that are similar to human pathogens, so they are considered to be potential emerging human pathogens. The exact nature of these symbionts and the benefit they represent for the amoebal host still have to be clarified.

These include *Legionella* and *Legionella*-like pathogens.

Giant viruses

The giant viruses Mimivirus, Megavirus and Pandoravirus infect *Acanthamoeba*.

Currently *Acanthamoeba* is the only species that is a host for such huge viruses (who have more than 1000 protein-coding genes; for instance, *Pandoravirus* has about 2500 protein-coding genes in its genome).

Diversity

Acanthamoeba can be distinguished from other genera of amoeba based on morphological characteristics. However, differentiating one species of *Acanthamoeba* from another by morphology has proven difficult. Based on 18S rDNA sequencing, known *Acanthamoeba* strains can be organized into 12 groups, denoted T1-T12. Most disease-causing isolates belong to type T4.

Below is a list of described species of *Acanthamoeba*, with sequence types noted where known. Species which have been identified in diseased patients are marked with *.

- *A. astronyxis** (T7)
- *A. byersi**
- *A. castellanii** (T4)
- *A. comandoni* (T9)
- *A. culbertsoni** (T10)
- *A. divionensis* (T4)
- *A. griffini* (T3)
- *A. hatchetti** (T11)
- *A. healyi* (T12)
- *A. jacobsi*
- *A. keratitis**
- *A. lenticulata* (T3)
- *A. lugdunensis** (T4)
- *A. mauritaniensis* (T4)
- *A. palestinensis** (T1)
- *A. paradivionensis* (T4)
- *A. pearcei*
- *A. polyphaga** (T4)
- *A. pustulosa* (T2)
- *A. quina**
- *A. rhysodes** (T4)
- *A. royreba*
- *A. stevensoni* (T11)
- *A. terricola* (renamed *A. castellanii* Poussard)
- *A. triangularis* (T4)
- *A. tubiashi* (T8)

Leishmania - causes Leishmaniasis

Leishmania is a genus of trypanosomes that are responsible for the disease leishmaniasis.

They are spread by sandflies of the genus *Phlebotomus* in the Old World, and of the genus *Lutzomyia* in the New World. At least 93 sandfly species are proven or probable vectors worldwide. Their primary hosts are vertebrates; *Leishmania* commonly infects hyraxes, canids, rodents, and humans.

Epidemiology

Leishmania currently affects 12 million people in 98 countries. About 2 million new cases occur each year, and 21 species are known to cause disease in humans.

Structure

Leishmania species are unicellular eukaryotes having a well-defined nucleus and other cell organelles including kinetoplasts and flagella. Depending on the stage of their lifecycle, they exist in two structural variants, as:

- The **amastigote** form is found in the mononuclear phagocytes and circulatory systems of humans. It is an intracellular and nonmotile form, being devoid of external flagella. The short flagellum is embedded at the anterior end without projecting out. It is oval in shape, and measures 3–6 µm in length and 1–3 µm in breadth. The kinetoplast and basal body lie towards the anterior end.
- The **promastigote** form is found in the alimentary tract of sandflies. It is an extracellular and motile form. It is considerably larger and highly elongated, measuring 15-30 µm in length and 5 µm in width. It is spindle-shaped, tapering at both ends. A long flagellum (about the body length) is projected externally at the anterior end. The nucleus lies at the centre, and in front of it are the kinetoplast and the basal body.

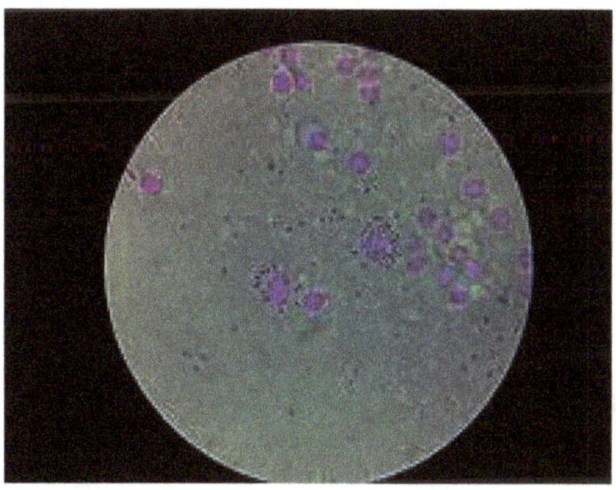

L. infantum amastigote forms

Evolution

The details of the evolution of this genus are debated, but *Leishmania* apparently evolved from an ancestral trypanosome lineage. The oldest lineage is that of the Bodonidae, followed by *Trypanosoma brucei*, the latter being confined to the African continent. *Trypanosoma cruzi* groups with trypanosomes from bats, South American mammals, and kangaroos suggest an origin in the Southern Hemisphere. These clades are only distantly related.

The remaining clades in this tree are *Blastocrithidia*, *Herpetomonas*, and *Phytomonas*. The four genera *Leptomonas*, *Crithidia*, *Leishmania*, and *Endotrypanum* form the terminal branches, suggesting a relatively recent origin. Several of these genera may be polyphyletic and may need further division.

The origins of genus *Leishmania* itself are unclear. One theory proposes an African origin, with migration to the Americas. Another proposes migration from the Americas to the Old World via the Bering Strait land bridge around 15 million years ago. A third theory proposes a palearctic origin. Such migrations would entail subsequent migration of vector and reservoir or successive adaptations along the way. A more recent migration is that of *L. infantum* from Mediterranean countries to Latin America (known as *L. chagasi*), since European colonization of the New World, where the parasites picked up their current New World vectors in their respective ecologies. This is the cause of the epidemics now evident. One recent New World epidemic concerns foxhounds in the USA.

Leishmania might have evolved in the Neotropics.

A large data set analysis suggests that *Lesihmania* evolved 90 million years ago-100 million years ago in Gondwana. The reptile infecting species originated in mammalian clades.

Sauroleishmania species were originally defined on the basis that they infected reptiles (lizards) rather than mammals. Molecular studies have cast doubts on this basis for classification and they have been moved to subgenus status within *Leishmania*. This subgenus probably evolved from a group that originally infected mammals.

Taxonomy

53 species are recognised in this genus. The status of several of these is disputed, so the final number may differ. At least 20 species infect humans. To make things more complex, hybrids might be involved, as it has been reported in Brazil with an hybrid between *Leishmania (V.) guyanensis* and *Leishmania (V.) shawi shawi*.

At least three subgenera exist: *Leishmania*, *Sauroleishmania*, and *Viannia*. The division into the two subgenera (*Leishmania* and *Viannia*) was made by Lainson and Shaw in 1987 on the basis of their location within the insect gut. The species in the *Viannia* subgenus develop in the hind gut: *L. (V.) braziliensis* has been proposed as the type species for this subgenus. This division has been confirmed by all subsequent studies.

Endotrypanum is also closely related and may also be moved to subgenus status within *Leishmania*. The subgenus *Endotypanum* is unique in that the parasites of this subgenus infect the erythrocytes of their hosts (sloths). The species in this subgenus are confined to Central and South America.

Sauroleishmania was originally described by Ranquein 1973 as a separate genus, but molecular studies suggest this is actually a subgenus rather than a separate genus.

A proposed division of the *Leishmania* is into *Euleishmania* and *Paraleishmania*. The proposed groups *Paraleishmania* would include all the species in the genus *Endotypanum* and *L. colomubensis*, *L. deanei*, *L. equatorensis*, and *L. hertigi*. The group *Euleishmania* would include those species currently placed in the subgenera *Leishmania* and *Viannia*. These groups may be accorded subgenus (or other) status at some point, but their positions remains undefined at present.

Five subgenera are recognised - *Leishmania*, *Paraleishmania*, *Sauroleishmania*, *Viannia* and the *L. enrittii* complex. The *Endotrypanum* genus is now recognised as a division of *Paraleishmania*.

L. archibaldi may be the same species as *L. dononani*. *L. herreri* may belong to the genus *Endotypanum* rather than to *Leishmania*.

The enzyme *Seltryp* which is involved in selenocysteine synthesis appears to be unique to this order. It has been lost in the subgenus *Viannia*.

Classification

- *Subgenus Leishmania*
- *Leishmania aethiopica*
- *Leishmania amazonensis*
- *Leishmania arabica*
- *Leishmania donovani*
- *Leishmania gerbilli*
- *Leishmania hertigi*
- *Leishmania infantum*
- *Leishmania killicki*
- *Leishmania major*
- *Leishmania mexicana*
- *Leishmania siamensis*
- *Leishmania tropica*
- *Leishmania turanica*

Subgenus Sauroleishmania

- *Leishmania adleri*
- *Leishmania agamae*
- *Leishmania ceramodactyli*
- *Leishmania deanei*
- *Leishmania garnhami*
- *Leishmania gulikae*
- *Leishmania gymnodactyli*
- *Leishmania hemidactyli*

- *Leishmania hoogstraali*
- *Leishmania nicollei*
- *Leishmania senegalensis*
- *Leishmania tarentolae*

Subgenus Viannia

- *Leishmania braziliensis*
- *Leishmania colombiensis*
- *Leishmania equatorensis*
- *Leishmania guyanensis*
- *Leishmania lainsoni*
- *Leishmania naiffi*
- *Leishmania panamensis*
- *Leishmania peruviana*
- *Leishmania pifanoi*
- *Leishmania shawi*
- *Leishmania utingensis*

The genus *Endotrypanum* is also included here as this may be reclassified as Leishmania

Genus Endotrypanum

- *Endotrypanum monterogeii*
- *Endotrypanum schaudinni*

L. enrittii complex

- *Leishmania enrittii*
- *Leishmania martiniquensis*

Biochemistry and Cell Biology

The biochemistry and cell biology of *Leishmania* is similar to that of other kinetoplastids. They share the same main morphological features; a single flagellum which has an invagination, the flagellar pocket, at its base, a kinetoplast which is found in the single mitochondrion and a subpelicular array of microtubules which make up the main part of the cytoskeleton.

Lipophosphoglycan coat

Leishmania possesses a lipophosphoglycan coat over the outside of the cell. Lipophosphoglycan is a trigger for toll-like receptor 2, a signalling receptor involved in triggering an innate immune response in mammals.

The precise structure of lipophosphoglycan varies depending on the species and lifecycle stage of the parasite. The glycan component is particularly variable and different lipophosphoglycan variants can be used as a molecular marker for different lifecycle stages. Lectins, a group of plant proteins which bind different glycans, are often used to detect these lipophosphoglycan variants. For example, peanut agglutinin binds a particular lipophosphoglycan found on the surface of the infective form of *L. major*.

Lipophosphoglycan is used by the parasite to promote its survival in the host and the mechanisms by which the parasite does this center around modulating the immune response of the host. This is vital, as the *Leishmania* parasites live within macrophages and need to prevent the macrophages from killing them. Lipophosphoglycan has a role in resisting the complement system, inhibiting the oxidative burst response, inducing an inflammation response and preventing natural killer T cells recognising that the macrophage is infected with the *Leishmania* parasite.

Type	Pathogen	Location
Cutaneous leishmaniasis (localised and diffuse) infections appear as obvious skin reactions.	The most common is the *Oriental Sore* (caused by Old World species *L. major*, *L. tropica*, and *L. aethiopica*). In the New World, the most common culprits is *L. mexicana*.	Cutaneous infections are most common in Afghanistan, Brazil, Iran, Peru, Saudi Arabia and Syria.
Mucocutaneous leishmaniasis infections start off as a reaction at the bite, and can go by metastasis into the mucous membrane and become fatal.	*L. braziliensis*	Mucocutaneous infections are most common in Bolivia, Brazil and Peru. Mucocutaneous infections are also found in Karamay, China Xinjiang Uygur Autonomous Region.
Visceral leishmaniasis infections are often recognised by fever, swelling of the liver and spleen, and anemia. They are known by many local names, of which the most common is probably *kala azar*,	Caused exclusively by species of the *L. donovani* complex (*L. donovani*, *L. infantum* syn. *L. chagasi*).	Found in tropical and subtropical areas of all continents except Australia, visceral infections are most common in Bangladesh, Brazil, India, Nepal, and Sudan. Visceral leishmaniasis also found in part of China, such as Sichuan Province, Gansu Province, and Xinjiang Uygur Autonomous Region.

Intracellular Mechanism of Infection

In order to avoid destruction by the immune system and thrive, the *Leishmania* 'hides' inside its host's cells. This location enables it to avoid the action of the humoral immune response (because the pathogen is safely inside a cell and outside the open bloodstream), and furthermore it may prevent the immune system from destroying its host through nondanger surface signals which discourage apoptosis. The primary cell types *Leishmania* infiltrates are phagocytotic cells such as neutrophils and macrophages.

Usually, a phagocytotic immune cell like a macrophage will ingest a pathogen within an enclosed endosome and then fill this endosome with enzymes which digest the pathogen. However, in the case of *Leishmania*, these enzymes have no effect, allowing the parasite to multiply rapidly. This uninhibited growth of parasites eventually overwhelms the host macrophage or other immune cell, causing it to die.

Transmitted by the sandfly, the protozoan parasites of *L. major* may switch the strategy of the first immune defense from eating/inflammation/killing to eating/no inflammation/ no killing of their host phagocyte and corrupt it for their own benefit. They use the willingly phagocytosing polymorphonuclear neutrophil granulocytes (PMNs) rigorously as a tricky hideout, where they proliferate unrecognized from the immune system and enter the long-lived macrophages to establish a "hidden" infection.

Uptake and Survival

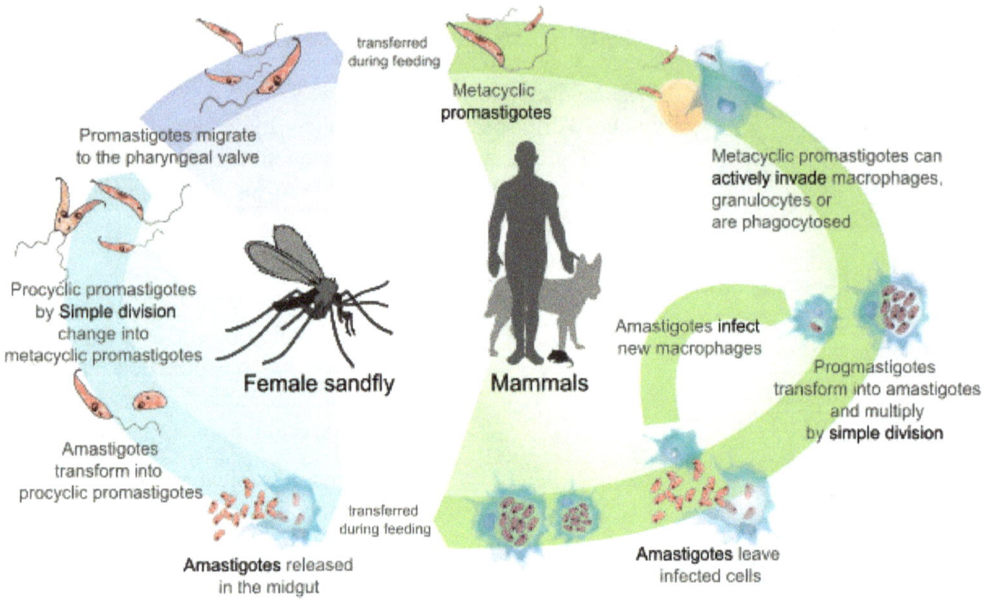

Lifecycle of *Leishmania*

Upon microbial infection, PMNs move out from the bloodstream through the vessels' endothelial layer, to the site of the infected tissue (dermal tissue after fly bite). They immediately initiate the first immune response and phagocytize the invader by recognition of foreign and activating surfaces on the parasite. Activated PMN secrete chemokines, IL-8 particularly, to attract further granulocytes and stimulate phagocytosis. Further, *L. major* increases the secretion of IL-8 by PMNs. This mechanism is observed during infection with other obligate intracellular parasites, as well. For microbes like these, multiple intracellular survival mechanisms exist. Surprisingly, the coinjection of apoptotic and viable pathogens causes by far a more fulminate course of disease than injection of only viable parasites. When the anti-inflammatory signal phosphatidylserine usually found on apoptotic cells, is exposed on the surface of dead parasites, *L. major* switches off the oxidative burst, thereby preventing killing and degradation of the viable pathogen.

In the case of *Leishmania*, progeny are not generated in PMNs, but in this way they can survive and persist untangled in the primary site of infection. The promastigote forms also release *Leishmania* chemotactic factor (LCF) to actively recruit neutrophils, but not other leukocytes, for instance monocytes or NK cells. In addition to that, the production of interferon gamma (IFNγ)-inducible protein 10 (IP10) by PMNs is blocked in attendance of *Leishmania*, what involves the shut down of inflammatory and protective immune response by NK and Th1 cell recruitment. The pathogens stay viable during phagocytosis since their primary hosts, the PMNs, expose apoptotic cell-associated molecular pattern (ACAMP) signaling "no pathogen".

The lifespan of neutrophil granulocytes is quite short. They circulate in bloodstream for about 6 to 10 hours after leaving bone marrow, whereupon they undergo spontaneous apoptosis. Microbial pathogens have been reported to influence cellular apoptosis by different strategies. Obviously because of the inhibition of caspase3-activation, *L. major* can induce the delay of neutrophils apoptosis and extend their lifespan for at least 2–3 days. The fact of extended lifespan is very beneficial for the development of infection because the final host cells for these parasites are macrophages, which normally migrate to the sites of infection within two or three days. The pathogens are not dronish; instead they take over the command at the primary site of infection. They induce the production by PMNs of the chemokines MIP-1α and MIP-1β (macrophage inflammatory protein) to recruit macrophages.

Silent Phagocytosis Theory

To save the integrity of the surrounding tissue from the toxic cell components and proteolytic enzymes contained in neutrophils, the apoptotic PMNs are silently cleared by macrophages. Dying PMNs expose the "eat me"-signal phosphatidylserine which is transferred to the outer leaflet of the plasma membrane during apoptosis. By reason of delayed apoptosis, the parasites that persist in PMNs are taken up into macrophages, employing an absolutely physiological and nonphlogistic process. The strategy of this "silent phagocytosis" has the following advantages for the parasite:

- Taking up apoptotic cells silences macrophage killing activity leading to a survival of the pathogens.
- Pathogens inside of PMNs have no direct contact to the macrophage surface receptors, because they can not see the parasite inside the apoptotic cell. So, the activation of the phagocyte for immune activation does not occur.

However, studies have shown this is unlikely, as the pathogens are seen to leave apoptopic cells and no evidence is known of macrophage uptake by this method.

Molecular Biology and Genomics

An important aspect of the *Leishmania* protozoan is its glycoconjugate layer of lipophosphoglycan (LPG). This is held together with a phosphoinositide membrane anchor, and has a tripartite structure consisting of a lipid domain, a neutral hexasaccharide, and a phosphorylated galactose-mannose, with a termination in a neutral cap. Not only do these parasites develop postphlebotomus digestion, but it is also thought to be essential to oxidative bursts, thus allowing passage for infection. Characteristics of intracellular digestion include an endosome fusing with a lysosome, releasing acid hydrolases which degrade DNA, RNA, proteins and carbohydrates.

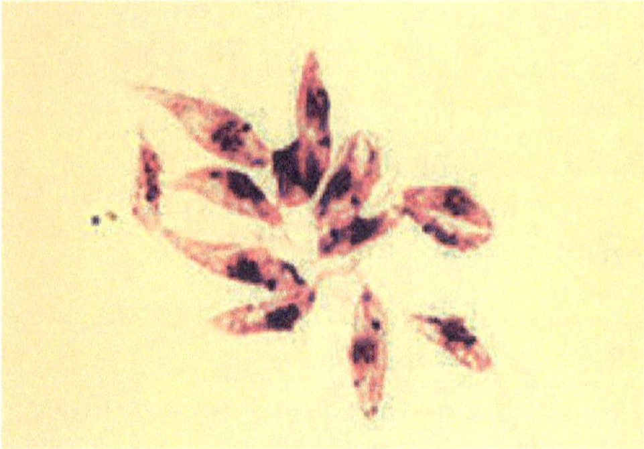

Leishmania tropica

The genomes of four *Leishmania* species (*L. major*, *L. infantum*, *L. donovani* and *L. braziliensis*) have been sequenced, revealing more than 8300 protein-coding and 900 RNA genes. Almost 40% of protein-coding genes fall into 662 families containing between two and 500 members. Most of the smaller gene families are tandem arrays of one to three genes, while the larger gene families are often dispersed in tandem arrays at different loci throughout the genome. Each of the 35 or 36 chromosomes is organized into a small number of gene clusters of tens-to-hundreds of genes on the same DNA strand. These clusters can be organized in head-to-head (divergent) or tail-to-tail (convergent) fashion, with the latter often separated by tRNA, rRNA and/or snRNA genes. Transcription of protein-coding genes initiates bidirectionally in the divergent strand-switch regions between gene clusters and extends polycistronically through each gene cluster before terminating in the strand-switch region separating convergent clusters. *Leishmania* telomeres are usually relatively small, consisting of a few different types of repeat sequence. Evidence can be found for recombination between several different groups of telomeres. The *L. major* and *L. infantum* genomes contain only about 50 copies of inactive degenerated *Ingi*/L1Tc-related elements (DIREs), while *L. braziliensis* also contains several telomere-associated transposable elements and spliced leader-associated retroelements. The *Leishmania* genomes share a conserved core proteome of about 6200 genes with the related trypanosomatids *Trypanosoma brucei* and *Trypanosoma cruzi*, but around 1000 *Leishmania*-specific genes are known, which are mostly randomly distributed throughout the genome. Relatively few (about 200) species-specific differences in gene content exist between the three sequenced *Leishmania* genomes, but about 8% of the genes appear to be evolving at different rates between the three species, indicative of different selective pressures that could be related to disease pathology. About 65% of protein-coding genes currently lack functional assignment.

Leishmania species produce several different heat shock proteins. These incluse Hsp83, a homolog of Hsp90. A regulatory element in the 3’ UTR of Hsp83 controls translation of Hsp83 in a temperature-sensitive manner. This region forms a stable RNA structure which melts at higher temperatures.

Sexual Reproduction

A microbial pathogen's reproductive system is one of the basic biologic processes that condition the micoroorganism's ecology and disease spread. Akopyants et al. demonstrated that *L. major* has a sexual cycle, including a meiotic process. Hybrid progeny are formed that have full genomic complements from both parents. Mating only occurs in the sand fly vector, and hybrids can be transmitted to the mammalian host by sand fly bite. In *L. braziliensis* matings in nature are predominantly between related individuals resulting in extreme inbreeding. The rate of outcrossing between different strains of *Leishmania* in the sand fly vector depends on the frequency of co-infection. Such outcrossing events appear to be rare in *L. major* and *L. donovani*.

L. infantum produces proteins BRCA1 and RAD51 that interact with each other to promote homologous recombinational repair. These proteins play a key role in meiosis. Thus, meiotic events provide the adaptive advantage of efficient recombinational repair of DNA damages even when they do not lead to outcrossing.

Classification

Babesia is a protozoan parasite of which *B. microti* and *B. divergens* are the two species most frequently found to infect humans. Infections from other species of *Babesia* have been documented in humans, but are not regularly seen. Babesiosis is also known as piroplasmosis. Due to historical misclassifications, this protozoan was labeled with many names that are no longer used. Common names of the disease include Texas cattle fever, redwater fever, tick fever, and Nantucket fever.

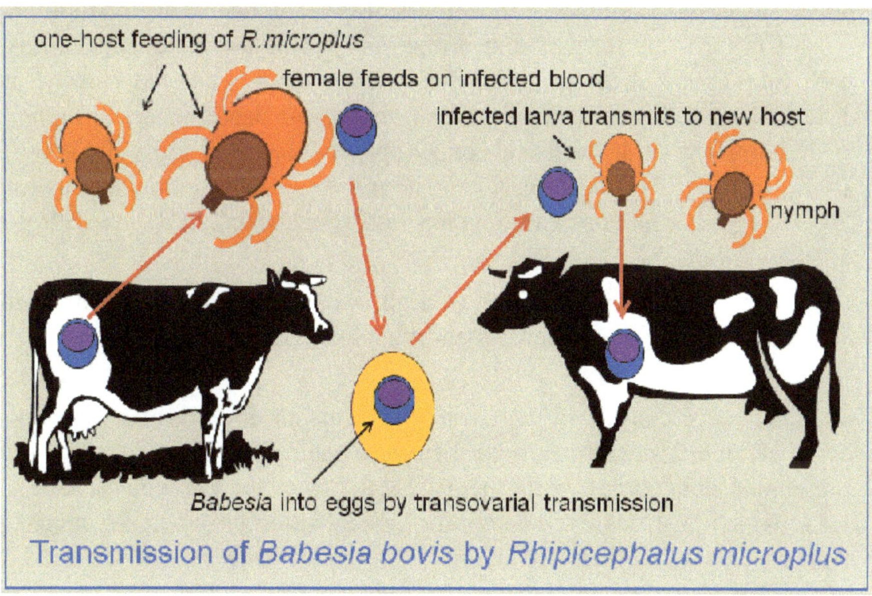

B. bovis transmission

Genomics

Although it was initially reported that the mitochondrial genome is circular unlike other sequenced Apicomplexa mitochondrial genomes, this has now been revised. The mitochondrial genome is actually linear.

Partial RNA sequencing of canine piroplams has identified a number of additional species.

The genome of *B. microti* has been sequenced. The sequence shows that this species does not belong to the either of the established genera — *Babesia* and *Theileria* — but instead belongs to a separate genus.

Clinical presentation

The severity of *B. microti* infections varies. For 25% of cases in adults and 50% of cases in children, the disease is asymptomatic or mild with flu-like symptoms. In other cases, symptoms are characterized by irregular fevers, chills, headaches, general lethargy, pain, and malaise. In severe cases, hemolytic anemia, jaundice, shortness of breath, and hemoglobinuria are documented due to the lytic effects of parasitic multiplication. Immunocompetent individuals with healthy spleens often recover without treatment. Splenectomized patients are more susceptible to contracting the disease and the course of infection often ends fatally within five to eight days of symptom onset. Parasitemia levels can reach up to 85% in patients without spleens compared to 1–10% in individuals with spleens and effective immune systems. Splenectomized patients suffer from severe hemolytic anemia with occasional incidences of hepatomegaly and splenomegaly documented.

Complications arising from *B. microti* infections include acute respiratory failure, congestive heart failure, and renal failure. Infections can be fatal in 5-10% of hospitalized patients, with increased risk of death in the immunosuppressed, the elderly, and those coinfected with Lyme disease. *B. divergens* infections have a much higher fatality rate (42%) and present with more severe symptoms. Infected individuals suffer from hemoglobinuria followed by jaundice, a persistently high fever, chills, and sweats. If left untreated, *B. divergens* infections can develop into shock-like symptoms with pulmonary edema and renal failure.

Signs of infection usually arise one to eight weeks after a bite from an infectious tick. Infections from *B. divergens* have a shorter latent period, usually ranging from one to three weeks.

Bovine babesiosis caused by *B. bovis* remains an important constraint for the development of cattle industries worldwide. Effective control can be achieved by vaccination with live attenuated phenotypes of the parasite. However, these vaccines have a number of drawbacks, which justifies the search for better, safer vaccines. In recent years, a number of parasite proteins with immunogenic potential have been discovered. Through polymerase chain reaction, genetic sequencing, and bioinformatics analysis of the genes, a high degree of conservation (98-100%) was found among Brazilian isolates of *B. bovis* and the T2Bo isolate. Thus, these genes are worth considering as viable candidates to be included in a recombinant cocktail vaccine for cattle babesiosis caused by *B. bovis*.

Transmission

Babesia species are spread through the saliva of a tick when it bites. At its nymphal stage, a tick bites into the skin for a blood meal. The tick, if not removed, stays attached for three to four days, with longer periods of feeding associated with a higher probability of acquiring the parasite. The parasite can survive in the tick as it molts through its various developmental stages, resulting in all stages being potentially infectious. Some species of *Babesia* can be transmitted from a female tick to its offspring before migrating to salivary glands for feeding. *B. microti*, the most common species in humans, though, has not been shown to transmit transovarially. Ticks of domestic animals that transmit *Babesia*, causing much disease, include the very widespread cattle ticks, *Rhipicephalus (Boophilus) microplus*, and *R.(B.) decoloratus*. These ticks have a strict one-host feeding cycle on cattle, so the *Babesia* can only be transmitted by the transovarial route.

In the Americas, *Ixodes scapularis* is the most common vector. This hard tick, commonly known as a deer tick, is also the vector for other tick-associated illnesses, such as Lyme disease. Many species of *Babesia* only infect nonhuman mammalian hosts, most commonly cattle, horses, and sheep. *B. microti* and *B. divergens* are the two main pathogenic species in humans. Their reservoirs are theorized to be the white-footed mouse (*Peromyscus leucopus*), microtus voles (*Microtus* spp.), and the white-tailed deer (*Odocoileus virginianus*). These woodland species are hypothesized reservoirs because although they are known to harbor the disease, complete reservoir competence has not yet been shown.

Most cases of transmission between humans are attributed to a tick vector. As of 2003, though, the Centers for Disease Control and Prevention (CDC) acknowledged more than 40 cases of babesiosis contracted from packed red blood cell (PRBC) transfusions and two infections documented from organ transplantation. PRBC transfusions that cause infections were identified through testing of the blood donor for *B. microti* antibodies. The occurrence of PRBC transfusions as a mechanism of *Babesia* transmission puts pressure on governmental organizations, such as the CDC, to heighten standard measures for screening blood donations.

Adaptations of Babesia and Rise of Genetic Diversity

Babesia show host specificity, allowing many different subspecies of Babesia to emerge, each infecting a different kind of vertebrae organism. Interestingly, while the different subspecies, such as *B. bovis* and *Babesia bigemina* prefer to infect cattle in tropical environments, they are capable of infecting other animals, such as the white-tailed deer. Therefore, while the organism has the capacity to display host specificity, and thus increase transmission effectiveness, it can also infect a variety of hosts.

The process by which Babesia achieves this is through mutations and natural selection. As the protozoa exposes itself to different environments, individuals within the population may develop mutations that increase their fitness within the current environment. These individuals exhibit greater fitness and thus the population evolves to increase their numbers. This also explains why there is such great genetic diversity for this organism.

Babesia persists long-term in the host's system and maintains a selfish relationship with it: the host gains no benefit from the parasite invasion but rather suffers by being infected. This allows the parasite to exploit all of the resources offered by the host, allowing it to increase in number, and eventually increase rate of transmission. Too lethal of an infection would result in the death of the host resulting in the parasite being unable to spread, which would ultimately be seen as a loss from an evolutionary standpoint. Different species of Babesia are able to withstand the stress of the host's immune system. Infection typically stimulates the innate, and not humoral, immune system. This results in control of the infection, but not clearance, allowing the organism to persist.

Lifecycle

Babesia species enter red blood cells (erythrocytes) at the sporozoite stage. Within the red blood cell, the protozoa become cyclical and develop into a trophozoite ring. The trophozoites moult into merozoites, which have a tetrad structure coined a Maltese-cross form. The tetrad morphology, which can be seen with Giemsa staining of a thin blood smear, is unique to *Babesia*, and serves as a distinguishing feature from *Plasmodium falciparum*, a protozoan of similar morphology that causes malaria. Trophozoite and merozoite growth ruptures the host erythrocyte, leading to the release of vermicules, the infectious parasitic bodies, which rapidly spread the protozoa throughout the blood.

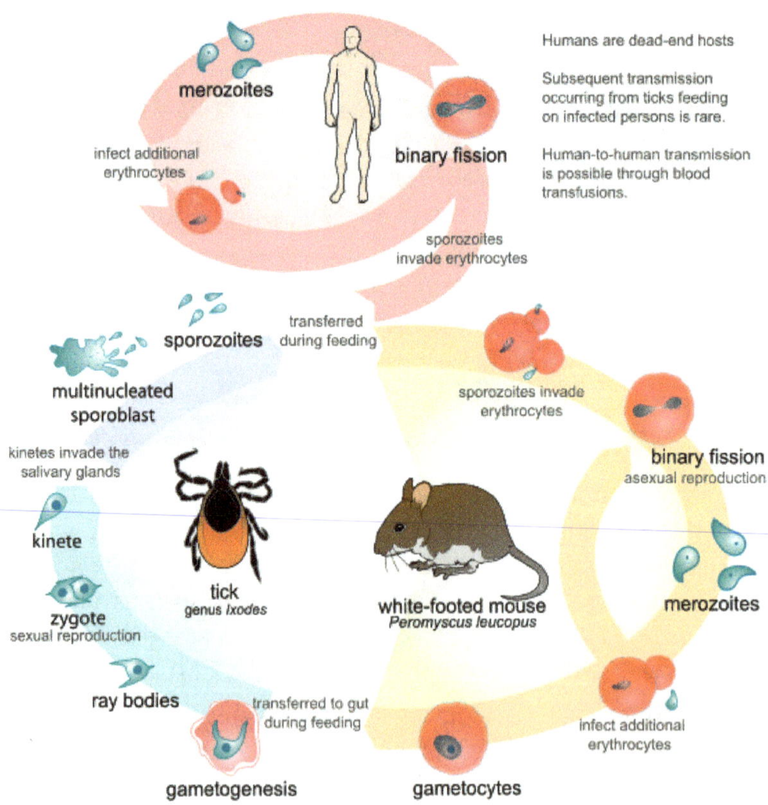

Lifecycle of *Babesia*

The lifecycle of *B. microti*, which is typical of parasites in that genus, requires a biological stage in a rodent or deer host, and is transmitted by ticks of the family Ixodidae between these hosts. To begin, the ticks introduce the sporozoites into the host when taking a blood meal. Sporozoites enter erythrocytes in the blood and begin the cyclical development between trophozoites and merozoites. Rather than producing more trophozoites, some merozoites produce gametocytes. The tick definitive host takes up the gametocytes when attached for a blood meal. The gametes are fertilized in the gut of the tick and develop into sporozoites in the salivary glands. The sporozoites are introduced into a human upon inoculation at the bite of an infected tick. Even as an incidental host, the phase changes which occur in the parasite are the same within humans as in the biological hosts. *Babesia* can be diagnosed at the trophozoite stage, and can be transmitted from human to human either through the tick vector or through blood transfusions.

Patterns of incidence

In the past, it was noticed that the emergence of tick-borne diseases coincided with climate change, but it is questionable whether or not climate change is a cause of the emergence. After much data collection, a correlation was found between climate change and the incidence of tick-borne diseases. However, the correlation is not strong enough to outright claim that climate change is a major factor of the increasing prevalence of tick-borne diseases.

High environmental temperature, humidity and rainfall have been correlated with fostering a more accommodating environment for the ticks carrying Babesia. This may explain why *B. bigemina* infection in cattle in the hilly region of Meghalaya has increased. It has also been noted that the life span and number of generations of *Babesia microplus* are affected by the climate, as warm weather has been correlated with increasing the longevity of larvae and number of annual generations.However, it is important to acknowledge what type of warm weather pertains to this claim. Dry warm weather results in interference with the life cycle of Babesia within the tick, and cold weather completely interrupts transmission. Warm, wet weather increases the intensity of infestation- the population is able to better able to thrive due to the relatively fluid environment being more accommodating by making water and nutrients more accessible.

Diagnosis and treatment

Diagnostic tests

As a protozoan parasite, the most effective way to identify *Babesia* infection is through blood sample testing. It is important to pay specific attention to particular morphologies of *Babesia* in blood smears because its substantial similarity to the malarial parasite *Plasmodium falciparum* results in many patients suffering from babesiosis being misdiagnosed. The few distinguishing factors for *Babesia* include protozoa with varying shapes and sizes, the potential to contain vacuoles, and the lack of pigment production. Trophozoites within an erythrocyte that appear in a tetrad formation are also indicative of *Babesia*. A trained eye is necessary to distinguish the two species.

Even with much study of babesiosis and malaria, misdiagnosis with blood smear can be frequent and problematic. To supplement a blood smear, diagnoses should be made with an indirect fluorescent antibody (IFA) test. IFA testing has a much higher specificity than stained blood smears with antibody detection in 88-96% of infected patients. Diagnostic measures through antibody testing are also particularly useful for identifying serum prevalence in asymptomatic individuals. Due to the transmissibility of *Babesia* through blood transfusions, IFA testing would be an effective means of screening for the disease in blood donations.

Historically, babesiosis diagnosis was carried out with xenodiagnosis in hamsters for *B. microti* and in gerbils for *B.divergens*.While successful at identifying the disease, this diagnostic technique has been abandoned for faster diagnostic measures.

Treatment

Several methods are available to manage and treat babesiosis in animals. In many cases, patients spontaneously recover, having only experienced mild symptoms undiagnosed as the disease. This occurrence is almost always seen in *B. microti* infections, which are generally more common in the United States. For *B. divergens* and more severe *B. microti* infections, the standard treatment historically for symptomatic individuals was oral or intravenous clindamycin with oral quinine. With the results of research completed in 2000, however, treatment regimens have been increasingly leaning towards oral atovaquone with oral azithromycin. The latter medications are preferred, as they are equally effective in all but the most severe cases and exhibit fewer associated adverse reactions. In severe cases, blood exchange transfusions have been performed to lower the parasitic load in the individual. Other rudimentary treatment measures include addressing and correcting abnormal clinical signals.

Epidemiology

Of the species to infect humans, *B. microti* is most common in the Americas, whereas *B. divergens* is the predominant strain found in Europe. Endemic areas are regions of tick habitat, including the forest regions of the northeastern United States and temperate regions of Europe. Ixodidae, the tick vectors of *B. microti*, also transmit the better-known *Borrelia burgdorferi*, causative agent of Lyme disease. For reasons that remain unclear, in areas endemic to both Lyme disease and babesiosis, Lyme disease transmission prevails and is more predominant in the region. Prevalence of babesiosis in malaria-endemic regions remains unknown due to the likelihood of misdiagnosis as malaria. As the disease results in a high number of asympomatic individuals, many populations can possess high seroprevalence without much documentation of illness. For example, in Rhode Island and Nantucket, seroprevalence has been measured to be 20-25%. Prevalence of babesiosis is mostly documented during the months of May to September when tick activity in endemic regions is high.

Prevention

The most effective public health measure for *Babesia* is avoidance of tick exposure. This can be performed through personal prevention strategies such as avoiding tick-infested areas (especially during high tick season between May and September), remaining covered with light clothing, searching for ticks after being outdoors, and removing discovered ticks from the skin.Other preventive measures include applying diethyltoluamide (DEET), a common repellent that is effective against ticks and insects. (For people who react adversely to DEET, alternative insect repellents should be used.) On a state level, if health departments are particularly motivated, tick elimination is a possibility. In 1906, efforts were made to eradicate the tick vector of the bovine disease form of babesiosis in the United States. This eradication was recorded as being successfully completed four decades later. Complete eradication efforts would be a long-term project, which would significantly reduce the prevalence of both babesiosis and Lyme disease. However, as public health departments are often short on funding, preventive measures seem to be more recommended over vector control. Due to the relatively low prevalence of the disease and the presence of several reservoirs, babesiosis is currently not a candidate for vaccine-based prevention. In regions where ticks of domestic animals are routinely controlled with chemical acaricides to reduce incidence of infection with *B. bovis* and *B. bigemina*, the risk to humans from these parasites will be reduced.

Characteristics

Balamuthia mandrillaris is a free-living, heterotrophic amoeba, consisting of a standard complement of organelles surrounded by a three-layered cell wall, and with an abnormally large cell nucleus. On average, a *Balamuthia* trophozoite is approximately 30 to 120 micrometres in diameter. The cysts fall approximately in this range as well.

Life cycle

Balamuthia's life cycle, like the *Acanthamoeba*, consists of a cystic stage and a trophozoite stage, both of which are infectious, and both of which can be identified as inclusions in the brain tissue on microscopic examination of brain biopsies performed on infected individuals. The trophozoite is pleomorphic and uninucleated, but binucleate forms are occasionally seen. Cysts are also uninucleated possessing three walls: an outer thin irregular ectocyst, an inner thick endocyst, and a middle amorphous fibrillar mesocyst.

Pathology

Balamuthia mandrillaris is larger than human leukocytes therefore making phagocytosis impossible. Instead, the immune system attempts to contain them at the portal of entry by mounting a type IV hypersensitivity reaction. They may enter the body through the lower respiratory tract or through open wounds. Upon introduction, the amoeba may form a skin lesion, or may migrate to the brain, causing a condition known as granulomatous amoebic encephalitis, (GAE), which is usually fatal. This granulomatous feature is mostly seen in immunocompetent patients; immunocompromised individuals exhibit a "peri-vascular cuffing". *Balamuthia*-induced GAE can cause focal paralysis, seizures, and brainstem symptoms such as facial paralysis, difficulty swallowing, and double vision.

Balamuthia may also cause a variety of non-neurological symptoms, including skin lesions, which can progress to GAE. Patients experiencing this particular syndrome may report a skin lesion (often similar to those caused by MRSA), which does not respond well to topical antibiotics. The lesion is usually localised and very slow to heal, or fails to heal altogether. In some presentations, the infection may be mistaken for certain forms of skin cancer or leishmaniasis. *Balamuthia* lesions on the face often cause swelling.

Diagnostic tests

Balamuthia is most easily identifiable in a brain biopsy performed on an individual suffering from GAE. The amoeba cannot be cultured on an agar plate coated with gram negative bacteria because unlike Naegleria, *Balamuthia mandrillaris* does not feed on bacteria. Instead *Balamuthia* must be cultured on primate liver or human brain microvascular endothelial cells (the cells that constitute the blood–brain barrier).

Treatment

Balamuthia infection has had successful treatments. In two cases, both were treated with a cocktail of antibiotics and antifungal drugs, although it is unclear if any or all of these medications played a part in treatment. Both victims suffered permanent neurological deficits as a result of their infection. Another two cases were presented and both of these individuals received successful treatments due to discovering the infection early. Two individuals, a five-year-old girl and a 64-year-old man, developed GAE. After diagnosis, they were given powerful antimicrobial therapy. Both patients recovered.

Organ transplantation

According to a MMWR report published in September 2010, two confirmed cases of *Balamuthia* transmission occurred through organ transplantation in December 2009 in Mississippi. Two kidney recipients, a 31-year-old woman and a 27-year-old man, suffered from post transplant encephalitis due to balamuthia. The woman died in February 2010 and the man survived with partial paralysis of right arm. The CDC was notified by a physician on December 14, 2009 about possible transplant transmission in these two patients. Histopathologic testing of donor and recipient tissues confirmed the transmission. Two other patients who received heart and liver transplants from the same donor but in different hospitals were placed on preemptive therapy and remain unaffected. A second cluster of transplant transmitted *Balamuthia* in Arizona was reported in the same weekly report. There were four recipients: two from Arizona (liver and kidney-pancreas), one from California (kidney) and another from Utah (heart). Recipients from Arizona—a 56-year-old male and a 24-year-old male—both succumbed to encephalitis within a span of 40 days from transplantation. The other two were placed on preemptive therapy after the first two were reported and remain unaffected.

General characteristics

Cryptosporidium causes cryptosporidiosis, an infection that may present as a diarrhoeal with or without a persistent cough in immunocompetent hosts.Other apicomplexan pathogens include the malaria parasite *Plasmodium*, and the toxoplasmosis parasite *Toxoplasma*. Unlike *Plasmodium*, which transmits via a mosquito vector, *Cryptosporidium* does not use an insect vector, and is capable of completing its lifecycle within a single host, resulting in cyst stages that are excreted in feces or through coughing fomites and are capable of transmission to a new host.

A number of *Cryptosporidium* species infect mammals. In humans, the main causes of disease are *C. parvum* and *C. hominis* (previously *C. parvum* genotype 1). *C. canis*, *C. felis*, *C. meleagridis*, and *C. muris* can also cause disease in humans.

Cryptosporidiosis is typically an acute, short-term infection, can be recurrent through reinfection in immunocompetent hosts, and become severe or life-threatening in immunocompromised individuals. In humans, it remains in the lower intestine and may remain for up to five weeks. The parasite is transmitted by environmentally hardy cysts (oocysts) that, once ingested, exist in the small intestine and result in an infection of intestinal epithelial tissue.Transmission by ingestion or inhalation of coughed fomites is a second, less likely route of infection.

The genome of *Cryptosporidium parvum*, sequenced in 2004, was found to be unusual amongst eukaryotes in that the mitochondria seem not to contain DNA. A closely related species, *C. hominis*, also has its genome sequence available.

Life cycle

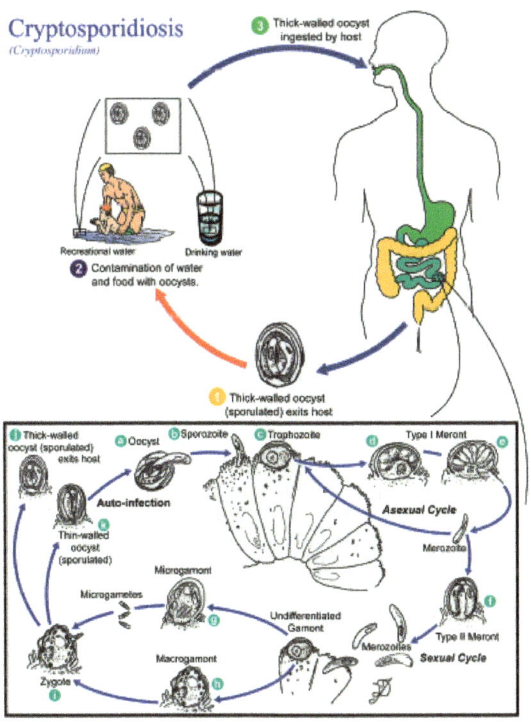

Life cycle of *Cryptosporidium* spp.

The *Cryptosporidium* spore phase (oocyst) can survive for lengthy periods outside a host. It can also resist many common disinfectants, notably chlorine-based disinfectants.

Water treatment and detection

Many treatment plants that take raw water from rivers, lakes, and reservoirs for public drinking water production use conventional filtration technologies. Direct filtration, which is typically used to treat water with low particulate levels, includes coagulation and filtration but not sedimentation. Other common filtration processes including slow sand filters, diatomaceous earth filter, and membranes will remove 99% of *Cryptosporidium*. Membranes and bag- and cartridge-filter products remove *Cryptosporidium* specifically.

Cryptosporidium is highly resistant to chlorine disinfection; but with high enough concentrations and contact time, *Cryptosporidium* inactivation will occur with chlorine dioxide and ozone treatment. In general, the required levels of chlorine preclude the use of chlorine disinfection as a reliable method to control *Cryptosporidium* in drinking water. Ultraviolet light treatment at relatively low doses will inactivate *Cryptosporidium*. Water Research Foundation-funded research originally discovered UV's efficacy in inactivating *Cryptosporidium*.

One of the largest challenges in identifying outbreaks is the ability to verify the results in a laboratory. The oocytes may be seen by microscopic examination of a stool sample, but they may be confused with other objects or artifacts similar in appearance. Most cryptosporidia are 3–6 μm in size, although some reports have described larger cells. Real-time monitoring technology is now able to detect *Cryptosporidium* with online systems versus the spot testing and batch testing methods used in the past.

For the end consumer of drinking water believed to be contaminated by *Cryptosporidium*, the safest option is to boil all water used for drinking.

Exposure Risks

The following groups have an elevated risk of being exposed to *Cryptosporidium*:

- People who swim regularly in pools with insufficient sanitation (Certain strains of *Cryptosporidium* are chlorine-resistant)
- Child-care workers
- Parents of infected children
- People caring for other people with cryptosporidiosis
- Backpackers, hikers, and campers who drink unfiltered, untreated water
- People, including swimmers, who swallow water from contaminated sources
- People handling infected cattle
- People exposed to human faeces

Cases of cryptosporidiosis can occur in a city with clean water; cases of cryptosporidiosis can have different origins. Like many fecal-oral pathogens, it can also be transmitted by contaminated food or poor hygiene. Testing of water, as well as epidemiological study, are necessary to determine the sources of specific infections. *Cryptosporidium* typically does not cause serious illness in healthy people. It may chronically sicken some children, as well as adults exposed and immunocompromised. A subset of the immunocompromised population is people with AIDS, amongst MSM with AIDS insertive anal sex is an increased risk factor. Analingus, oral–genital sex after anal–genital sex are known transmission routes.

Other transmission routes include exposure to laboratory specimens.

Life cycle

Naegleria fowleri is a thermophilic (heat-loving), free-living amoeba. It is found in warm and hot freshwater ponds, lakes and rivers, and in the very warm water of hot springs. As the water temperature rises, its numbers increase. It was first discovered in 1965, and first identified in Australia. *N. fowleri* occurs in three forms – as a cyst, a trophozoite (ameboid), and a biflagellate (it has two flagella). It does not form a cyst in human tissue, where only the amoeboid trophozoite stage exists. The flagellate form can exist in the cerebrospinal fluid.

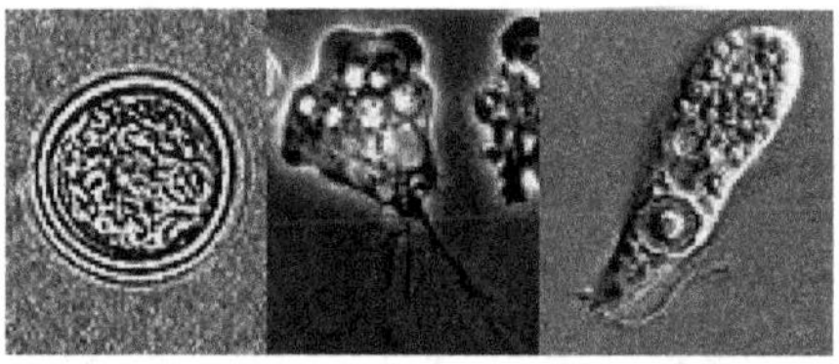

Biotic phases: cyst, trophozoite, flagellate

Cellular stages

Cyst stage

The cyst form is spherical and about 7-15 μm in diameter. They are smooth, and have a single-layered wall with a single nucleus. Cysts are naturally resistant to environmental factors, so as to increase the chances of survival until better conditions occur. Trophozoites encyst due to unfavorable conditions. Factors that induce cyst formation include a lack of food, overcrowding, desiccation, accumulation of waste products, and cold temperatures. When conditions improve, the amoeba can escape through the pore, or ostiole, seen in the middle of the cyst. *N. fowleri* has been found to encyst at temperatures below 10 °C (50 °F).

Trophozoite stage

The trophozoite is the feeding, dividing, and infective stage for humans. The trophozoite attaches to olfactory epithelium, where it follows the olfactory cell axon through the cribriform plate (in the nasal cavity) to the brain. This reproductive stage of the protozoan organism, which transforms near 25 °C (77 °F) and grows fastest around 42 °C (106.7

°F), proliferates by binary fission. The trophozoites are characterized by a nucleus and a surrounding halo. They travel by pseudopodia, which means that they extend parts of their body's cell membrane (the pseudopods) and then fill them with plasma to force locomotion. The pseudopods form at different points along the cell, thus allowing the trophozoite to change directions. In their free-living state, trophozoites feed on bacteria. In tissues, they phagocytize (consume by enclosing and then digesting prey) red blood cells and white blood cells, destroying tissue.

Flagellate

The flagellate is pear-shaped and biflagellate: this means that it has two flagella. This stage can be inhaled into the nasal cavity during swimming or diving. This biflagellate form occurs when trophozoites are exposed to a change in ionic concentration, such as placement in distilled water. The flagellate form does not exist in human tissue, but can exist in the cerebrospinal fluid. Once inside the nasal cavity, the flagellated form transforms into a trophozoite. The transformation of trophozoite to flagellate occurs within a few hours.

Ecology

Naegleria fowleri are amoeboflagellates that inhabit soil and water. *Naegleria fowleri* is more sensitive to drying and pH (acid levels) than other amoeboflagellates. It cannot survive in sea water. This amoeba is able to grow best at moderately elevated temperatures making summer month cases more likely. *N. fowleri* is thermotolerant and able to survive 45 °C (113 °F). Warm, fresh water with a sufficient supply of bacterial food provide a habitat for amoebae. Man-made bodies of water, disturbed natural habitats, or areas with soil and unchlorinated/unfiltered water are locations where many amoebic infections have happened. *N. fowleri* seems to thrive during periods of disturbance; the flagellate-empty hypothesis explains that Naglerias success may be due to decreased competition from decreased amount of the normal, thermosensitive protozoal fauna. In other words, *N. fowleri* thrives in the absence of other predators consuming its food supply. This hypothesis suggests that human disturbances such as thermal pollution increase *N. fowleri* abundance by removing their resource competitors. Ameoboflagellates have a motile flagellate stage that is designed for dispersal which is advantageous if an environment has been cleared out of competing organisms.

Pathogenicity

N. fowleri can cause an often lethal infection of the brain called naegleriasis (also known as primary amoebic meningoencephalitis (PAM), amoebic encephalitis/meningitis, or simply *Naegleria* infection). Infections most often occur when water containing *N. fowleri* is inhaled through the nose, where it then enters the nasal and olfactory nerve tissue, traveling to the brain through the cribriform plate. *N. fowleri* normally eat bacteria, but during human infections, the trophozoites consume astrocytes and neurons. The reason why *N. fowleri* prefers to pass across the cribriform plate has remained unknown, but the neurotransmitter acetylcholine has been suggested to act as a stimulus, as a structural homolog of animal CHRM1 has been shown to present in Naegleria and Acanthamoeba.

It takes up to 5 days (1–12 days average) for symptoms to appear after nasal exposure to *N. fowleri* flagellates. Initial symptoms are may include headache, fever, nausea, or vomiting. Later symptoms can include stiff neck, confusion, lack of attention, loss of balance, seizures, and hallucinations. Once symptoms begin to appear, death will usually occur within two weeks. A person infected with *N. fowleri* cannot spread the infection to another person.

The core antimicrobial treatment consists of antifungal drug amphotericin B, but the fatality rate even with this treatment is greater than 95%. New treatments are being sought. Miltefosine, an antiparasitic, has been used in a few cases with mixed results.

Lifecycle

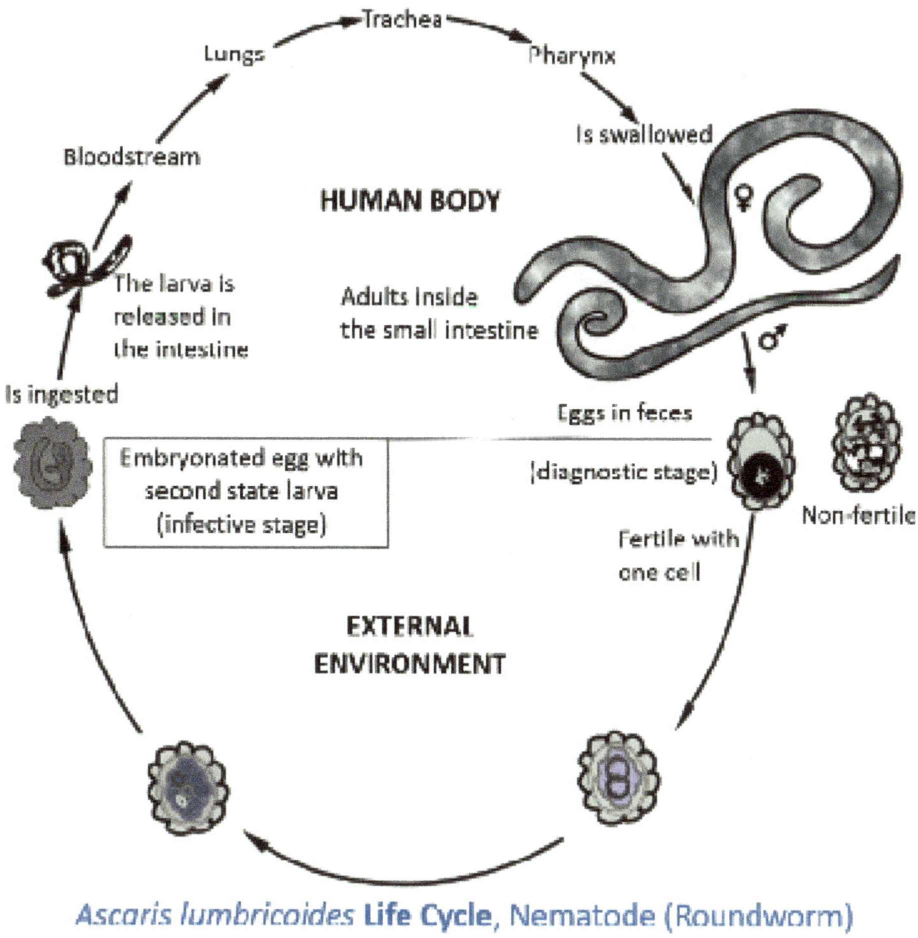

Image showing lifecycle inside and outside of the human body of one fairly well described helminth: *A. lumbricoides*

Ascaris lumbricoides, a roundworm, infects humans when an ingested fertilised egg becomes a larval worm (called rhabditiform larva) that penetrates the wall of the duodenum and enters the blood stream. From there, it is carried to the liver and heart, and enters pulmonary circulation to break free in the alveoli, where it grows and molts. In three weeks, the larva passes from the respiratory system to be coughed up, swallowed, and thus returned to the small intestine, where it matures to an adult male or female worm. Fertilization can now occur and the female produces as many as 200,000 eggs per day for a year. These fertilized eggs become infectious after two weeks in soil; they can persist in soil for 10 years or more.

The eggs have a lipid layer which makes them resistant to the effects of acids and alkalis, as well as other chemicals. This resilience helps to explain why this nematode is such a ubiquitous parasite.

Characteristics

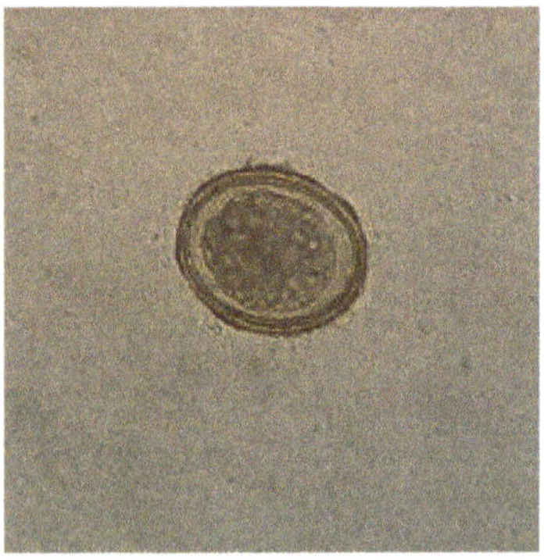

Fertile egg as can be seen in a microscope

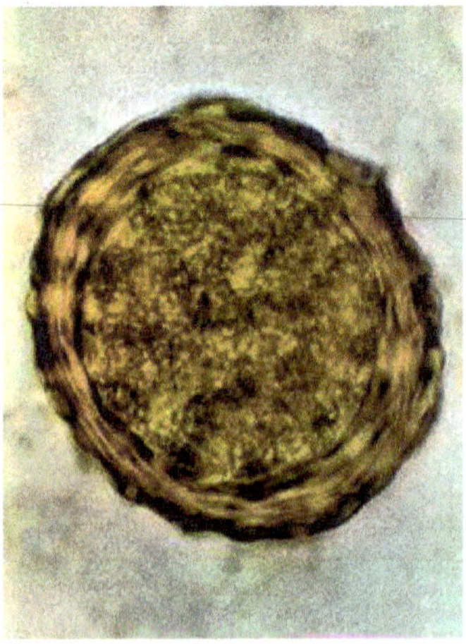

Fertile egg in human faeces (detail)

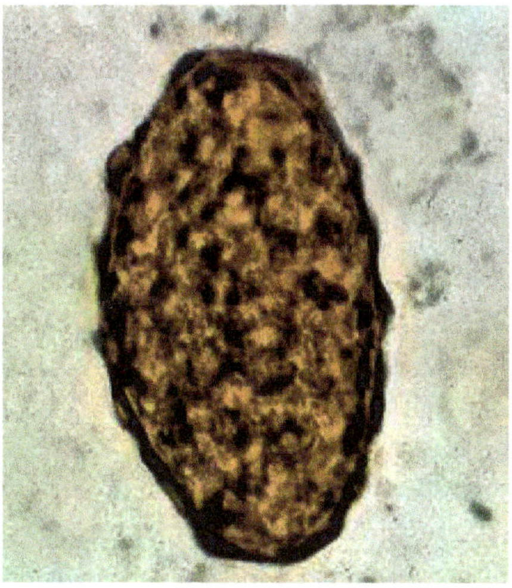

Infertile egg

Ascaris lumbricoides is characterized by its great size. Males are 2–4 mm (0.08–0.2 in) in diameter and 15–31 cm (5.9–12 in) long. The male's posterior end is curved ventrally and has a bluntly pointed tail. Females are 3–6 mm (0.1–0.2 in) wide and 20–49 cm (7.9–19 in) long. The vulva is located in the anterior end and accounts for about one-third of its body length. Uteri may contain up to 27 million eggs at a time, with 200,000 being laid per day. Fertilized eggs are oval to round in shape and are 45–75 μm (0.0018–0.0030 in) long and 35–50 μm (0.0014–0.0020 in) wide with a thick outer shell. Unfertilized eggs measure 88–94 μm (0.0035–0.0037 in) long and 44 μm (0.0017 in) wide.

Epidemiology

An estimated 1 billion people are infected with *A. lumbricoides* worldwide. While infection occurs throughout most of the world, *A. lumbricoides* infection is most common in sub-Saharan Africa, the Americas, China, and east Asia.

Ascaris lumbricoides eggs are extremely resistant to strong chemicals, desiccation, and low temperatures. The eggs can remain viable in the soil for several months or even years. Eggs of *A. lumbricoides* have been identified in archeological coprolites in the Americas, Europe, Africa, the Middle East, and New Zealand, the oldest ones being more than 24,000 years old.

Infection and Prevention

Infections with these parasites are more common where sanitation is poor, and raw human feces are used as fertilizer.

Often, no symptoms are seen with an *A. lumbricoides* infection. However, in the case of a particularly bad infection, symptoms may include bloody sputum, cough, fever, abdominal discomfort, intestinal ulcer, and passing worms. Ascariasis is also the most common cause of Löffler's syndrome worldwide. Accompanying symptoms include pulmonary infiltration, eosinophilia, and radiographic opacities. Significant increases in fertility are observed in infected women.

Preventing any fecal-borne disease requires educated hygienic habits/culture and effective fecal treatment systems. This is particularly important with *A. lumbricoides* because its eggs are one of the most difficult pathogens to kill (second only to prions), and the eggs commonly survive 1–3 years. *A. lumbricoides* lives in the intestine where it lays eggs. Infection occurs when the eggs, too small to be seen by the unaided eye, are eaten. The eggs may get onto vegetables when improperly processed human feces of infected people are used as fertilizer for food crops. Infection may occur when food is handled without removing or killing the eggs on the hands, clothes, hair, raw vegetables/fruit, or cooked food that is (re)infected by handlers, containers, etc. Bleach does not readily kill *A. lumbricoides* eggs, but it will remove their sticky film, to allow the eggs to be rinsed away. *A. lumbricoides* eggs can be reduced by hot composting methods, but to completely kill them may require rubbing alcohol, iodine, specialized chemicals, cooking heat, or "unusually" hot composting (for example, over 50 °C (122 °F) for 24 hours).

Details of infection

Infections happen when a human swallows water or food contaminated with unhatched eggs, which hatch into juveniles in the duodenum. They then penetrate the mucosa and submucosa and enter venules or lymphatics. Next, they pass through the right heart and into pulmonary circulation. They then break out of the capillaries and enter the air spaces. Acute tissue reaction occurs when several worms get lost during this migration and accumulate in other organs of the body. The juveniles migrate from the lung up the respiratory tract to the pharynx where they are swallowed. They begin producing eggs within 60–65 days of being swallowed. These are produced within the small intestine, where the juveniles mature. It might seem odd that the worms end up in the same place where they began. One hypothesis to account for this behavior is that the migration mimics an intermediate host, which would be required for juveniles of an ancestral form to develop to the third stage. Another possibility is that tissue migration enables faster growth and larger size, which increases reproductive capacity.

Signs and Symptoms

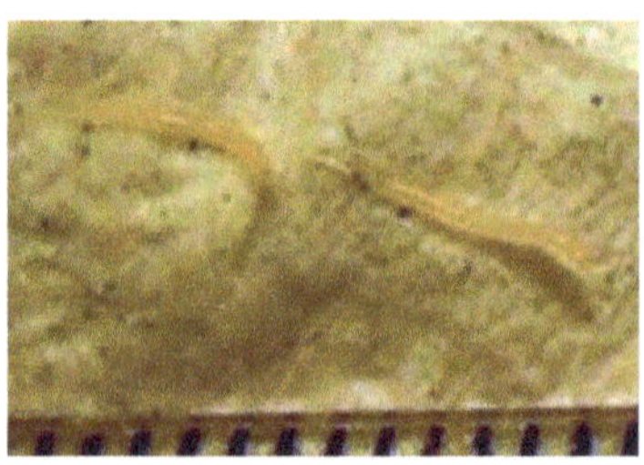

Two female pinworms next to a ruler. The markings are one millimeter apart.

One third of individuals with pinworm infection are totally asymptomatic.The main symptoms are pruritus ani and perineal pruritus, i.e., itching in and around the anus and around the perineum. The itching occurs mainly during the night, and is caused by the female pinworms migrating to lay eggs around the anus. Both the migrating females and the clumps of eggs are irritating, but the mechanisms causing the intense pruritus have not been explained. The intensity of the itching varies, and it can be described as tickling, crawling sensations, or even acute pain. The itching leads to continuously scratching the area around the anus, which can further result in tearing of the skin and complications such as secondary bacterial infections, including bacterial dermatitis (i.e., skin inflammation) and folliculitis (i.e., hair follicle inflammation). General symptoms are insomnia (i.e., persistent difficulties to sleep) and restlessness. A considerable proportion of children suffer from loss of appetite, weight loss, irritability, emotional instability, and enuresis (i.e., inability to control urination).

Pinworms cannot damage the skin, and they do not normally migrate through tissues. However, in women they may move onto the vulva and into the vagina, from there moving to the external orifice of the uterus, and onwards to the uterine cavity, fallopian tubes, ovaries, and peritoneal cavity. This can cause vulvovaginitis, i.e. an inflammation of the vulva and vagina. This causes vaginal discharge and pruritus vulvae, i.e., itchiness of the vulva. The pinworms can also enter the urethra, and presumably, they carry intestinal bacteria with them. According to Gutierrez (2000), a statistically significant correlation between pinworm infection and urinary tract infections has been shown; however, Burkhart & Burkhart (2005) maintain that the incidence of pinworms as a cause of urinary tract infections remains unknown. Incidentally, one report indicated that 36% of young girls with a urinary tract infection also had pinworms. Dysuria (i.e., painful urination) has been associated with pinworm infection.

The relationship between pinworm infestation and appendicitis has been researched, but there is a lack of clear consensus in the matter: while Gutierres (2005) maintains that there exists a consensus that pinworms do not produce the inflammatory reaction, Cook (1994) states that it is controversial whether pinworms are causatively related to acute appendicitis, and Burkhart & Burkhart (2004) state that pinworm infection causes symptoms of appendicitis to surface.

Cause

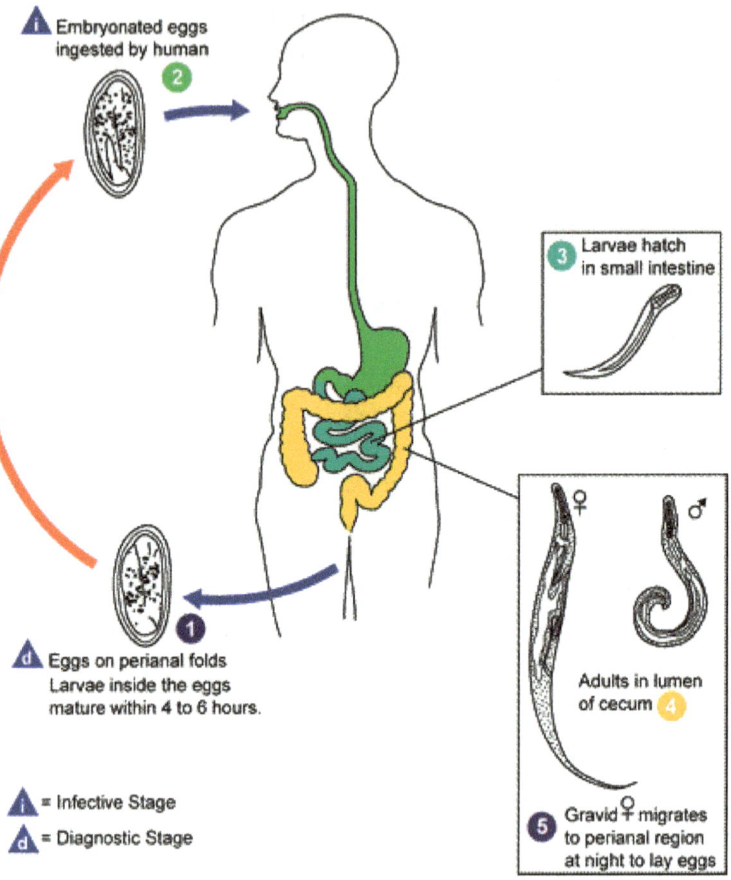

Life cycle.

The cause of a pinworm infection is the worm *Enterobius vermicularis*. The entire lifecycle — from egg to adult — takes place in the human gastrointestinal tract of a single human host. Cook *et al.* (2009) and Burkhart & Burkhart (2005) disagree over the length of this process, with Cook *et al.* stating two to four weeks, while Burkhart & Burkhart states that it takes from four to eight weeks.

Lifecycle

The lifecycle begins with eggs being ingested. The eggs hatch in the duodenum (i.e., first part of the small intestine). The emerging pinworm larvae grow rapidly to a size of 140 to 150 micrometers in size, and migrate through the small intestine towards the colon. During this migration they moult twice and become adults. Females survive for 5 to 13 weeks, and males about 7 weeks. The male and female pinworms mate in the ileum (i.e., last part of the small intestine), whereafter the male pinworms usually die, and are passed out with stool. The gravid female pinworms settle in the ileum, caecum (i.e., beginning of the large intestine), appendix and ascending colon, where they attach themselves to the mucosa and ingest colonic contents. Almost the entire body of a gravid female becomes filled with eggs. The estimations of the number of eggs in a gravid female pinworm ranges from about 11,000 to 16,000. The egg-laying process begins approximately five weeks after initial ingestion of pinworm eggs by the human host. The gravid female pinworms migrate through the colon towards the rectum at a rate of 12 to 14 centimeters per hour. They emerge from the anus, and while moving on the skin near the anus, the female pinworms deposit eggs either through (1) contracting and expelling the eggs, (2) dying and then disintegrating, or (3) bodily rupture due to the host scratching the worm. After depositing the eggs, the female becomes opaque and dies. The reason the female emerges from the anus is to obtain the oxygen necessary for the maturation of the eggs.

Spread

Pinworm infection spreads through human-to-human transmission, by ingesting (i.e., swallowing) infectious pinworm eggs. The eggs are hardy and can remain viable (i.e., infectious) in a moist environment for up to three weeks. They do not tolerate heat well, but can survive in low temperatures: two-thirds of the eggs are still viable after 18 hours at −8 degrees Celsius (18 °F).

After the eggs have been initially deposited near the anus, they are readily transmitted to other surfaces through contamination. The surface of the eggs is sticky when laid, and the eggs are readily transmitted from their initial deposit near the anus to fingernails, hands, night-clothing and bed linen. From here, eggs are further transmitted to food, water, furniture, toys, bathroom fixtures and other objects. Household pets often carry the eggs in their fur, while not actually being infected. Dust containing eggs can become airborne and widely dispersed when dislodged from surfaces, for instance when shaking out bed clothes and linen. Consequently, the eggs can enter the mouth and nose through inhalation, and be swallowed later. Although pinworms do not strictly multiply inside the body of their human host, some of the pinworm larvae may hatch on the anal mucosa, and migrate up the bowel and back into the gastrointestinal tract of the original host. This process is called *retroinfection*. According to Burkhart (2005), when this retroinfection occurs, it leads to a heavy parasitic load and ensures that the pinworm infestation continues. This statement is contradictory to a statement by Caldwell, who contends that retroinfection is rare and not clinically significant.Despite the limited, 13 week lifespan of individual pinworms, autoinfection (i.e., infection from the original host to itself), either through the anus-to-mouth route or through retroinfection, causes the pinworms to inhabit the same host indefinitely.

Diagnosis

Diagnosis depends on finding the eggs or the adult pinworms. Individual eggs are invisible to the naked eye, but they can be seen using a low-power microscope. On the other hand, the light-yellowish thread-like adult pinworms are clearly visually detectable, usually during the night when they move near the anus, or on toilet paper. Transparent adhesive tape (e.g. Scotch Tape) applied on the anal area will pick up deposited eggs, and diagnosis can be made by examining the tape with a microscope. This test is most successful if done every morning for several days, because the females do not lay eggs every day, and the number of eggs vary.

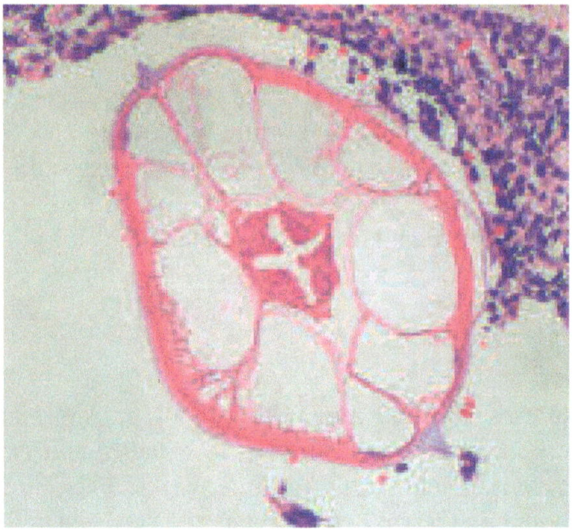

High magnification micrograph of a pinworm in cross section in the appendix. H&E stain.

Pinworms do not lay eggs in the feces, but sometimes eggs are deposited in the intestine. As such, routine examination of fecal material gives a positive diagnosis in only 5 to 15% of infected subjects, and is therefore of little practical diagnostic use. In a heavy infection, female pinworms may adhere to stools that pass out through the anus, and they may thus be detected on the surface on the stool. Adult pinworms are occasionally seen during colonoscopy. On a microscopic level, pinworms have an identifying feature of alae (i.e., protruding ridges) running the length of the worm.

Prevention

Pinworm infection cannot be totally prevented under most circumstances. This is due to the prevalence of the parasite and the ease of transmission through soiled night clothes, airborne eggs, contaminated furniture, toys and other objects.Infection may occur in the highest strata of society, where hygiene and nutritional status are typically high. The stigma associated with pinworm infection is hence considered a possible over-emphasis. Counselling is sometimes needed for upset parents that have discovered their children are infected, as they may not realize how prevalent the infection is.

Preventative action revolves around personal hygiene and the cleanliness of the living quarters. The *rate* of reinfection can be reduced through hygienic measures, and this is recommended especially in recurring cases. The main measures are keeping fingernails short, and washing and scrubbing hands and fingers carefully, especially after defecation and before meals. Under ideal conditions, bed covers, sleeping garments, and hand towels should be changed daily. Simple laundering of clothes and linen disinfects them.

Children should wear gloves while asleep, and the bedroom floor should be kept clean. Food should be covered to limit contamination with dust-borne parasite eggs. Household detergents have little effect on the viability of pinworm eggs, and cleaning the bathroom with a damp cloth moistened with an antibacterial agent or bleach will merely spread the still-viable eggs. Similarly, shaking clothes and bed linen will detach and spread the eggs.

Treatment

Medication is the primary treatment for pinworm infection. They are so effective that many medical scientists regard hygienic measures as impractical. However, reinfection is frequent regardless of the medication used. Total elimination of the parasite in a household may require repeated doses of medication for up to a year or more. Because the drugs kill the adult pinworms, but not the eggs, the first retreatment is recommended in two weeks. Also, if one household member spreads the eggs to another, it will be a matter of two or three weeks before those eggs become adult worms and thus amenable to treatment. Asymptomatic infections, often in small children, can serve as reservoirs of infection, and therefore the entire household should be treated regardless of whether or not symptoms are present.

The benzimidazole compounds albendazole (brand names e.g., *Albenza*, *Eskazole*, *Zentel* and *Andazol*) and mebendazole (brand names e.g., *Ovex*, *Vermox*, *Antiox* and *Pripsen*) are the most effective. They work by inhibiting the microtubule function in the pinworm adults, causing glycogen depletion, thereby effectively starving the parasite. A single 100 milligram dose of mebendazole with one repetition after a week, is considered the safest, and is usually effective with cure rate of 96%. Mebendazole has no serious side effects, although abdominal pain and diarrhea have been reported. Pyrantel pamoate (also called pyrantel embonate, brand names e.g., *Reese's Pinworm Medicine*, *Pin-X*, *Combantrin*, *Anthel*, *Helmintox*, and *Helmex*) kills adult pinworms through neuromuscular blockade, and is considered as effective as the benzimidazole compounds and is used as a second-line medication. Other medications are piperazine, which causes flaccid paralysis in the adult pinworms, and pyrvinium pamoate (also called pyrvinium embonate), which works by inhibiting oxygen uptake of the adult pinworms. Pinworms located in the genitourinary system (in this case, female genital area) may require other drug treatments.

Epidemiology

Pinworm infection occurs worldwide, and is the most common helminth (i.e., parasitic worm) infection in the United States and Western Europe. In the United States, a study by the Center of Disease Control reported an overall incidence rate of 11.4% among people of all ages. Pinworms are particularly common in children, with prevalence rates in this age group having been reported as high as 61% in India, 50% in England, 39% in Thailand, 37% in Sweden, and 29% in Denmark.Finger sucking has been shown to increase both incidence and relapse rates, and nail biting has been similarly associated. Because it spreads from host to host through contamination, enterobiasis is common among people living in close contact, and tends to occur in all people within a household. The prevalence of pinworms is not associated with gender, nor with any particular social class, race, or culture. Pinworms are an exception to the tenet that intestinal parasites are uncommon in affluent communities.

Geographic distribution

S. stercoralis has a very low prevalence in societies where fecal contamination of soil or water is rare. Hence, it is a very rare infection in developed economies. In developing countries, it is less prevalent in urban areas than in rural areas (where sanitation standards are poor). *S. stercoralis* can be found in areas with tropical and subtropical climates.

Strongyloidiasis was first described in the 19th century in French soldiers returning home from expeditions in Indochina. Today, the countries of the old Indochina (Vietnam, Cambodia, and Laos) still have endemic strongyloidiasis, with the typical prevalences being 10% or less. Regions of Japan used to have endemic strongyloidiasis, but control programs have eliminated the disease. Strongyloidiasis appears to have a high prevalence in some areas of Brazil and Central America. It is endemic in Africa, but the prevalence is typically low (1% or less). Pockets have been reported from rural Italy, but current status is unknown. In the Pacific islands, strongyloidiasis is rare, although some cases have been reported from Fiji. In tropical Australia, some rural and remote Australian Aboriginal communities have very high prevalences of strongyloidiasis.

In some African countries (e.g., Zaire), *S. fuelleborni* was more common than *S. stercoralis* in parasite surveys from the 1970s, but current status is unknown. In Papua New Guinea, *S. stercoralis* is endemic, but prevalence is low. However, in some areas, another species, *S. kellyi*, is a very common parasite of children in the New Guinea Highlands and Western Province.

Knowledge of the geographic distribution of strongyloidiasis is of significance to travelers who may acquire the parasite during their stays in endemic areas.

Because strongyloidiasis is transmittable by textiles, such as bedclothes and clothing, care must be taken never to use hotel bed sheets in endemic areas. Personal sleeping bags and using plastic slippers when showering are very important when travelling in tropical regions.

Life cycle

The strongyloid's life cycle is heterogonic—it is more complex than that of most nematodes, with its alternation between free-living and parasitic cycles, and its potential for autoinfection and multiplication within the host. The parasitic cycle is homogenic, while the free-living cycle is heterogonic. The heterogonic life cycle is advantageous to the parasite because it allows reproduction for one or more generations in the absence of a host.

In the free-living cycle, the rhabditiform larvae passed in the stool can either molt twice and become infective filariform larvae (direct development) or molt four times and become free-living adult males and females that mate and produce eggs from which rhabditiform larvae hatch. In the direct development, first-stage larvae (L1) transform into infective larvae (IL) via three molts. The indirect route results first in the development of free-living adults that mate; the female lays eggs, which hatch and then develop into IL. The direct route gives IL faster (three days) versus the indirect route (seven to 10 days). However, the indirect route results in an increase in the number of IL produced. Speed of development of IL is traded for increased numbers. The free-living males and females of *S. stercoralis* die after one generation; they do not persist in the soil. The latter, in turn, can either develop into a new generation of free-living adults or develop into infective filariform larvae. The filariform larvae penetrate the human host skin to initiate the parasitic cycle.

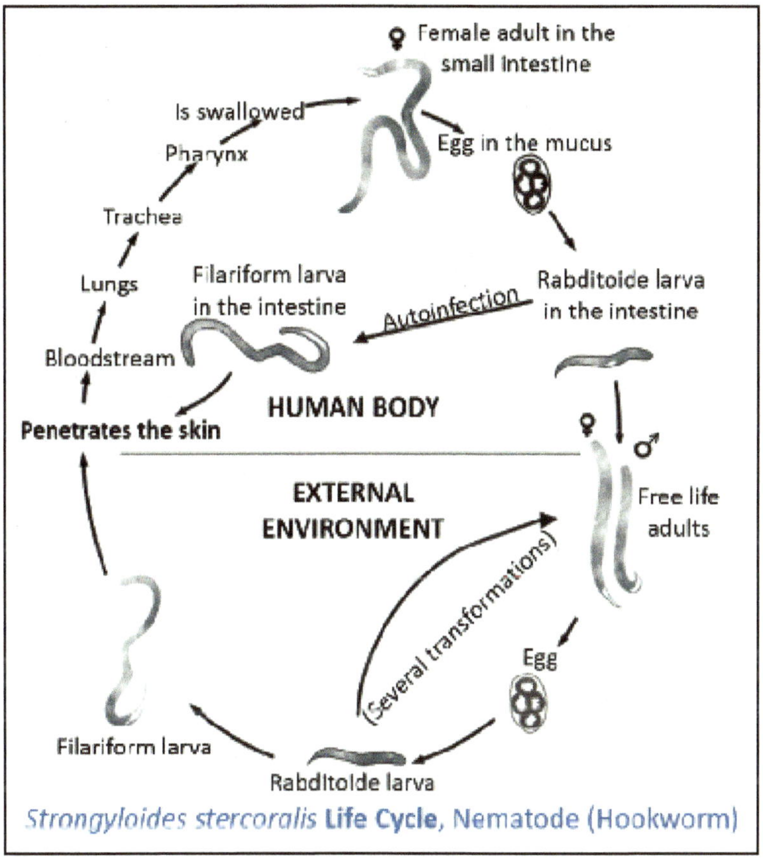

Life Cycle of *Strongyloides stercoralis* inside and outside of the human body

The infectious larvae penetrate the skin when it contacts soil. While *S. stercoralis* is attracted to chemicals such as carbon dioxide or sodium chloride, these chemicals are not specific. Larvae have been thought to locate their hosts via chemicals in the skin, the predominant one being urocanic acid, a histidine metabolite on the uppermost layer of skin that is removed by sweat or the daily skin-shedding cycle. Urocanic acid concentrations can be up to five times greater in the foot than any other part of the human body. Some of them enter the superficial veins and are carried in the blood to the lungs, where they enter the alveoli. They are then coughed up and swallowed into the gut, where they parasitise the intestinal mucosa of the duodenum and jejunum. In the small intestine, they molt twice and become adult female worms. The females live threaded in the epithelium of the small intestine and, by parthenogenesis, produce eggs, which yield rhabditiform larvae. Only females will reach reproductive adulthood in the intestine. Female strongyloids reproduce through parthenogenesis. The eggs hatch in the intestine and young larvae are then excreted in the feces. It takes about two weeks to reach egg development from the initial skin penetration. By this process, *S. stercoralis* can cause both respiratory and gastrointestinal symptoms. The worms also participate in autoinfection, in which the rhabditiform larvae become infective filariform larvae, which can penetrate either the intestinal mucosa (internal autoinfection) or the skin of the perianal area (external autoinfection); in either case, the filariform larvae may follow the previously described route, being carried successively to the lungs, the bronchial tree, the pharynx, and the small intestine, where they mature into adults; or they may disseminate widely in the body. To date, occurrence of autoinfection in humans with helminthic infections is recognized only in *Strongyloides stercoralis* and *Capillaria philippinensis* infections. In the case of *Strongyloides*, autoinfection may explain the possibility of persistent infections for many years in persons not having been in an endemic area and of hyperinfections in immunodepressed individuals.

Characteristics

Whereas males grow to only about 0.9 mm (0.04 in) in length, females can grow from 2.0 to 2.5 mm (0.08 to 0.10 in). Both sexes also possess a tiny buccal capsule and cylindrical esophagus without a posterior bulb. In the free-living stage, the esophagi of both sexes are rhabditiform. Males can be distinguished from females by two structures: the spicules and gubernaculum.

An unusual feature of *S. stercoralis* is autoinfection. Only one other species in the *Strongyloides* genus, *S. felis*, has this trait. Autoinfection is the development of L1 into small infective larvae in the gut of the host. These autoinfective larvae penetrate the wall of the lower ileum or colon or the skin of the perianal region, enter the circulation again, travel to the lungs, and then to the small intestine, thus repeating the cycle. Autoinfection makes strongyloidiasis due to *S. stercoralis* an infection with several unusual features.

Persistence of infection is the first of these important features. Because of autoinfection, humans have been known to still be infected up to 65 years after they were first exposed to the parasite (e.g., World War II or Vietnam War veterans). Once a host is infected with *S. stercoralis*, infection is lifelong unless effective treatment eliminates all adult parasites and migrating autoinfective larvae.

Symptoms

Many people infected are asymptomatic at first. Symptoms include dermatitis: swelling, itching, larva currens, and mild hemorrhage at the site where the skin has been penetrated. Spontaneous scratch-like lesions may be seen on the face or elsewhere. If the parasite reaches the lungs, the chest may feel as if it is burning, and wheezing and coughing may result, along with pneumonia-like symptoms (Löffler's syndrome). The intestines could eventually be invaded, leading to burning pain, tissue damage, sepsis, and ulcers. Stools may have yellow mucus with a recognizable smell. Chronic diarrhea can be a symptom. In severe cases, edema may result in obstruction of the intestinal tract, as well as loss of peristaltic contractions.

Strongyloidiasis in immunocompetent individuals is usually an indolent disease. However, in immunocompromised individuals, it can cause a hyperinfective syndrome (also called disseminated strongyloidiasis) due to the reproductive capacity of the parasite inside the host. This hyperinfective syndrome can have a mortality rate close to 90% if disseminated.

Immunosuppressive drugs, especially corticosteroids and agents used for tissue transplantation, can increase the rate of autoinfection to the point where an overwhelming number of larvae migrate through the lungs, which in many cases can prove fatal. In addition, diseases such as human T-lymphotropic virus 1, which enhance the Th1 arm of the immune system and lessen the Th2 arm, increase the disease state. Another consequence of autoinfection is the autoinfective larvae can carry gut bacteria back into the body. About 50% of people with hyperinfection present with bacterial disease due to enteric bacteria. Also, a unique effect of autoinfective larvae is larva currens due to the rapid migration of the larvae through the skin. Larva currens appears as a red line that moves rapidly (more than 5 cm or 2 in per day), and then quickly disappears. It is pathognomonic for autoinfective larvae and can be used as a diagnostic criterion for strongyloidiasis due to *S. stercoralis*.

Diagnosis

Locating juvenile larvae, either rhabditiform or filariform, in recent stool samples will confirm the presence of this parasite.Other techniques used include direct fecal smears, culturing fecal samples on agar plates, serodiagnosis through ELISA, and duodenal fumigation. Still, diagnosis can be difficult because of the day-to-day variation in juvenile parasite load.

Treatment

Ideally, prevention, by improved sanitation (proper disposal of feces), practicing good hygiene (washing of hands), etc., is used before any drug regimen is administered.

Ivermectin is the drug of first choice for treatment because of higher tolerance in patients. Thiabendazole was used previously, but, owing to its high prevalence of side effects (dizziness, vomiting, nausea, malaise) and lower efficacy, it has been superseded by ivermectin and as second-line albendazole. However, these drugs have little effect on the majority of these autoinfective larvae during their migration through the body. Hence, repeated treatments with ivermectin must be administered to kill adult parasites that develop from the autoinfective larvae. This means at least two weeks treatment, then a weeks pause, then again treatment. Follow-up treatment and blood tests are necessary for decades following infection.

In the UK, mebendazole and piperazine are currently (2007) preferred. Mebendazole has a much higher failure rate in clinical practice than albendazole, thiabendazole, or ivermectin.

Chemoattractant

This parasite depends on chemical cues to find a potential host. It uses sensor neurons of class AFD to identify cues excreted by the host.*S. stercoralis* is attracted to nonspecific attractants of warmth, carbon dioxide, and sodium chloride. Urocanic acid, a component of skin secretions in mammals, is a major chemoattractant. Larvae of *S. stercoralis* are strongly attracted to this compound. This compound can be suppressed by metal ions, suggesting a possible strategy for preventing infection.

Infection

Infection by *T. canis* or *T. cati* can cause various clinical manifestations. One of these is visceral larva migrans, wherein the larvae are unable to develop in humans as they do in cats and dogs, their natural hosts. Arrested development leaves the larvae to wander aimlessly in the body, causing inflammation, most commonly in the liver and lungs.

Eggs are introduced into the body through ingestion. This can occur when eggs are deposited on the hands or face, after handling infected dogs or cats. In children without exposure to animals, eggs can be introduced by directly ingesting egg-contaminated soil while playing in a yard or on a playground. Usually, the scenario involves a young child with a new puppy. Unfortunately, many young children who have been infected with these larvae, causing ocular larva migrans in the eye, have been misdiagnosed to have retinoblastoma and have had their eyes erroneously removed.

Diagnosis

Direct identification of larvae in human disease is not feasible, so the diagnosis relies on history supported by serologic ELISA assay. The most sensitive assay, called excretory/secretory (E/S), contains 96 immunogenic antigens isolated from cultured *T. canis* larvae.

Prevention

A number of products supplied by veterinarians can prevent or treat infections with this parasite. A great deal of information on this subject can be found on the computer sites maintained by the Companion Animal Parasite Council.

Treatment

Visceral toxocariasis in humans (or dogs) can be treated with antiparasitic drugs such as albendazole or mebendazole, usually in combination with anti-inflammatory medications. Treatment for ocular larva migrans is to kill the larvae with a laser to prevent further damage, although some loss of vision in the affected eye is irreversible.

Association with asthma

Infection with *Toxocara* has been shown to stimulate atopic disease, specifically asthma. Infection with this parasite causes asthma-like symptoms such as accumulation of eosinophils, an inflammatory response, and production of IgE, the immunoglobulins associated with allergic responses. People with asthma are shown to have a higher prevalence of *Toxocara* seropositivity. Research suggests that the IgE production stimulated by infection with *Toxocara* may contribute to the onsets of allergic asthma in children. The effects of how parasite load, frequency of exposure, and influence of genetics affect this relationship between *Toxocara* infection and allergic asthma are still unknown, yet important in understanding how to prevent asthma and other atopic diseases around the globe.

Life cycle

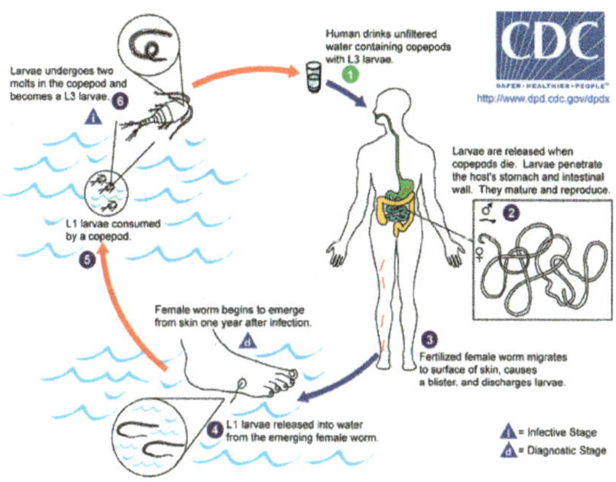

General life cycle of *Dracunculus medinensis* in humans

D. medinensis larvae are found in freshwater, where they are ingested by copepods of the genus *Cyclops*. Within the copepod, the *D. medinensis* larvae develop to an infective stage within 14 days. When the infected copepod is ingested by a mammalian host, the copepod is dissolved by stomach acid and the *D. medinensis* larvae migrate through the wall of the mammalian intestine, and mature into adults. 100 days after infection, a male and female *D. medinensis* meet and sexually reproduce within the host tissue. The male dies in the host tissue while the female migrates to the host subcutaneous tissue. Approximately one year after infection, the female causes the formation of a blister on the skin's surface, generally on the lower extremities, though occasionally on the hand or scrotum. When the blister ruptures, the female slowly emerges over the course of several days or weeks. This causes extreme pain and irritation to the host. When the host submerges the affected body part in water, the female expels thousands of larvae into the water. From here, the larvae infect copepods, continuing the life cycle.

Treatment

The female guinea worm slowly starts to emerge from the host's skin after the blister ruptures. The most common method for removing the worm involves submerging the affected body part in water to help coax the worm out. The site is then cleaned thoroughly. Then, slight pressure is applied to the worm as it is slowly pulled out of the wound. To avoid breaking the worm, pulling should stop when resistance is met. Full extraction of the female guinea worm usually takes several days. After each day's worth of extraction, the exposed portion of the worm is wrapped around a piece of rolled-up gauze or small stick to maintain tension. This method of wrapping the worm around a stick or gauze is speculated to be the source for the Rod of Asclepius, the symbol of medicine. Once secure, topical antibiotics are applied to affected region to help prevent secondary infections due to bacteria and then is wrapped in gauze to protect the wound. The same steps are repeated each day until the whole worm has been successfully removed from the lesion.

Guinea worm cases by year		
Year	**Reported Cases**	**Countries**
1989	892,055	16
1995	129,852	19
2000	75,223	16
2001	63,717	16
2002	54,638	14
2003	32,193	13
2004	16,026	13
2005	10,674	12
2006	25,217	10
2007	9,585	9
2008	4,619	7
2009	3,190	5
2010	1,797	6
2011	1,060	4
2012	542	4
2013	148	5
2014	126	4
2015	22	4

In the 1980s, the Carter Center initiated a program to eradicate guinea worm. The Guinea Worm Eradication campaign began in 1980 at the US Centers for Disease Control and Prevention. In 1984, the CDC was appointed as the World Health Organization Collaborating Center for research, training, and eradication of *Dracunculus medinensis*. There were 20 countries in 1986 that were affected by guinea worms. That year, WHO started the eradication program and the Carter Center took the lead on the effort. The program included education of people in affected areas that the disease was caused by larvae in drinking water, isolation and support for sufferers, and – crucially – widespread distribution of net filters and pipe filters for drinking water, and education about the importance of using them.

As of 2015, the species has been reported to be near eradication. The International Commission for the Certification of Dracunculus Eradication (ICCDE) has certified 198 countries, territories, and other WHO represented areas. In January 2015, eight countries remained to be certified as *Dracunculus medinensis* free. These eight countries include Angola, Democratic Republic of the Congo, Kenya, Sudan, Chad, Ethiopia, Mali, and South Sudan. Of these, Chad, Ethiopia, Mali, and South Sudan are the only remaining endemic countries. Not coincidentally, all four are affected by civil wars which affect the safety of health workers.

Other animals

However, as of 2016 there have been more than 500 dogs in Chad, 13 in Ethiopia and one dog in Mali and South Sudan, respectively, diagnosed with guinea worm. Furthermore, it has been possible to infect frogs under laboratory conditions and recently natural infection has been reported in wild frogs in Chad. These findings are a potential problem for the eradication programme.

Etymology

Dracunculus medinensis (*little dragon from Medina*) is a parasitic nematode that infects humans and domestic animals through contaminated water. D. medinensis was described in Egypt as early as the 15th century BCE and may have been the "fiery serpent" of the Israelites described in the Bible.

Terminology

The term *hookworm* is sometimes used to refer to hookworm infection. A hookworm is a type of parasitic worm (helminth).

Signs and symptoms

There are no specific symptoms or signs of hookworm infection, but they give rise to a combination of intestinal inflammation and progressive iron-deficiency anemia and protein deficiency. Coughing, chest pain, wheezing, and fever will sometimes result from severe infection. Epigastric pains, indigestion, nausea, vomiting, constipation, and diarrhea can occur early or in later stages as well, although gastrointestinal symptoms tend to improve with time. Signs of advanced severe infection are those of anemia and protein deficiency, including emaciation, cardiac failure and abdominal distension with ascites. Larval invasion of the skin (mostly in the Americas) can produce a skin disease called cutaneous larva migrans also known as *creeping eruption*. The hosts of these worms are not human and the larvae can only penetrate the upper five layers of the skin, where they give rise to intense, local itching, usually on the foot or lower leg, known as *ground itch*. This infection is due to larvae from the *A. Braziliense* hookworm. The larvae migrate in tortuous tunnels between the *stratum basale* and *stratum corneum* of the skin, causing serpiginous vesicular lesions. With advancing movement of the larvae, the rear portions of the lesions become dry and crusty. The lesions are typically intensely itchy.

Characteristics

A. duodenale worms are grayish white or pinkish with the head slightly bent in relation to the rest of the body. This bend forms a definitive hook shape at the anterior end for which hookworms are named. They possess well-developed mouths with two pairs of teeth. While males measure approximately one centimeter by 0.5 millimeter, the females are often longer and stouter. Additionally, males can be distinguished from females based on the presence of a prominent posterior copulatory bursa.

N. americanus is very similar in morphology to *A. duodenale*. *N. americanus* is generally smaller than *A. duodenale* with males usually 5 to 9 mm long and females about 1 cm long. Whereas *A. duodenale* possesses two pairs of teeth, *N. americanus* possesses a pair of cutting plates in the buccal capsule. Additionally, the hook shape is much more defined in *Necator* than in *Ancylostoma*.

Pathology

Hookworm infection is generally considered to be asymptomatic, but as Norman Stoll described in 1962, hookworm infection is an extremely dangerous infection because its damage is "silent and insidious." There are general symptoms that an individual may experience soon after infection. Ground-itch, which is an allergic reaction at the site of parasitic penetration and entry, is common in patients infected with *N. americanus*. Additionally, cough and pneumonitis may result as the larvae begin to break into the alveoli and travel up the trachea. Then once the larvae reach the small intestine of the host and begin to mature, the infected individual will suffer from diarrhea and other gastrointestinal discomfort. However, the "silent and insidious" symptoms referred to by Stoll are related to chronic, heavy-intensity hookworm infections. Major morbidity associated with hookworm infection is caused by intestinal blood loss, iron deficiency anemia, and protein malnutrition. They result mainly from adult hookworms in the small intestine ingesting blood, rupturing erythrocytes, and degrading hemoglobin in the host. This long-term blood loss can manifest itself physically through facial and peripheral edema; eosinophilia and pica caused by iron deficiency anemia are also experienced by some hookworm-infected patients. Recently, more attention has been given to other important outcomes of hookworm infection that play a large role in public health. It is now widely accepted that children who suffer from chronic hookworm infection can suffer from growth retardation as well as intellectual and cognitive impairments. Additionally, recent research has focused on the potential of adverse maternal-fetal outcomes when the mother is infected with hookworm during pregnancy.

The disease was linked to nematode worms (*Ankylostoma duodenalis*) from one-third to half an inch long in the intestine chiefly through the labours of Theodor Bilharz and Griesinger in Egypt (1854).

The symptoms can be linked to inflammation in the gut stimulated by feeding hookworms, such as nausea, abdominal pain and intermittent diarrhea, and to progressive anemia in prolonged disease: capricious appetite, pica (or dirt-eating), obstinate constipation followed by diarrhea, palpitations, thready pulse, coldness of the skin, pallor of the mucous membranes, fatigue and weakness, shortness of breath and in cases running a fatal course, dysentery, hemorrhages and edema.

Blood tests in early infection often show a rise in numbers of eosinophils, a type of white blood cell that is preferentially stimulated by worm infections in tissues (large numbers of eosinophils are also present in the local inflammatory response). Falling blood hemoglobin levels will be seen in cases of prolonged infection with anemia.

In contrast to most intestinal helminthiases, where the heaviest parasitic loads tend to occur in children, hookworm prevalence and intensity can be higher among adult males. The explanation for this is that hookworm infection tends to be occupational, so that coworkers and other close groups maintain a high prevalence of infection among themselves by contaminating their work environment. However, in most endemic areas, adult women are the most severely affected by anemia, mainly because they have much higher physiological needs for iron (menstruation, repeated pregnancy).

An interesting consequence of this in the case of *Ancylostoma duodenale* infection is translactational transmission of infection: the skin-invasive larvae of this species do not all immediately pass through the lungs and on into the gut, but spread around the body via the circulation, to become dormant inside muscle fibers. In a pregnant woman, after childbirth some or all of these larvae are stimulated to re-enter the circulation (presumably by sudden hormonal changes), then to pass into the mammary glands, so that the newborn baby can receive a large dose of infective larvae through its mother's milk. This accounts for otherwise inexplicable cases of very heavy, even fatal, hookworm infections in children a month or so of age, in places such as China, India and northern Australia. An identical phenomenon is much more commonly seen with *Ancylostoma caninum* infections in dogs, where the newborn pups can even die of hemorrhaging from their intestines caused by massive numbers of feeding hookworms. This also reflects the close evolutionary link between the human and canine parasites, which probably have a common ancestor dating back to when humans and dogs first started living closely together. Filariform larvae is the infective stage of the parasite, infection occurs when larvae in soil penetrate the skin, or when they are ingested through contaminated food and water following skin penetration, larvae

Life cycle

See the image for the biological life cycle of the hookworm where it thrives in warm earth where temperatures are over 18 °C. They exist primarily in sandy or loamy soil and cannot live in clay or muck. Rainfall averages must be more than 1000 mm (40 inches) a year for them to survive. Only if these conditions exist can the eggs hatch. Infective larvae of *Necator americanus* can survive at higher temperatures, whereas those of *Ancylostoma duodenale* are better adapted to cooler climates. Generally, they live for only a few weeks at most under natural conditions, and die almost immediately on exposure to direct sunlight or desiccation.

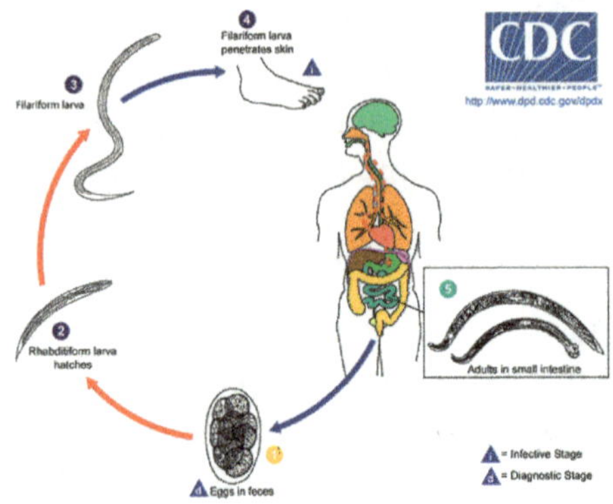

Hookworm life cycle

Infection of the host is by the larvae, not the eggs. While *A. duodenale* can be ingested, the usual method of infection is through the skin; this is commonly caused by walking barefoot through areas contaminated with fecal matter. The larvae are able to penetrate the skin of the foot, and once inside the body, they migrate through the vascular system to the lungs, and from there up the trachea, and are swallowed. They then pass down the esophagus and enter the digestive system, finishing their journey in the intestine, where the larvae mature into adult worms.

Once in the host gut, *Necator* tends to cause a prolonged infection, generally 1–5 years (many die within a year or two of infecting), though some adult worms have been recorded to live for 15 years or more. On the other hand, *Ancylostoma* adults are short lived, surviving on average for only about 6 months. However, infection can be prolonged because dormant larvae can be "recruited" sequentially from tissue "stores" (see Pathology, above) over many years, to replace expired adult worms. This can give rise to seasonal fluctuations in infection prevalence and intensity (apart from normal seasonal variations in transmission).

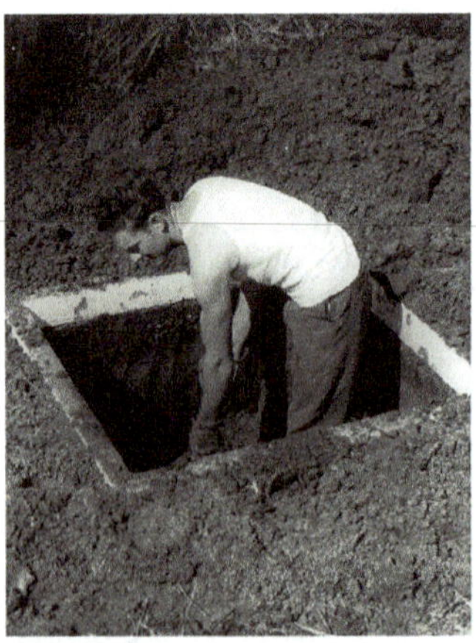

Civilian Public Service workers built and installed 2065 outhouses for hookworm eradication in Mississippi and Florida from 1943 to 1947.

They mate inside the host, females laying up to 30,000 eggs per day and some 18 to 54 million eggs during their lifetime, which pass out in feces. Because it takes 5–7 weeks for adult worms to mature, mate and produce eggs, in the early stages of very heavy infection, acute symptoms might occur without any eggs being detected in the patient's feces. This can make diagnosis very difficult.

Cellular stages

N. americanus and *A. duodenale* eggs can be found in warm, moist soil where they will eventually hatch into first stage larvae, or L1. L1, the feeding non-infective rhabditoform stage, will feed on soil microbes and eventually molt into second stage larvae, L2. L2, which is also in the rhabditoform stage, will feed for approximately 7 days and then molt into the third stage larvae, or L3. L3 is the filariform stage of the parasite, that is, the non-feeding infective form of the larvae. The L3 larvae are extremely motile and will seek higher ground to increase their chances of penetrating the skin of a human host. The L3 larvae can survive up to 2 weeks without finding a host. While *N. americanus* larvae only infect through penetration of skin, *A. duodenale* can infect both through penetration as well as orally. After the L3 larvae have successfully entered the host, the larvae then travel through the subcutaneous venules and lymphatic vessels of the human host. Eventually, the L3 larvae enter the lungs through the pulmonary capillaries and break out into the alveoli. They will then travel up the trachea to be coughed and swallowed by the host. After being swallowed, the L3 larvae are then found in the small intestine where they molt into the L4, or adult worm stage. The entire process from skin penetration to adult development takes about 5–9 weeks. The female adult worms will release eggs (*N. americanus* about 9,000–10,000 eggs/day and *A. duodenale* 25,000–30,000 eggs/day) which are passed in the feces of the human host. These eggs will hatch in the environment within several days and the cycle will start anew.

Infection and Diagnosis

The incubation period can vary between a few weeks to many months and is largely dependent on the number of Hookworm parasites an individual is infected with.

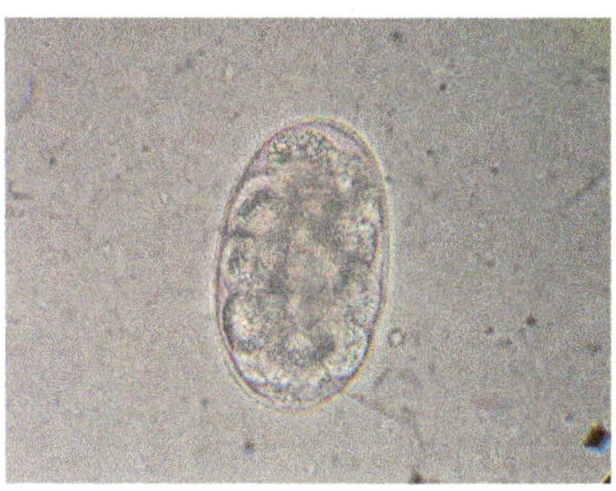

Hookworm egg

Diagnosis depends on finding characteristic worm eggs on microscopic examination of the stools, although this is not possible in early infection. Early signs of infection in most dogs include limbular limping and anal itching. The eggs are oval or elliptical, measuring 60 μm by 40 μm, colourless, not bile stained and with a thin transparent hyaline shell membrane. When released by the worm in the intestine, the egg contains an unsegmented ovum. During its passage down the intestine, the ovum develops and thus the eggs passed in feces have a segmented ovum, usually with 4 to 8 blastomeres. As the eggs of both *Ancylostoma* and *Necator* (and most other hookworm species) are indistinguishable, to identify the genus, they must be cultured in the lab to allow larvae to hatch out. If the fecal sample is left for a day or more under tropical conditions, the larvae will have hatched out, so eggs might no longer be evident. In such a case, it is essential to distinguish hookworms from *Strongyloides* larvae, as infection with the latter has more serious implications and requires different management. The larvae of the two hookworm species can also be distinguished microscopically, although this would not be done routinely, but usually for research purposes. Adult worms are rarely seen (except via endoscopy, surgery or autopsy), but if found, would allow definitive identification of the species. Classification can be performed based on the length of the buccal cavity, the space between the oral opening and the esophagus: hookworm rhabditoform larvae have long buccal cavities whereas *Strongyloides* rhabditoform larvae have short buccal cavities.

Recent research has focused on the development of DNA-based tools for diagnosis of infection, specific identification of hookworm, and analysis of genetic variability within hookworm populations. Because hookworm eggs are often indistinguishable from other parasitic eggs, PCR assays could serve as a molecular approach for accurate diagnosis of hookworm in the feces.

The infective larvae develop and survive in an environment of damp dirt, particularly sandy and loamy soil. They cannot survive in clay or muck. The main lines of precaution are those dictated by good hygiene behaviors:

- Do not defecate in the open, but rather in toilets.
- Do not use untreated human excreta or raw sewage as fertilizer in agriculture
- Do not walk barefoot in known infected areas.
- Deworm pet dogs and cats. Canine and feline hookworms rarely develop to adulthood in humans. *Ancylostoma caninum*, the common dog hookworm, occasionally develops into an adult to cause eosinophilic enteritis in people, but their invasive larvae can cause an itchy rash called cutaneous larva migrans.

Moxidectin has been released in the United States as part of Advantage Multi (imidacloprid + moxidectin) topical solution for dogs and cats. It utilizes moxidectin for control and prevention of roundworms, hookworms, heartworms, and whipworms.

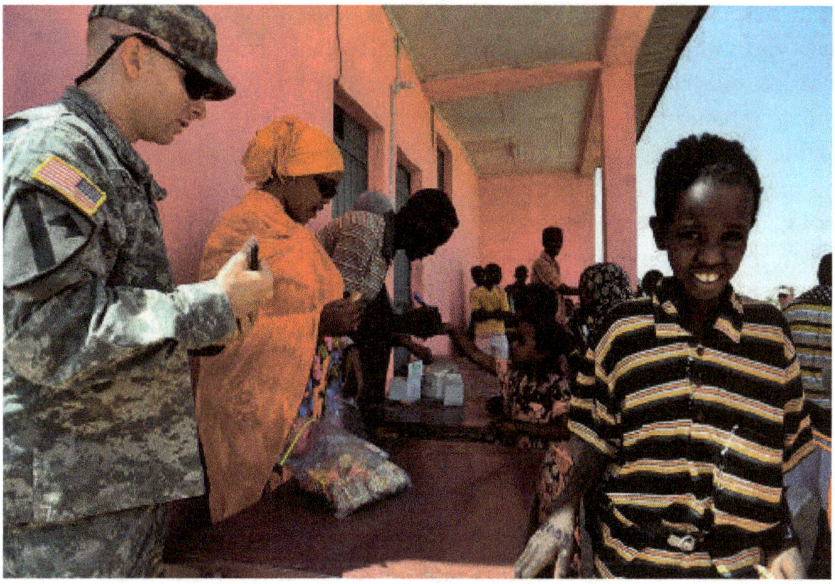

Ethiopian children treated for schistosoma and hookworms.

Treatment in Children

Most of these public health concerns have focused on children who are infected with hookworm. This focus on children is largely due to the large body of evidence that has demonstrated strong associations between hookworm infection and impaired learning, increased absences from school, and decreased future economic productivity. In 2001, the 54th World Health Assembly passed a resolution demanding member states to attain a minimum target of regular deworming of at least 75% of all at-risk school children by the year 2010. A 2008 World Health Organization publication reported on these efforts to treat at-risk school children. Some of the interesting statistics were as follows: 1) only 9 out of 130 endemic countries were able to reach the 75% target goal; and 2) less than 77 million school-aged children (of the total 878 million at risk) were reached, which means that only 8.78% of at-risk children are being treated for hookworm infection.

School-based Mass Deworming

School-based mass deworming programs have been the most popular strategy to address the issue of hookworm infection in children. School-based programs are extremely cost effective as schools already have an available, extensive, and sustained infrastructure with a skilled workforce that has a close relationship with the community. With little training from a local health system, teachers can easily administer the drugs which often cost less than US$0.50 per child per year.

Recently, many people have begun to question if the school-based programs are necessarily the most effective approach. An important concern with school-based programs is that they often do not reach children who do not attend school, thus ignoring a large amount of at-risk children. A 2008 study by Massa *et al.* continued the debate regarding school-based programs. They examined the effects of community-directed treatments versus school-based treatments in the Tanga Region of Tanzania. A major conclusion was that the mean infection intensity of hookworm was significantly lower in the villages employing the community-directed treatment approach than the school-based approach. The community-directed treatment model used in this specific study allowed villagers to take control of the child's treatment by having villagers select their own community drug distributors to administer the antihelminthic drugs. Additionally, villagers organized and implemented their own methods for distributing the drugs to all children. The positive results associated with this new model highlight the need for large-scale community involvement in deworming campaigns.

Public Health Education

Many mass deworming programs also combine their efforts with a public health education. These health education programs often stress important preventative techniques such as: washing your hands before eating, and staying away from water/areas contaminated by human faeces. These programs may also stress that shoes must be worn, however these come with their own health risks and may not be effective. Shoe wearing patterns in towns and villages across the globe are determined by cultural beliefs, and the levels of education within that society. The wearing of shoes will prevent the entry of hookworm infections from the surrounding soils into tender skin regions; such as areas between the toes.

Sanitation

Historical examples, such as the hookworm campaigns in Mississippi and Florida from 1943 to 1947 have shown that the primary cause of hookworm infection is poor sanitation, which can be solved by building and maintaining toilets. But while these may seem like simple tasks, they raise important public health challenges. Most infected populations are from poverty-stricken areas with very poor sanitation. Thus, it is most likely that at-risk children do not have access to clean water to wash their hands and live in environments with no proper sanitation infrastructure. Health education, therefore, must address preventive measures in ways that are both feasible and sustainable in the context of resource-limited settings.

Integrated Approaches

Evaluation of numerous public health interventions have generally shown that improvement in each individual component ordinarily attributed to poverty (for example, sanitation, health education and underlying nutrition status) often have minimal impact on transmission. For example, one study found that the introduction of latrines into a resource-limited community only reduced the prevalence of hookworm infection by four percent. However, another study in Salvador, Brazil found that improved drainage and sewerage had a significant impact ($p<0.0001$) on the prevalence of hookworm infection but no impact at all on the intensity of hookworm infection. This seems to suggest that environmental control alone has a limited but incomplete effect on the transmission of hookworms. It is imperative, therefore, that more research be performed to understand the efficacy and sustainability of integrated programs that combine numerous preventive methods including education, sanitation, and treatment.

Anthelmintic Drugs

The most common treatment for hookworm are benzimidazoles, specifically albendazole and mebendazole. BZAs kill adult worms by binding to the nematode's β-tubulin and subsequently inhibiting microtubule polymerization within the parasite. In certain circumstances, levamisole and pyrantel pamoate may be used. A 2008 review found that the efficacy of single-dose treatments for hookworm infections were as follows: 72% for albendazole, 15% for mebendazole, and 31% for pyrantel pamoate. This substantiates prior claims that albendazole is much more effective than mebendazole for hookworm infections. Also of note is that the World Health Organization does recommend anthelmintic treatment in pregnant women after the first trimester. It is also recommended that if the patient also suffers from anemia that ferrous sulfate (200 mg) be administered three times daily at the same time as anthelmintic treatment; this should be continued until hemoglobin values return to normal which could take up to 3 months.

Hookworm infection can be treated with local cryotherapy when the hookworm is still in the skin.

Albendazole is effective both in the intestinal stage and during the stage the parasite is still migrating under the skin.

In case of anemia, iron supplementation can cause relief symptoms of iron deficiency anemia. However, as red blood cell levels are restored, shortage of other essentials such as folic acid or vitamin B12 may develop, so these might also be supplemented.

Reinfection and Drug Resistance

Other important issues related to the treatment of hookworm are reinfection and drug resistance. It has been shown that reinfection after treatment can be extremely high. Some studies even show that 80% of pretreatment hookworm infection rates can be seen in treated communities within 30–36 months. While reinfection may occur, it is still recommended that regular treatments be conducted as it will minimize the occurrence of chronic outcomes. There are also increasing concerns about the issue of drug resistance. Drug resistance has appeared in front-line anthelmintics used for livestock nematodes. Generally human nematodes are less likely to develop resistance due to longer reproducing times, less frequent treatment, and more targeted treatment. Nonetheless, the global community must be careful to maintain the effectiveness of current anthelmintic as no new anthelmintic drugs are in the late-stage development.

Epidemiology

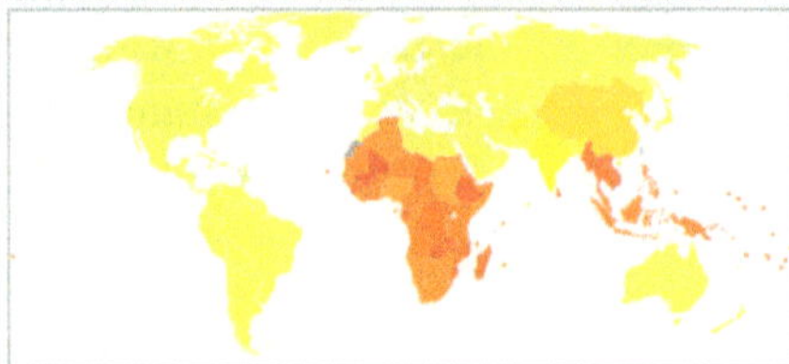

Disability-adjusted life year for hookworm disease per 100,000 inhabitants in 2002.

- no data
- less than 10
- 10–15
- 15–20
- 20–25
- 25–30
- 30–35
- 35–40
- 40–45
- 45–50
- 50–55
- 55–60
- more than 60

It is estimated that between 576–740 million individuals are infected with hookworm. Of these infected individuals, about 80 million are severely affected. The major etiology of hookworm infection is *N. americanus* which is found the Americas, sub-Saharan Africa, and Asia. *A. duodenale* is found in more scattered focal environments, namely Europe and the Mediterranean. Most infected individuals are concentrated in sub-Saharan Africa and East Asia/the Pacific Islands with each region having estimates of 198 million and 149 million infected individuals, respectively. Other affected regions include: South Asia (50 million), Latin America and the Caribbean (50 million), South Asia (59 million), Middle East/North Africa (10 million). A majority of these infected individuals live in poverty-stricken areas with poor sanitation. Hookworm infection is most concentrated among the world's poorest who live on less than $2 a day.

While hookworm infection may not directly lead to mortality, its effects on morbidity demand immediate attention. When considering disability-adjusted life years (DALYs), neglected tropical diseases, including hookworm infection, rank among diarrheal diseases, ischemic heart disease, malaria, and tuberculosis as one of the most important health problems of the developing world.

It has been estimated that as many as 22.1 million DALYs have been lost due to hookworm infection. Recently, there has been increasing interest to address the public health concerns associated with hookworm infection. For example, the Bill & Melinda Gates Foundation recently donated US$34 million to fight Neglected Tropical Diseases including hookworm infection.Former US President Clinton also announced a mega-commitment at the Clinton Global Initiative (CGI) 2008 Annual Meeting to de-worm 10 million children. Many of the numbers regarding the prevalence of hookworm infection are estimates as there is no international surveillance mechanism currently in place to determine prevalence and global distribution. Some prevalence rates have been measured through survey data in endemic regions around the world. The following are some of the most recent findings on prevalence rates in regions endemic with hookworm.

Darjeeling, Hooghly District, West Bengal, India (Pal *et al.* 2007)

- 42.8% infection rate of predominantly *N. americanus* although with some *A. duodenale* infection.
- Both hookworm infection load and degree of anemia in the mild range

Xiulongkan Village, Hainan Province, China (Gandhi *et al.* 2001)

- 60% infection rate of predominantly *N. americanus*
- Important trends noted were that prevalence increased with age (plateau of about 41 years) and women had higher prevalence rates than men

Hoa Binh, Northwest Vietnam (Verle *et al.* 2003)

- 52% of a total of 526 tested households infected
- Could not identify species, but previous studies in North Vietnam reported *N. americanus* in more than 95% of hookworm larvae

Minas Gerais, Brazil (Fleming *et al.* 2006)

- 62.8% infection rate of predominantly *N. americanus*

KwaZulu-Natal, South Africa (Mabaso *et al.* 2004)

- Inland areas had a prevalence rate of 9.3% of *N. americanus*
- Coastal plain areas had a prevalence rate of 62.5% of *N. americanus*

There have also been recent technological developments that will hopefully facilitate more accurate mapping of hookworm prevalence. Some researchers have begun to use geographical information systems (GIS) and remote sensing (RS) to examine helminth ecology and epidemiology. Brooker *et al.* utilized this technology to create helminth distribution maps of sub-Saharan Africa. By relating satellite derived environmental data with prevalence data from school-based surveys, they were able to create detailed prevalence maps. The study focused on a wide range of helminths, but interesting conclusions about hookworm specifically were found. As compared to other helminths, hookworm is able to survive in much hotter conditions and was highly prevalent throughout the upper end of the thermal range. Hopefully this information along with more detailed prevalence maps can lead to more effective public health measures. Improved molecular diagnostic tools are another technological advancement that could help improve existing prevalence statistics. Recent research has focused on the development of DNA-based tool that can be used for diagnosis of infection, specific identification of hookworm, and analysis of genetic variability in hookworm populations. Again this can serve as a major tool for different public health measures against hookworm infection. Most research regarding diagnostic tools is now focused on the creation of a rapid and cost-effective assay for the specific diagnosis of hookworm infection. Many are hopeful that its development can be achieved within the next 5 years.

History

The symptoms now attributed to hookworm appear in papyrus papers of ancient Egypt (c. 1500 BC), described as a derangement characterized by anemia. Avicenna, a Persian physician of the eleventh century, discovered the worm in several of his patients and related it to their disease. In later times, the condition was noticeably prevalent in the mining industry in England, France, Germany, Belgium, North Queensland, and elsewhere.

Italian physician Angelo Dubini was the modern-day discoverer of the worm in 1838 after an autopsy of a peasant woman. Dubini published details in 1843 and identified the species as *A. duodenale*. Working in the Egyptian medical system in 1852 German physician Theodor Bilharz, drawing upon the work of colleague Wilhelm Griesinger, found these worms during autopsies and went a step further in linking them to local endemic occurrences of chlorosis, which would probably be called iron deficiency anemia today.

A breakthrough came 25 years later following a diarrhea and anemia epidemic that took place among Italian workmen employed on the Gotthard Rail Tunnel. In an 1880 paper, physicians Camillo Bozzolo, Edoardo Perroncito, and Luigi Pagliani correctly hypothesized that hookworm was linked to the fact that workers had to defecate inside the 15 km tunnel, and that many wore worn-out shoes. In 1897, it was established that the skin was the principal avenue of infection and the biological life cycle of the hookworm was clarified.

Eradication Programmes

In 1899, American zoologist Charles Wardell Stiles identified progressive pernicious anemia seen in the southern United States as being caused by the hookworm *A. duodenale*. Testing in the 1900s revealed very heavy infestations in school-age children. In Puerto Rico, Dr. Bailey K. Ashford, a US Army physician, organized and conducted a parasite treatment campaign, which cured approximately 300,000 people (one-third of the Puerto Rican population) and reduced the death rate from this anemia by 90 percent during the years 1903–1904.

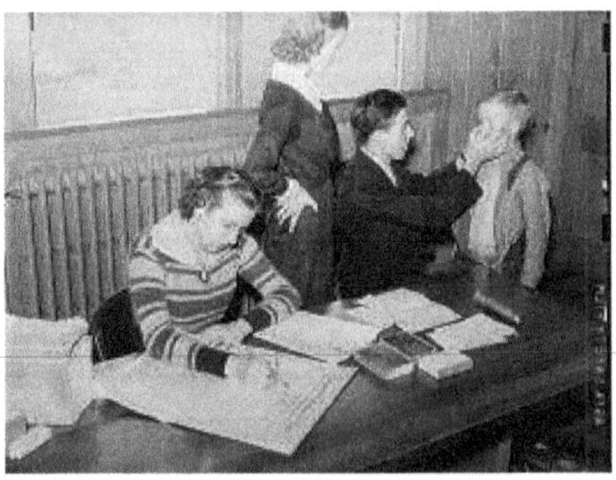

A doctor examines a boy for signs of hookworm in Coffee County, Alabama, 1939.

On October 26, 1909 the Rockefeller Sanitary Commission for the Eradication of Hookworm Disease was organized as a result of a gift of US$1 million from John D. Rockefeller, Sr. The five-year program was a remarkable success and a great contribution to United States public health, instilling public education, medication, field work and modern government health departments in eleven southern states. The hookworm exhibit was a prominent part of the 1910 Mississippi state fair.

The Commission found that an average of 40% of school-aged children were infected with hookworm. Areas with higher levels of hookworm infection prior to the eradication programme experienced greater increases in school enrolment, attendance and literacy after the intervention. Econometric studies have shown that this effect cannot be explained by a variety of alternative factors, including differential trends across areas, changing crop prices, shifts in certain educational and health policies and the effect of malaria eradication. No significant contemporaneous results were found for adults who should have benefited less from the intervention owing to their substantially lower (prior) infection rates. The program nearly eradicated hookworm and would flourish afterwards with new funding as the Rockefeller Foundation International Health Division. The RF's hookworm campaign in Mexico showed how science and politics play a role in developing health policies. It brought together government officials, health officials, public health workers, Rockefeller officials and the community. This campaign was launched to eradicate hookworms in Mexico. Although the campaign did not focus on long-term treatments, it did set the terms of the relationship between Mexico and the Rockefeller Foundation. The scientific knowledge behind this campaign helped shaped public health policies, improved public health and built a strong relationship between USA and Mexico.

In the 1920s, hookworm eradication reached the Caribbean and Latin America, where great mortality was reported among people in the West Indies towards the end of the 18th century, as well as through descriptions sent from Brazil and various other tropical and sub-tropical regions.

Treatments

Early treatment relied on the use of Epsom salt to reduce protective mucus, followed by thymol to kill the worms. Later tetrachloroethylene was the leading method. It was not until later in the mid-20th century when new organic drug compounds were developed.

Disease

Anemia in Pregnancy

It is estimated that a third of all pregnant women in developing countries are infected with hookworm, 56% of all pregnant women in developing countries suffer from anemia, 20% of all maternal deaths are either directly or indirectly related to anemia. Numbers like this have led to an increased interest in the topic of hookworm-related anemia during pregnancy.With the understanding that chronic hookworm infection can often lead to anemia, many people are now questioning if the treatment of hookworm could effect change in severe anemia rates and thus also on maternal and child health as well. Most evidence suggests that the contribution of hookworm to maternal anemia merits that all women of child-bearing age living in endemic areas be subject to periodic anthelmintic treatment. The World Health Organization even recommends that infected pregnant women be treated after their first trimester. Regardless of these suggestions, only Madagascar, Nepal and Sri Lanka have added deworming to their antenatal care programs.

This lack of deworming of pregnant women is explained by the fact that most individuals still fear that anthelmintic treatment will result in adverse birth outcomes. But a 2006 study by Gyorkos et al. found that when comparing a group of pregnant women treated with mebendazole with a control placebo group, both illustrated rather similar rates in adverse birth outcomes. The treated group demonstrated 5.6% adverse birth outcomes, while the control group had 6.25% adverse birth outcomes.Furthermore, Larocque et al. illustrated that treatment for hookworm infection actually led to positive health results in the infant. This study concluded that treatment with mebendazole plus iron supplements during antenatal care significantly reduced the proportion of very low birth weight infants when compared to a placebo control group. Studies so far have validated recommendations to treat infected pregnant women for hookworm infection during pregnancy.

A review of effects of antihelminths (anti-worm drugs) given in pregnancy found that there was not enough evidence to support treating pregnant women in their second or third trimesters. The women who were treated in the second trimester and the women who had no treatment showed no difference in numbers of maternal anaemia, low birth weight, preterm birth or deaths of babies.

The intensity of hookworm infection as well as the species of hookworm have yet to be studied as they relate to hookworm-related anemia during pregnancy. Additionally, more research must be done in different regions of the world to see if trends noted in completed studies persist.

Malaria co-Infection

Co-infection with hookworm and *Plasmodium falciparum* is common in Africa. Although exact numbers are unknown, preliminary analyses estimate that as many as a quarter of African schoolchildren (17.8–32.1 million children aged 5–14 years) may be coincidentally at-risk of both *P. falciparum* and hookworm. While original hypotheses stated that co-infection with multiple parasites would impair the host's immune response to a single parasite and increase susceptibility to clinical disease, studies have yielded contrasting results. For example, one study in Senegal showed that the risk of clinical malaria infection was increased in helminth-infected children in comparison to helminth-free children while other studies have failed to reproduce such results, and even among laboratory mouse experiments the effect of helminths on malaria is variable.Some hypotheses and studies suggest that helminth infections may protect against cerebral malaria due to the possible modulation of pro-inflammatory and anti-inflammatory cytokines responses. Furthermore, the mechanisms underlying this supposed increased susceptibility to disease are unknown. For example, helminth infections cause potent and highly polarized immune response characterized by increased T-helper cell type 2 (T_h2) cytokine and Immunoglobulin E(IgE) production.However, the effect of such responses on the human immune response is unknown. Additionally, both malaria and helminth infection can cause anemia, but the effect of co-infection and possible enhancement of anemia is poorly understood.

Hygiene Hypothesis

The hygiene hypothesis states that infants and children who lack exposure to infectious agents are more susceptible to allergic diseases via modulation of immune system development. As Mary Ruebush writes in her book *Why Dirt is Good*, "what a child is doing when he puts things in his mouth is allowing his immune response to explore his environment. Not only does this allow for 'practice' of immune responses, which will be necessary for protection, but it also plays a critical role in teaching the immature immune response what is best ignored." The theory was first proposed by David P. Strachan who noted that hay fever and eczema were less common in children who belonged to large families. Since then, studies have noted the effect of gastrointestinal worms on the development of allergies in the developing world. For example, a study in Gambia found that eradication of worms in some villages led to increased skin reactions to allergies among children.

Although the exact mechanism is unknown, scientists hypothesize that the helper T cells are key players. Allergic diseases, which are immunological responses to normally harmless antigens, are driven by a TH2-mediated immune response. Bacteria, viruses, and parasites, on the other hand, elicit a TH1-mediated immune response which inhibits or down-regulates the TH2 response. TH1 also inhibits the activity of TH17 which is heightened in numerous inflammatory diseases including multiple sclerosis and asthma. More research is currently being performed to better understand the possible mechanism for the hygiene hypothesis.

Vaccines

While annual or semi-annual mass antihelminthic administration is a critical aspect of any public health intervention, many have begun to realize how unsustainable it is due to aspects such as poverty, high rates of re-infection, and diminished efficacy of drugs with repeated use. Current research, therefore, has focused on the development of a vaccine that could be integrated into existing control programs. The goal of vaccine development is not necessarily to create a vaccine with sterilizing immunity or complete protection against immunity. A vaccine that reduces the likelihood of vaccinated individuals developing severe infections and thus reduced blood and nutrient levels could still have a significant impact on the high burden of disease throughout the world.

Current research focuses on targeting two stages in the development of the worm: the larval stage and the adult stage. Research on larval antigens has focused on proteins that are members of the pathogenesis-related protein superfamily, *Ancylostoma* Secreted Proteins. Although they were first described in *Anyclostoma*, these proteins have also been successfully isolated from the secreted product of *N. americanus*. *N. americanus* ASP-2 (Na-ASP-2) is currently the leading larval-stage hookworm vaccine candidate. A randomized, double-blind, placebo-controlled study has already been performed; 36 healthy adults without a history of hookworm infection were given three intramuscular injections of three different concentrations of Na-ASP-2 and observed for six months after the final vaccination. The vaccine induced significant anti-Na-ASP-2 IgG and cellular immune responses. In addition, it was safe and produced no debilitating side effects. The vaccine is now in a phase one trial; healthy adult volunteers with documented evidence of previous infection in Brazil are being given the same dose concentration on the same schedule used in the initial study. If this study is successful, the next step would be to conduct a phase two trial to assess the rate and intensity of hookworm infection among vaccinated persons. Because the Na-ASP-2 vaccine only targets the larval stage, it is critical that all subjects enrolled in the study be treated with antihelminthic drugs to eliminate adult worms prior to vaccination.

Adult hookworm antigens have also been identified as potential candidates for vaccines. When adult worms attach to the intestinal mucosa of the human host, erythrocytes are ruptured in the worm's digestive tract which causes the release of free hemoglobin which is subsequently degraded by a proteolytic cascade. Several of these proteins that are responsible for this proteolytic cascade are also essential for the worm's nutrition and survival. Therefore, a vaccine that could induce antibodies for these antigens could interfere with the hookworm's digestive pathway and impair the worm's survival. Three proteins have been identified: the aspartic protease-hemoglobinase APR-1, the cysteine protease-hemoglobinase CP-2, and a glutathione S-transferase. Vaccination with APR-1 and CP-2 led to reduced host blood loss and fecal egg counts in dogs. With APR-1, vaccination even led to reduced worm burden. Research is currently stymied at the development of at least one of these antigens as a recombinant protein for testing in clinical trials.

Hookworm in Therapy

Moderate hookworm infections have been demonstrated to have beneficial effects on hosts suffering from diseases linked to overactive immune systems. This is possibly explained by the hygiene hypothesis. Research at the University of Nottingham conducted in Ethiopia observed a small subset of people with hookworm infections were half as likely to experience asthma or hay fever. Potential benefits have also been hypothesized in cases of multiple sclerosis,Crohn's Disease and diabetes.

Some research conducted has shown favourable results using hookworms to treat coeliac disease. Though research points to anti-allergenic properties associated with hook worm infections, the FDA does not currently recognize hookworms as a treatment.

Structure

Scolex

The worm's scolex ("head") attaches to the intestine of the definitive host. In some species, the scolex is dominated by bothria, or "sucking grooves" that function like suction cups. Other species have hooks and suckers that aid in attachment. Cyclophyllid cestodes can be identified by the presence of four suckers on their scolices.

While the scolex is often the most distinctive part of an adult tapeworm, it is often unnoticed in a clinical setting, as it is inside the host. Therefore, identifying eggs and proglottids in feces is the simplest way to diagnose an infection.

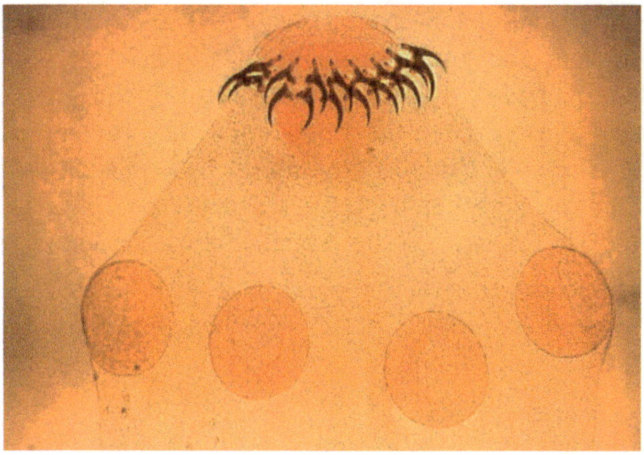

Scolex of *Taenia solium* with hooks and suckers.

Body Systems

The main nerve centre of a cestode is a cerebral ganglion in its scolex. Motor and sensory innervation depends on the number of nerves in and complexity of the scolex. Smaller nerves emanate from the ganglion to supply the general body muscular and sensory ending. The cirrus and vagina are innervated, and sensory endings around the genital pore are more plentiful than other areas. Sensory function includes both tactoreception (touch) and chemoreception (smell or taste). Some nerves are only temporary.

Proglottids

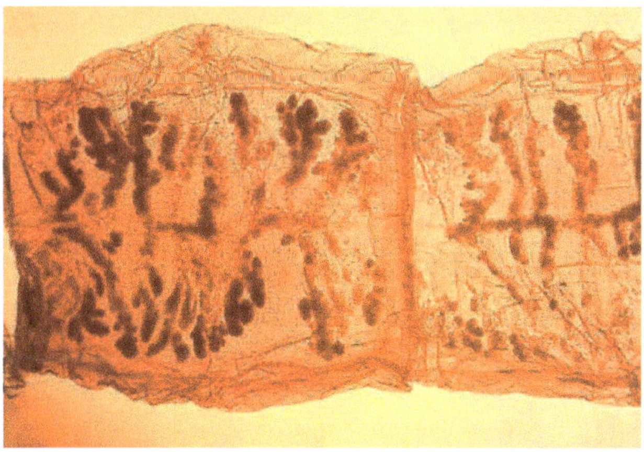

Two proglottids of *Taenia solium*

The body is composed of successive segments called proglottids. The sum of the proglottids is called a strobila, which is thin, and resembles a strip of tape. From this is derived the common name "tapeworm". Proglottids are continually produced by the neck region of the scolex, as long as the scolex is attached and alive. Like some other flatworms, cestodes use flame cells (protonephridia), located in the proglottids, for excretion. Mature proglottids are released from the tapeworm's end segment and leave the host in feces or migrate as independent motile proglottids. The proglottids farthest away from the scolex are the mature ones containing eggs. Mature proglottids are essentially bags of eggs, each of which is infective to the proper intermediate host.

The layout of proglottids comes in two forms: craspedote, meaning any given proglottid is overlapped by the previous proglottid, and acraspedote, indicating the proglottids are not overlapping.

Cestodes are unable to synthesise lipids and are entirely dependent on their host, although lipids are not used as an energy reserve, but for reproduction. Once anchored to the host's intestinal wall, the tapeworm absorbs nutrients through its skin as the food being digested by the host flows over and around it. Soon, it begins to grow a tail composed of a series of segments, with each segment containing an independent digestive system and reproductive tract. Older segments are pushed toward the tip of the tail as new segments are produced by the neckpiece. By the time a segment has reached the end of the worm's tail, only the reproductive tract is left. The segment then separates, carrying the tapeworm eggs out of the definitive host as what is basically a sack of eggs.

Lifecycle

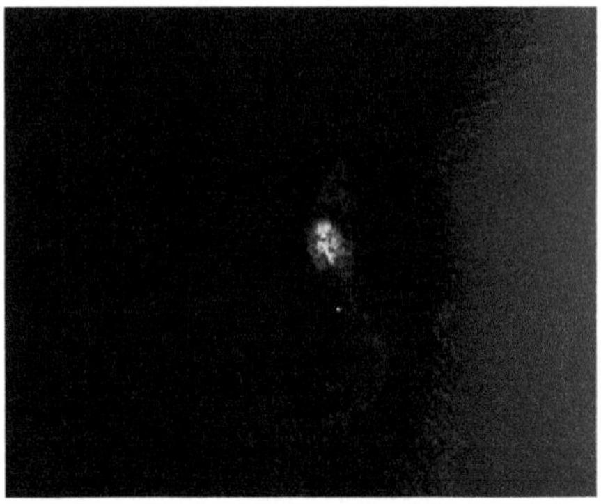

Image of a tapeworm proglottid leaving its definitive host

True tapeworms are exclusively hermaphrodites; they have both male and female reproductive systems in their bodies. The reproductive system includes one or more testes, cirri, vas deferens, and seminal vesicles as male organs, and a single lobed or unlobed ovary with the connecting oviduct and uterus as female organs. The common external opening for both male and female reproductive systems is known as the genital pore, which is situated at the surface opening of the cup-shaped atrium.Though they are sexually hermaphroditic, self-fertilization is a rare phenomenon. To permit hybridization, cross-fertilization between two individuals is often practiced for reproduction. During copulation, the cirri of one individual connect with those of the other through the genital pore, and then spermatozoa are exchanged.

The lifecycle of tapeworms is simple in the sense that no asexual phases occur as in other flatworms, but complicated in that at least one intermediate host is required as well as the definitive host. This lifecycle pattern has been a crucial criterion for assessing evolution among Platyhelminthes. Many tapeworms have a two-phase lifecycle with two types of hosts. The adult *Taenia saginata* lives in the gut of a primate such as a human, but more alarming is *Taenia solium*, which can form cysts in the human brain. Proglottids leave the body through the anus and fall onto the ground, where they may be eaten with grass by an animal such as a cow. If the tapeworm is compatible with the eating animal, this animal becomes an intermediate host. The juvenile form of the worm enters through the mouth, but then migrates and establishes as a cyst in the intermediate host's body tissues such as muscles, rather than the gut. This can cause more damage to the intermediate host than it does to its definitive host. The parasite completes its lifecycle when the intermediate host passes on the parasite to the definitive host. This is usually done by the definitive host eating a suitably infected intermediate host, e.g., a human eating raw or undercooked meat.

Infection and Treatment

Symptoms vary widely, as do treatment options, and these issues are discussed in detail in the individual articles on each worm. Praziquantel is an effective treatment for tapeworm infection, and is preferred over the older niclosamide. Cestodes can also be treated with certain kinds of antibiotics. While accidental tapeworm infections in developed countries are quite rare, some US dieters have risked intentional infection for the purpose of weight loss.

Certain medicines are used to remove it, such as praziquantel or albendazole. Physicians also give enema treatment to the patient to completely remove intestinal flatworms.

Taxonomy

The taxonomy of the Cestoda has been clarified with molecular data. The Gyrocotylidea are a sister group to all other Cestoda (Nephroposticophora): the Amphilinidea form the sister group to the Eucestoda. The Caryophyllidea are the sister group to Spathebothriidea and remaining Eucestoda. The Haplobothriidea are the sister group to Diphyllobothriidae. The Diphyllidea and Trypanorhyncha may be sister groups, but this is not definite.

At the more derived groups, the taxonomy appears to be:

- Bothriocephalidea
- Litobothriidea
- Lecanicephalidea
- Rhinebothriidea
- Tetraphyllidea
- Acanthobothrium, Proteocephalidea
- Cyclophyllidea, Mesocestoididae, Nippotaeniidea, Tetrabothriidea
- The Tetraphyllidea appear to be paraphyletic. The relations between Nippotaeniidea,

Mesocestoididae, Tetrabothriidea, and Cyclophyllidea require further clarification.

- The taxonomy of the Eucestoda has been also clarified. The current taxonomy is
- Monogenea
- Amphilinidea
- Caryophyllidea
- Spathebothriidea
- Trypanorhyncha
- Pseudophyllidea
- Tetraphyllidea
- Diphyllidea, Proteocephalidea
- Nippotaeniidea
- Cyclophyllidea, Tetrabothriidea

The Tetraphyllidea, Pseudophyllidea (because of the Diphyllobothriidae) and Cyclophyllidea (because of the Mesocestoididae) are paraphyletic.

The Taeniidae may be the most basal of the 12 orders of the Cyclophyllidea.

The Tetraphyllidea, Lecanicephalidea, Proteocephalidea, Nippotaeniidea, Tetrabothriidea, and Cyclophyllidea are considered to be the 'higher' tapeworms.

The 277 known species in the marine order Trypanorhyncha are placed in five superfamilies - Tentacularioidea, Gymnorhynchoidea, Otobothrioidea, Eutetrarhynchidae, and Lacistorhynchidae.

Life cycle

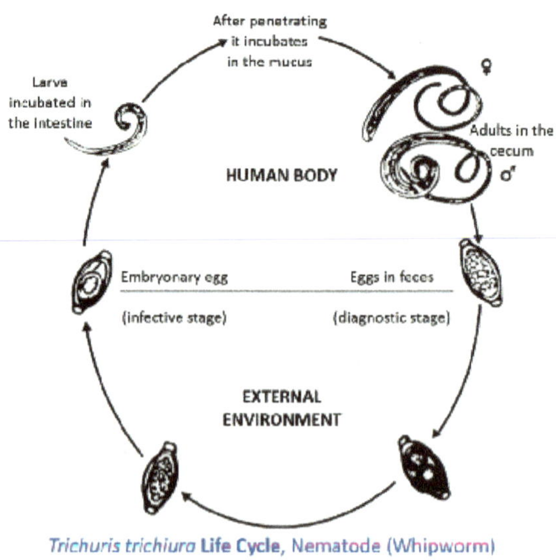

Life cycle of Trichuris trichiura inside and outside the human body

The female T. trichiura produces 2,000–10,000 single-celled eggs per day. Eggs are deposited from human feces to soil where, after two to three weeks, they become embryonated and enter the "infective" stage. These embryonated infective eggs are ingested and hatch in the human small intestine exploiting the intestinal microflora as hatching stimulus. This is the location of growth and molting. The infective larvae penetrate the villi and continue to develop in the small intestine. The young worms move to the caecum and penetrate the mucosa and there they complete development to adult worms in the large intestine. The life cycle from time of ingestion of eggs to development of mature worms takes approximately three months. During this time, there may be limited signs of infection in stool samples due to lack of egg production and shedding. The female T. trichiura begin to lay eggs after three months of maturity. Worms can live up to five years, during which time females can lay up to 20,000 eggs per day.

Recent studies using genome-wide scan revealed two quantitative trait loci on chromosome 9 and chromosome 18 may be responsible for genetic predisposition or susceptibility to infection of *T. trichiura* **by some individuals.**

Characteristics

Trichuris trichiura has a narrow anterior esophageal end and shorter and thicker posterior anus. These pinkish-white worms are threaded through the mucosa. They attach to the host through their slender anterior end and feed on tissue secretions instead of blood. Females are larger than males; approximately 35–50 mm long compared to 30–45 mm. The females have a bluntly round posterior end compared to their male counterparts with a coiled posterior end. Their characteristic eggs are barrel-shaped and brown, and have bipolar protuberances..

Infection

Infection occurs through ingestion of eggs and is more common in warmer areas. Whipworms eggs are passed in the feces of infected persons, and if an infected person defecates outside or if untreated human feces as used as fertilizer, eggs are deposited on soil where they can mature into an infective stage. Ingestion of these eggs "can happen when hands or fingers that have contaminated dirt on them are put in the mouth or by consuming vegetables or fruits that have not been carefully cooked, washed or peeled." The eggs hatch in the small intestine, and then move into the wall of the small intestine and develop. On reaching adulthood, the thinner end (the front of the worm) burrows into the large intestine and the thicker end hangs into the lumen and mates with nearby worms. The females can grow to 50 mm (2.0 in) long. Neither the male nor the female has much of a visible tail past the anus.

Whipworm commonly infects patients also infected with *Giardia*, *Entamoeba histolytica*, *Ascaris lumbricoides*, and hookworms.

Epidemiology

There is a worldwide distribution of *Trichuris trichiura*, with an estimated 1 billion human infections. However, it is chiefly tropical, especially in Asia and, to a lesser degree, in

Africa and South America. Within the United States, infection is rare overall but may be common in the rural Southeast, where 2.2 million people are thought to be infected. Poor hygiene is associated with trichuriasis as well as the consumption of shaded moist soil, or food that may have been fecally contaminated. Children are especially vulnerable to infection due to their high exposure risk. Eggs are infective about 2–3 weeks after they are deposited in the soil under proper conditions of warmth and moisture, hence its tropical distribution.

Other Animals

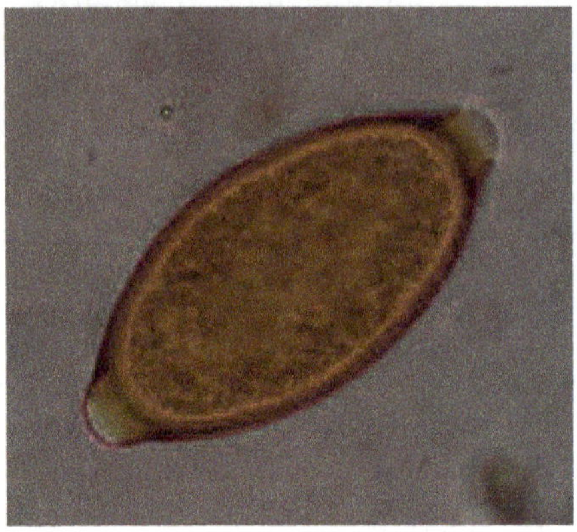

Egg of *Trichuris vulpis*

Whipworms develop when a dog swallows whipworm eggs, passed from an infected dog. Symptoms may include diarrhea, anemia, and dehydration. The dog whipworm (*Trichuris vulpis*) is commonly found in the U.S. It is hard to detect at times, because the numbers of eggs shed are low, and they are shed in waves. Centrifugation is the preferred method. There are several preventives available by prescription from a veterinarian to prevent dogs from getting whipworm.

The cat whipworm is a rare parasite. In Europe, it is represented mostly by Trichuris campanula, and in North America it is Trichuris serrata more often. Whipworm eggs found in cats in North America must be differentiated from lungworms, and from mouse whipworm eggs just passing through.

Treatment of inflammatory disorders

The hygiene hypothesis suggests that various immunological disorders that have been observed in humans only within the last 100 years, such as Crohn's disease, or that have become more common during that period as hygienic practices have become more widespread, may result from a lack of exposure to parasitic worms (also called helminths) during childhood. The use of Trichuris suis ova (TSO, or pig whipworm eggs) by Weinstock, et al., as a therapy for treating Crohn's disease and to a lesser extent ulcerative colitis are two examples that support this hypothesis. There is also anecdotal evidence that treatment of inflammatory bowel disease (IBD) with TSO decreases the incidence of asthma, allergy, and other inflammatory disorders. Some scientific evidence suggests that the course of multiple sclerosis may be very favorably altered by helminth infection; TSO is being studied as a treatment for this disease.

And some other Parasitism are listed below

REFERENCES

1. Cross, John H. (1996). "Enteric Nematodes of Humans". In Baron, Samuel. Medical Microbiology (4th ed.). Galveston: University of Texas Medical Branch at Galveston. ISBN 0-9631172-1-1.
2. Hayes, K. S.; Bancroft, A. J.; Goldrick, M.; Portsmouth, C.; Roberts, I. S.; Grencis, R. K. (2010). "Exploitation of the Intestinal Microflora by the Parasitic Nematode Trichuris muris". Science. 328 (5984): 1391–4. doi:10.1126/science.1187703. PMC 3428897Freely accessible. PMID 20538949.
3. "Trichuris trichiura definition - Medical Dictionary definitions of popular medical terms easily defined on MedTerms". Medterms.com. 2000-04-15. Retrieved 2009-05-19.
4. Crompton, DW (1999). "How much human helminthiasis is there in the world?". The Journal of Parasitology. 85 (3): 397–403. doi:10.2307/3285768. PMID 10386428.
5. de Silva, Nilanthi R; Brooker, Simon; Hotez, Peter J; Montresor, Antonio; Engels, Dirk; Savioli, Lorenzo (2003). "Soil-transmitted helminth infections: updating the global picture". Trends in Parasitology. 19 (12): 547–51. doi:10.1016/j.pt.2003.10.002. PMID 14642761.
6. "Whipworms". VeterinaryPartner.com. 24 September 2007.
7. Hendrix CM, Blagburn BL, Lindsay DS (1987). "Whipworms and intestinal threadworms". Vet. Clin. North Am. Small Anim. Pract. 17 (6): 1355–75. PMID 3328393.
8. Hunter MM, McKay DM (2004). "Review article: helminths as therapeutic agents for inflammatory bowel disease". Aliment. Pharmacol. Ther. 19 (2): 167–77. doi:10.1111/j.0269-2813.2004.01803.x. PMID 14723608.
9. Summers RW, Elliott DE, Urban JF, Thompson R, Weinstock JV (2005). "Trichuris suis therapy in Crohn's disease". Gut. 54 (1): 87–90. doi:10.1136/gut.2004.041749. PMC 1774382Freely accessible. PMID 15591509.
10. Jump up ^ Summers RW, Elliott DE, Qadir K, Urban JF, Thompson R, Weinstock JV (2003). "Trichuris suis seems to be safe and possibly effective in the treatment of inflammatory bowel disease". Am. J. Gastroenterol. 98 (9): 2034–41. doi:10.1111/j.1572-0241.2003.07660.x. PMID 14499784.
11. Buning, J; et al. (March 2008). "Helminths as governors of inflammatory bowel disease". Gut. 57 (8): 1182–1183. doi:10.1136/gut.2008.152355. PMID 18628388. Retrieved 2010-12-10. in our patient Treg [regulatory T cells] activated by helminthosis [T. suis infestation] were most likely the key element protecting a

host with latent ulcerative colitis against development of a severe protcocolitis. (1183)

12. "Helminthic Therapy: How to put your Asthma, Colitis, IBD, Crohn's or Multiple Sclerosis into remission with hookworm". Asthmahookworm.com. Retrieved 2009-05-19.
13. "Allergies: Trichuris suis Ova (TSO) Therapy to Treat Food Allergies". Allergizer.com. Retrieved 2009-05-19.
14. Correale J, Farez M (2007). "Association between parasite infection and immune responses in multiple sclerosis". Annals of Neurology. 61 (2): 97–108. doi:10.1002/ana.21067. PMID 17230481.
15. "Asphelia Announces Initiation of an Independent TSO Trial for Multiple Sclerosis". redOrbit. 2008-04-07.
16. Klaver, Elsenoor J.; Kuijk, Loes M.; Laan, Lisa C.; Kringel, Helene; van Vliet, Sandra J.; Bouma, Gerd; Cummings, Richard D.; Kraal, Georg; van Die, Irma (2013). "Trichuris suis-induced modulation of human dendritic cell function is glycan-mediated". International Journal for Parasitology. 43 (3-4): 191–200. doi:10.1016/j.ijpara.2012.10.021. PMID 23220043.

CHAPTER 3

Protozoan Parasites

Chapter Contents

- **Introduction**
- **History And Terminology**
- **Characteristics**
- **Classification**
- **Ecological Role**
- **Apicomplexa**
- **Taxonomy**
- **Phylum**

The group of organisms known as 'protozoa' are defined by a few of their shared characteristics. Protozoa are non-phototrophic, unicellular, eukaryotic microorganisms with no cell walls. This diverse group of over 65,000 species generally share these basic attributes. Looking deeper, this group can be extremely complex and variable. In fact, the protozoa are often described as the pinnacle of unicellular complexity.

Unlike the relatively simple bacteria, protozoa can have many different intracellular organelles performing specific tasks. Some species of protozoa have structures that are analogous to mouths, GI tracts, and anuses. This probably goes against everything you've been taught about microbes being simply bags of proteins and enzymes.

INTRODUCTION

In some systems of biological classification, the Protozoa are a diverse group of unicellular eukaryotic organisms. Historically, protozoa were defined as single-celled organisms with animal-like behaviors, such as motility and predation. The group was regarded as the zoological counterpart to the "protophyta", which were considered to be plant-like, as they are capable of photosynthesis. The terms *protozoa* and *protozoans* are also used informally to designate single-celled, non-photosynthetic protists, such as ciliates, amoebae and flagellates.

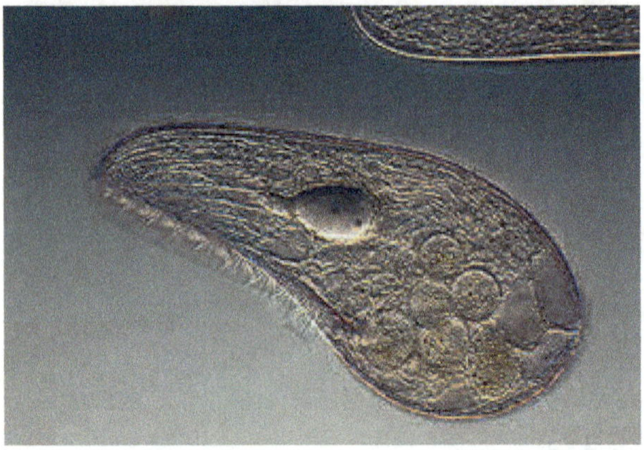

Blepharisma japonicum, a free-living ciliated protozoan.

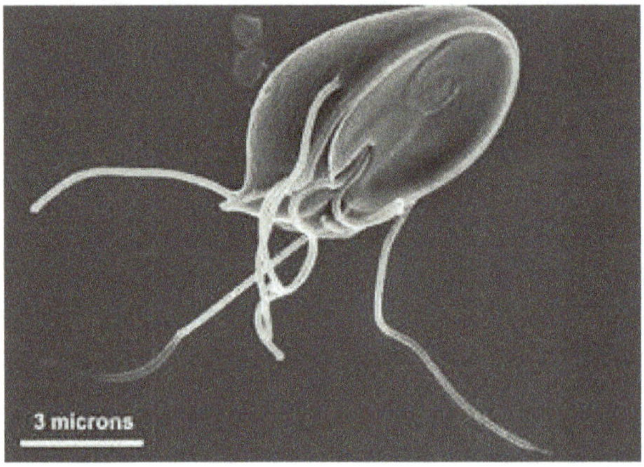

Giardia muris, a flagellate protozoan, is an intestinal parasite found in rodents, birds and reptiles.

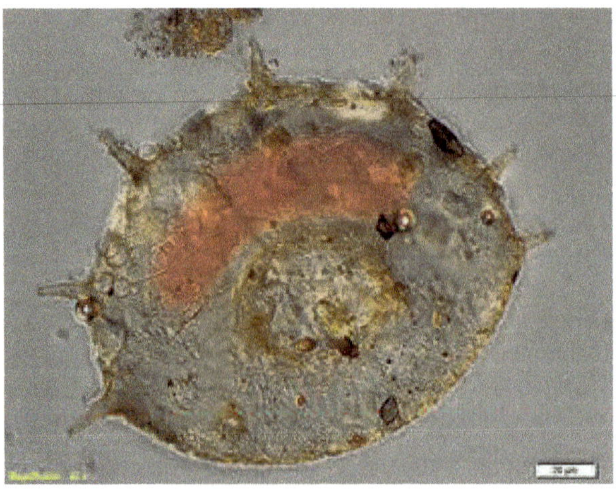

Centropyxis aculeata, a testate (shelled) amoeba

The term Protozoa was introduced in 1818 for a taxonomic class, but in later classification schemes the group was elevated to higher ranks, including phylum, subkingdom and kingdom. In several classification systems proposed by Thomas Cavalier-Smith and his collaborators since 1981, Protozoa is ranked as a kingdom. The seven-kingdom scheme proposed by Ruggiero et al. in 2015, places eight phyla under Protozoa: Euglenozoa, Amoebozoa, Metamonada, Choanozoa, Loukozoa, Percolozoa, Microsporidia and Sulcozoa. This kingdom does not form a clade, but an evolutionary grade or paraphyletic group, from which the fungi and animals are specifically excluded.

The use of Protozoa as a formal taxon has been discouraged by some researchers, mainly because the term, which is formed from the Greek *protos* "first" + *zoia*, plural of *zoion*, "animal", misleadingly implies kinship with animals (metazoa) and promotes an arbitrary separation of "animal-like" from "plant-like" organisms. Modern ultrastructural, biochemical, and genetic techniques have shown that protozoa, as traditionally defined, belong to widely divergent lineages, and can no longer be regarded as "primitive animals." For this reason, the terms "protists," "Protista" or "Protoctista" are sometimes preferred for the high-level classification of eukaryotic microbes. In 2005, members of the Society of Protozoologists voted to change the name of that organization to the International Society of Protistologists.

HISTORY AND TERMINOLOGY

The word "protozoa" (singular *protozoon* or *protozoan*) was coined in 1818 by zoologist Georg August Goldfuss, as the Greek equivalent of the German *Urthiere*, meaning „primitive, or original animals" (*ur-* 'proto-' + *Thier* 'animal'). Goldfuss erected Protozoa as a class containing what he believed to be the simplest animals. Originally, the group included not only microbes, but also some "lower" multicellular animals, such as rotifers, corals, sponges, jellyfish, bryozoa and polychaete worms.

In 1848, in light of advancements in cell theory pioneered by Theodore Schwann and Matthias Schleiden, the anatomist and zoologist C.T. von Siebold proposed that the bodies of microbial organisms such as ciliates and amoebae were made up of single cells, similar to those from which the multicellular tissues of plants and animals were constructed. Von Siebold redefined Protozoa to include only such unicellular forms, to the exclusion of all metazoa. At the same time, he raised the group to the level of a phylum containing two broad classes of microbes: Infusoria (mostly ciliates and flagellated algae), and Rhizopoda (amoeboid organisms). The definition of Protozoa as a phylum or sub-kingdom made up of "unicellular animals" was adopted by the zoologist Otto Bütschli—celebrated at his centenary as the "architect of protozoology"—and the term came into wide use.

As a phylum under Animalia, the Protozoa were firmly rooted in the old "two-kingdom" classification of life, according to which all living beings were classified as either animals or plants. As long as this scheme remained dominant, the protozoa were understood to be animals and studied in departments of Zoology, while photosynthetic microbes and microscopic fungi—the so-called Protophyta—were assigned to the Plants, and studied in departments of Botany.

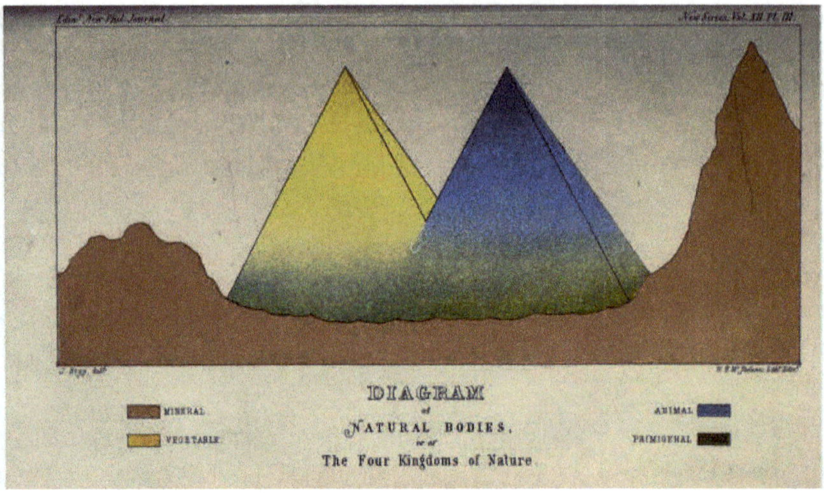

John Hogg's illustration of the Four Kingdoms of Nature, showing "Primigenal" as a greenish haze at the base of the Animals and Plants, 1860

Criticism of this system began in the latter half of the 19th century, with the realization that many organisms met the criteria for inclusion among both plants and animals. For example, the algae *Euglena* and *Dinobryon* have chloroplasts for photosynthesis, but can also feed on organic matter and are motile. In 1860, John Hogg argued against the use of "protozoa", on the grounds that "naturalists are divided in opinion—and probably some will ever continue so—whether many of these organisms, or living beings, are animals or plants." As an alternative, he proposed a new kingdom called Primigenum, consisting of both the protozoa and unicellular algae (protophyta), which he combined together under the name "Protoctista". In Hoggs's conception, the animal and plant kingdoms were likened to two great "pyramids" blending at their bases in the Kingdom Primigenum.

Six years later, Ernst Haeckel also proposed a third kingdom of life, which he named Protista. At first, Haeckel included a few multicellular organisms in this kingdom, but in later work he restricted the Protista to single-celled organisms, or simple colonies whose individual cells are not differentiated into different kinds of tissues.

Despite these proposals, Protozoa emerged as the preferred taxonomic placement for heterotrophic microbes such as amoebae and ciliates, and remained so for more than a century. In the course of the 20th century, however, the old "two kingdom" system began to weaken, with the growing awareness that fungi did not belong among the plants, and that most of the unicellular protozoa were no more closely related to the animals than they were to the plants. By mid-century, some biologists, such as Herbert Copeland, Robert H. Whittaker and Lynn Margulis, advocated the revival of Haeckel's Protista or Hogg's Protoctista as a kingdom-level eukaryotic group, alongside Plants, Animals and Fungi. A variety of multi-kingdom systems were proposed, and Kingdoms Protista and Protoctista became well established in biology texts and curricula.

While many taxonomists have abandoned Protozoa as a high-level group, Thomas Cavalier-Smith has retained it as a kingdom in the various classifications he has proposed. As of 2015, Cavalier-Smith's Protozoa excludes several major groups of organisms traditionally placed among the protozoa, including the ciliates, dinoflagellates and foraminifera (all members of the SAR supergroup). In its current form, his kingdom Protozoa is a paraphyletic group which includes a common ancestor and most of its descendents, but excludes two important clades that branch within it: the animals and fungi.

CHARACTERISTICS

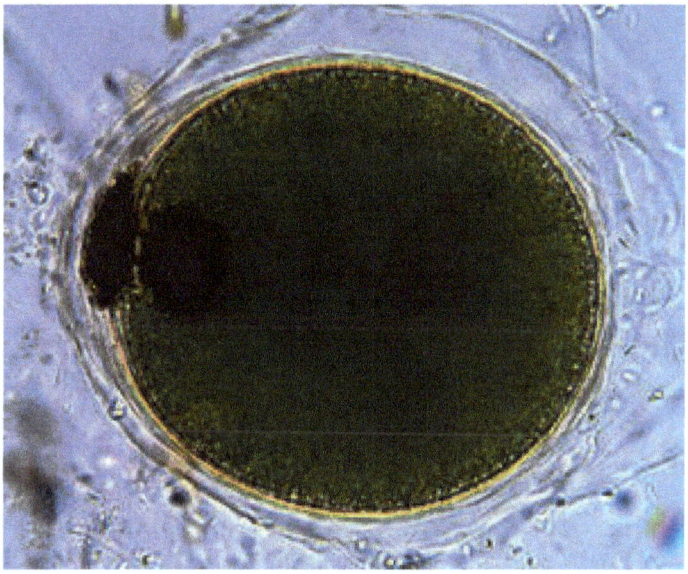

Resting cyst of ciliated protozoan *Dileptus viridis*.

Protozoa, as traditionally defined, are mainly microscopic organisms, ranging in size from 10 to 52 micrometers. Some, however, are significantly larger. Among the largest are the deep-sea–dwelling xenophyophores, single-celled foraminifera whose shells can reach 20 cm in diameter. Free-living forms are restricted to moist environments, such as soils, mosses and aquatic habitats, although many form resting cysts which enable them to survive drying. Many protozoan species are symbionts, some are parasites, and some are predators of bacteria, algae and other protists.

Motility and Feeding

Organisms traditionally classified as protozoa are abundant in aqueous environments and soil, occupying a range of trophic levels. The group includes flagellates (which move with the help of whip-like structures called flagella), ciliates (which move by using hair-like structures called cilia) and amoebae (which move by the use of foot-like structures called pseudopodia). Some protozoa are sessile, and do not move at all.

Protozoa may take in food by osmotrophy, absorbing nutrients through their cell membranes; or they may feed by phagocytosis, either by engulfing particles of food with pseudopodia (as amoebae do), or taking in food through a mouth-like aperture called a cytostome. All protozoa digest their food in stomach-like compartments called vacuoles.

Pellicle

The pellicle is a thin layer supporting the cell membrane in various protozoa, such as ciliates, protecting them and allowing them to retain their shape, especially during locomotion, allowing the organism to be more hydrodynamic. The pellicle varies from flexible and elastic to rigid. Although somewhat stiff, the pellicle is also flexible and allows the protist to fit into tighter spaces. In ciliates and Apicomplexa, it is formed from closely packed vesicles called alveoli. In euglenids, it is formed from protein strips arranged spirally along the length of the body. Familiar examples of protists with a pellicle are the euglenoids and the ciliate *Paramecium*. In some protozoa, the pellicle hosts epibiotic bacteria that adhere to the surface by their fimbriae (attachment pili).

Life Cycle

Some protozoa have life phases alternating between proliferative stages (e.g., trophozoites) and dormant cysts. As cysts, protozoa can survive harsh conditions, such as exposure to extreme temperatures or harmful chemicals, or long periods without access to nutrients, water, or oxygen for periods of time. Being a cyst enables parasitic species to survive outside of a host, and allows their transmission from one host to another. When protozoa are in the form of trophozoites (Greek *tropho* = to nourish), they actively feed. The conversion of a trophozoite to cyst form is known as encystation, while the process of transforming back into a trophozoite is known as excystation. Protozoa reproduce asexually by binary fission or multiple fission. Many protozoan species exchange genetic material by sexual means (typically, through conjugation); however, sexuality is generally decoupled from the process of reproduction, and does not immediately result in increased population.

CLASSIFICATION

The classification of protozoa has been and remains a problematic area of taxonomy. Where they are available, DNA sequences are used as the basis for classification; however, for the majority of described protozoa, such material is not available. Protozoa have been and still are organized mostly on the basis of their morphology, means of locomotion, and for the parasitic species their hosts.

- Flagellates (e.g., *Giardia lamblia*)
- Amoeboids (e.g., *Entamoeba histolytica*)
- Sporozoans (e.g., *Plasmodium knowlesi*)
    - Apicomplexa (now in Alveolata)
    - Microsporidia (now in Fungi)
    - Ascetosporea (now in Rhizaria)
    - Myxosporidia (now in Cnidaria)
- Ciliates (e.g., *Balantidium coli*)

As a phylum the Protozoa were, historically, divided into four subphyla reflecting the means of locomotion:

- Subphylum Sarcomastigophora
    - Superclass Mastigophora (includes flagellates)
    - Superclass Sarcodina
    - Superclass Opalinata
- Subphylum Sporozoa (includes apicomplexans)
- Subphylum Cnidospora
    - Class Microsporidea
- Subphylum Ciliophora (includes ciliates)

These systems are no longer considered to be valid.

Entamoeba

Entamoeba is a genus of Amoebozoa found as internal parasites or commensals of animals.

In 1875, Fedor Lösch described the first proven case of amoebic dysentery in St. Petersburg, Russia. He referred to the amoeba he observed microscopically as 'Amoeba coli'; however it is not clear whether he was using this as a descriptive term or intended it as a formal taxonomic name. The genus *Entamoeba* was defined by Casagrandi and Barbagallo for the species *Entamoeba coli*, which is known to be a commensal organism. Lösch's organism was renamed *Entamoeba histolytica* by Fritz Schaudinn in 1903; he later died, in 1906, from a self-inflicted infection when studying this amoeba. For a time during the first half of the 20th century the entire genus *Entamoeba* was transferred to *Endamoeba*, a genus of amoebas infecting invertebrates about which little is known. This move was reversed by the International Commission on Zoological Nomenclature in the late 1950s, and *Entamoeba* has stayed 'stable' ever since.

Trypanosoma Brucei

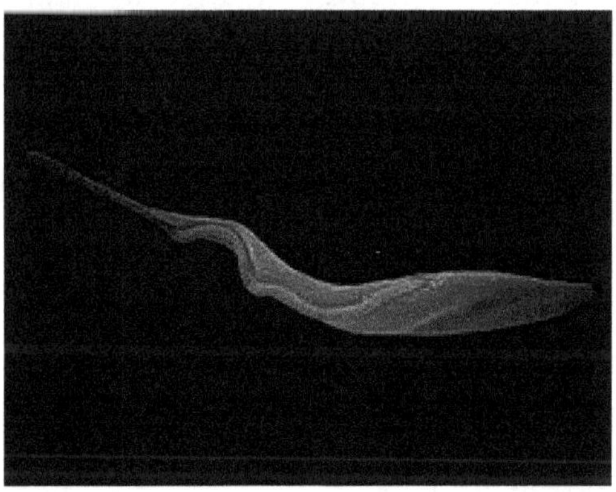

False colour SEM micrograph of procyclic form *Trypanosoma brucei* as found in the tsetse fly midgut. The cell body is shown in orange and the flagellum is in red. 84 pixels/µm.

Trypanosoma brucei is a species of parasitic protozoa belonging to the genus *Trypanosoma*. It causes African trypanosomiasis, known also as sleeping sickness in humans and nagana in other animals. *T. brucei* has traditionally been grouped into three subspecies: *T. b. brucei*, *T. b. gambiense* and *T. b. rhodesiense*. The latter two are typically parasites of humans, while the first is that of other animals. Only rarely can the *T.b.brucei* infect a human.

T. brucei is transmitted between mammal hosts by an insect vector belonging to the species of tsetse fly. Transmission occurs by biting during the insect's blood meal. The parasites undergo complex morphological changes as they move between insect and mammal over the course of their life cycle. The mammalian bloodstream forms are notable for their variant surface glycoprotein coats, which undergo remarkable antigenic variation, enabling persistent evasion of host adaptive immunity and chronic infection. *T. brucei* is one of only a few pathogens that can cross the blood brain barrier. There is an urgent need for the development of new drug therapies, as current treatments can prove fatal to the patient.

Whilst not historically regarded as *T. brucei* subspecies due to their different means of transmission, clinical presentation, and loss of kinetoplast DNA, genetic analyses reveal that *T. equiperdum* and *T. evansi* are evolved from parasites very similar to *T. b. brucei*, and are thought to be members of the *brucei* clade.

The parasite was discovered in 1894 by Sir David Bruce, after whom the scientific name was given in 1899.

Toxoplasma gondii - ***causes Toxoplasmosis***

Toxoplasma gondii is an obligate intracellular, parasiticprotozoan that causes the disease toxoplasmosis. Found worldwide, *T. gondii* is capable of infecting virtually all warm-blooded animals, but felids such as domestic cats are the only known definitive hosts in which the parasite can undergo sexual reproduction.

In humans, *T. gondii* is one of the most common parasites in developed countries;serological studies estimate that 30–50% of the global population has been exposed to and may be chronically infected with *T. gondii*, although infection rates differ significantly from country to country. For example, previous estimates have shown the highest prevalence of persons infected to be in France, at 84%. Although mild, flu-like symptoms occasionally occur during the first few weeks following exposure, infection with *T. gondii* produces no readily observable symptoms in healthy human adults. This asymptomatic state of infection is referred to as a latent infection and has recently been associated with numerous subtle adverse or pathological behavioral alterations in humans. In infants, HIV/AIDS patients, and others with weakened immunity, infection can cause a serious and occasionally fatal illness, toxoplasmosis.

T. gondii has been shown to alter the behavior of infected rodents in ways thought to increase the rodents' chances of being preyed upon by cats. Support for this "manipulation hypothesis" stems from studies showing *T. gondii*-infected rats have a decreased aversion to cat urine. Because cats are the only hosts within which *T. gondii* can sexually reproduce to complete and begin its lifecycle, such behavioral manipulations are thought to be evolutionary adaptations that increase the parasite's reproductive success. The rats would not shy away from areas where cats live and would also be less able to escape should a cat try to prey on them. The primary mechanisms of *T. gondii*–induced behavioral changes in rodents is now known to occur through epigenetic remodeling in neurons which govern the associated behaviors; for example, it modifies epigenetic methylation to cause hypomethylation of arginine vasopressin-related genes in the medial amygdala to greatly decrease predator aversion. Widespread histone-lysine acetylation in cortical astrocytes appears to be another epigenetic mechanism employed by *T. gondii*. Differences in aversion to cat urine are observed between non-infected and infected humans and sex differences within these groups were apparent, as well.

A number of studies have suggested that subtle behavioral or personality changes may occur in infected humans, and infection with the parasite has recently been associated with a number of neurological disorders, particularly schizophrenia.A 2015 study also found cognitive deficits in adults to be associated with joint infection by both *T. gondii* and *Helicobacter pylori* in a regression model with controls for race-ethnicity and educational attainment. However, although a causal relationship between latent toxoplasmosis with these neurological phenomena has not yet been established, preliminary evidence suggests that *T. gondii* infection can induce some of the same alterations in the human brain as those observed in mice.

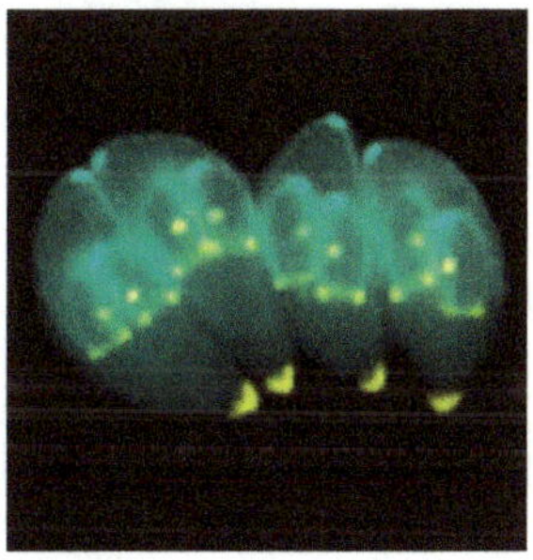

Dividing *T. gondii* parasites

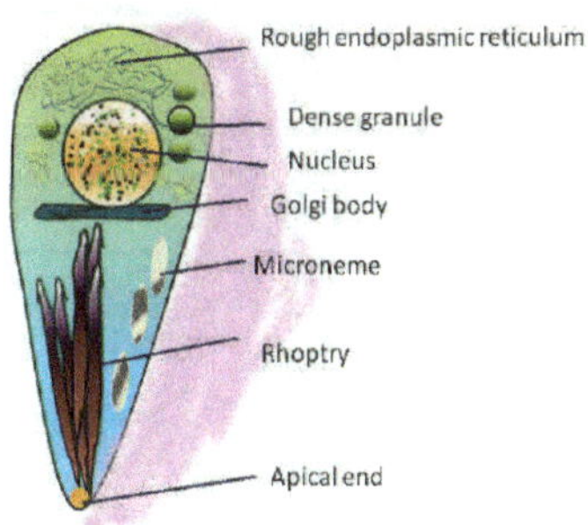

Diagram of *T. gondii* structure

Strongyloides stercoralis - ***causes Strongyloidiasis***

Strongyloides stercoralis is a human pathogenic parasitic roundworm causing the disease strongyloidiasis. Its common name is threadworm. In the UK and Australia, however, the term *threadworm* can also refer to nematodes of the genus *Enterobius*, otherwise known as pinworms.

The *Strongyloides stercoralis* nematode can parasitize humans. The adult parasitic stage lives in tunnels in the mucosa of the small intestine. The genus *Strongyloides* contains 53 species, and *S. stercoralis* is the type species. *S. stercoralis* has been reported in other mammals, including cats and dogs. However, it seems that the species in dogs is typically not *S. stercoralis*, but the related species *S. canis*. Non-human primates are more commonly infected with *S. fuelleborni* and *S. cebus*, although *S. stercoralis* has been reported in captive primates. Other species of *Strongyloides*, naturally parasitic in humans, but with restricted distributions, are *S. fuelleborni* in central Africa and *S. kellyi* in Papua New Guinea.

Toxocara - ***causes Toxocariasis***

The **Toxocaridae** are a zoonotic family of parasitic nematodes that infect canids and felids and which cause toxocariasis in humans (visceral larva migrans and ocular larva migrans). The worms are unable to reproduce in humans.

Four important species include:

- *Toxocara canis*, which infects dogs.
- *Toxocara cati*, which infects cats and lacks intermediate hosts.
- *Toxascaris leonina*, which infects mostly cats, but also dogs.
- *Toxocara vitulorum*, which infects buffalo and cattle.

Guinea Worm - causes Dracunculiasis

Dracunculus medinensis or Guinea worm is a nematode that causes dracunculiasis, also known as guinea worm disease. The disease is caused by the female which, at up to 800 mm (31 in) in length, is among the longest nematodes infecting humans. In contrast, the longest recorded male Guinea worm is only 40 mm (1.6 in).

The common name “guinea worm” is derived from the Guinea region of Western Africa.

Ascaris lumbricoides - ***cause Ascariasis***

Ascaris lumbricoides is the “giant roundworm” of humans, growing to a length of up to 35 cm (14 in). It is one of several species of Ascaris. An ascarid nematode of the phylum Nematoda, it is the most common parasitic worm in humans. This organism is responsible for the disease ascariasis, a type of helminthiasis and one of the group of neglected tropical diseases. An estimated one-sixth of the human population is infected by *A. lumbricoides* or another roundworm.Ascariasis is prevalent worldwide, especially in tropical and subtropical countries.

ECOLOGICAL ROLE

As components of the micro- and meiofauna, protozoa are an important food source for microinvertebrates. Thus, the ecological role of protozoa in the transfer of bacterial and algal production to successive trophic levels is important. As predators, they prey upon unicellular or filamentous algae, bacteria, and microfungi. Protozoan species include both herbivores and consumers in the decomposer link of the food chain. They also control bacteria populations and biomass to some extent. On average, protozoa eat ~ 100 to 1,000 bacteria per hour. Protozoa can stimulate decomposition of organic matter, digest cellulose in the rumen of cows and termite guts, and can play a role in nutrient mobilization.

Diseases

In Humans

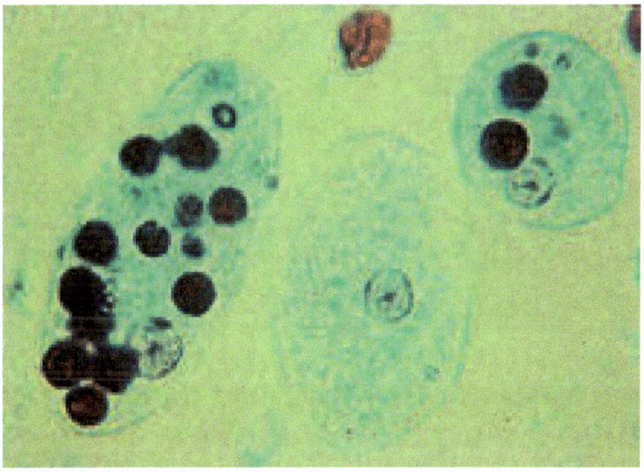

Trophozoites of the amoebic dysentery pathogen *Entamoeba histolytica* with ingested human red blood cells (dark circles)

Main article: Protozoan infection

A number of protozoan pathogens are human parasites, causing diseases such as malaria (by *Plasmodium*), amoebiasis, giardiasis, toxoplasmosis, cryptosporidiosis, trichomoniasis, Chagas disease, leishmaniasis, African trypanosomiasis (sleeping sickness), amoebic dysentery, acanthamoeba keratitis, and primary amoebic meningoencephalitis (naegleriasis).

In other Animals

The protozoan *Ophryocystis elektroscirrha* is a parasite of butterfly larvae, passed from female to caterpillar. Severely infected individuals are weak, unable to expand their wings, or unable to eclose, and have shortened lifespans, but parasite levels vary in populations. Infection creates a culling effect, whereby infected migrating animals are less likely to complete the migration. This results in populations with lower parasite loads at the end of the migration.This is not the case in laboratory or commercial rearing, where after a few generations, all individuals can be infected.

Acanthamoeba - causes Acanthamoeba keratitis

Acanthamoeba is a genus of amoebae, one of the most common protozoa in soil, and frequently found in fresh water and other habitats. *Acanthamoeba* has two evolutive forms, the metabolically active trophozoite and a dormant, stress resistant cyst. Trophozoites are small, usually 15 to 35 μm in length and amoeboid in shape. In nature, *Acanthamoeba* species are free-living bacterivores, but in certain situations they can cause infections (Acanthamebiasis) in humans and other animals.

Cyclospora - causes Cyclosporiasis

Cyclospora is a genus of apicomplexan parasites. It includes the species *Cyclospora cayetanensis*, the causative agent of cyclosporiasis.

Naegleria fowleri - causes Primary amoebic meningoencephalitis

Naegleria fowleri, colloquially known as the "brain-eating amoeba", is a species of the genus *Naegleria*, belonging to the phylum Percolozoa. It is a free-living, bacteria-eating amoeba that can be pathogenic, causing a fulminant (sudden and severe) brain infection called naegleriasis, also known as *primary amoebic meningoencephalitis* (PAM). This microorganism is typically found in bodies of warm freshwater, such as ponds, lakes, rivers, and hot springs. It is also found in the soil near warm-water discharges of industrial plants, and in unchlorinated or minimally-chlorinated swimming pools. It can be seen in either an amoeboid or temporary flagellate stage.

Pinworm - causes Enterobiasis

Pinworm infection, also known as **enterobiasis**, is a human parasitic disease caused by the pinworm. The most common symptom is itching in the anal area. This can make sleeping difficult. The period of time from swallowing eggs to the appearance of new eggs around the anus is 4 to 8 weeks. Some people who are infected do not have symptoms.

The disease is spread between people by pinworm eggs. The eggs initially occur around the anus and can survive for up to three weeks in the environment. They may be swallowed following contamination of the hands, food, or other articles. Those at risk are those who go to school, are institutionalized, or take care of people who are infected. Other animals do not spread the disease. Diagnosis is by seeing the worms which are about one centimeter or the eggs under a microscope.

Treatment is typically with two doses of the medications mebendazole, pyrantel pamoate, or albendazole two weeks apart. Everyone who lives with or takes care of an infected person should be treated at the same time. Washing personal items in hot water after each dose of medication is recommended. Good handwashing, daily bathing in the morning, and daily changing of underwear can help prevent reinfection.

Pinworm infections commonly occur in all parts of the world. It is most common worm infection in the developed world. School aged children are the most commonly infected. In the United States about 20% of people at one point in time develop pinworm. Infection rates among high risk groups may be as high as 50%. It is not considered a serious disease. Pinworms are believed to have affected humans throughout history.

APICOMPLEXA

The Apicomplexa (also called Apicomplexia) are a large phylum of parasitic protists. Most of them possess a unique form of organelle that comprises a type of plastid called an apicoplast, and an apical complex structure. The organelle is an adaptation that the apicomplexan applies in penetration of a host cell.

The Apicomplexa are unicellular and spore-forming. All species are obligateendoparasites of animals, except *Nephromyces*, a symbiont in marine animals, originally classified as a chytrid fungus. Motile structures such as flagella or pseudopods are present only in certain gamete stages.

The Apicomplexa are a diverse group that includes organisms such as the coccidia, gregarines, piroplasms, haemogregarines, and plasmodia. Diseases caused by Apicomplexa include:

- Babesiosis (*Babesia*)
- Malaria (*Plasmodium*)
- Cryptosporidiosis (*Cryptosporidium parvum*)
- Cyclosporiasis (*Cyclospora cayetanensis*)
- Isosporiasis (*Isospora belli*)
- Toxoplasmosis (*Toxoplasma gondii*)

The name of the taxon Apicomplexa derives from two Latin words *apex* (top) and *complexus* (infolds) — and refers to a set of organelles in the sporozoite. The Apicomplexa comprise the bulk of what used to be called the Sporozoa, a group of parasitic protozoans, in general without flagella, cilia, or pseudopods. Most of the Apicomplexa are motile, however, by use of a gliding mechanism that uses adhesions and small static myosin motors. The other main lines were the Ascetosporea (now in Rhizaria), the Myxozoa (now known to be derived from animals), and the Microsporidia (now known to be derived from fungi). Sometimes, the name Sporozoa is taken as a synonym for the Apicomplexa, or occasionally as a subset.

General Features of the Apicomplexa

All members of this phylum have an infectious stage — the sporozoite — which possesses three distinct structures in an apical complex. The apical complex consists of a set of spirally arranged microtubules (the conoid), a secretory body (the rhoptry) and one or more polar rings. Additional slender electron-dense secretory bodies (micronemes) surrounded by one or two polar rings may also be present. This structure gives the phylum its name.

A further group of spherical organelles is distributed throughout the cell rather than being localized at the apical complex and are known as the dense granules. These typically have a mean diameter around 0.7 μm. Secretion of the dense-granule content takes place after parasite invasion and localization within the parasitophorous vacuole and persists for several minutes.

Other morphological findings common to all members of this phylum include:

- The nucleus is haploid.
- Flagella are found only in the motile gamete. These are posteriorly directed and vary in number (usually one to three).
- Basal bodies are present. Although hemosporidians and piroplasmids have normal triplets of microtubules in their basal bodies, coccidians and gregarines have nine singlets.
- The mitochondria have tubular cristae.
- A Golgi apparatus is present.
- Centrioles, chloroplasts, ejectile organelles, and inclusions are absent.
- Colourless plastids are present in some species.
- The cell is surrounded by a pellicle of three membrane layers (the alveolar structure) penetrated by micropores.

Replication:

- Mitosis is usually closed, with an intranuclear spindle; in some species, it is open at the poles.
- Cell division is usually by schizogony.
- Meiosis occurs in the zygote.

Mobility:

Apicomplexans have a unique gliding capability which enables them to cross through tissues and enter and leave their host cells. This gliding ability is made possible by the use of adhesions and small static myosin motors.

Other features common to this phylum are a lack of cilia, sexual reproduction, use of micropores for feeding, and the production of oocysts containing sporozoites as the infective form.

Most apicomplexans have an apicoplast, (a nonphotosynthetic plastid) and mitochondrial and nuclear genomes, although *Cryptosporidium* species and gregarines are possible exceptions, as they are thought to have lost their plastids after the diverging last common ancestor of apicomplexans.

General Features of the Subgroups

Within this phylum are three groups — coccidians, gregarines, and haemosporidians. The coccidians and gregarines appear to be relatively closely related.

Perkinsus , while once considered a member of the Apicomplexa, has been moved to a new phylum —Perkinsozoa.

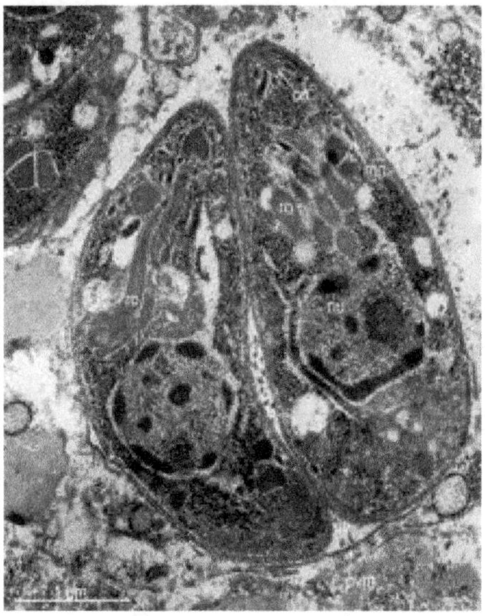

Two tachyzoites of *Toxoplasma gondii*, transmission electron microscopy

Gregarines

The gregarines are generally parasites of annelids, arthropods, and mollusks. They are often found in the guts of their hosts, but may invade the other tissues. In the typical gregarine lifecycle, a trophozoite develops within a host cell into a schizont. This then divides into a number of merozoites by schizogony. The merozoites are released by lysing the host cell, which in turn invade other cells. At some point in the apicomplexan lifecycle, gametocytes are formed. These are released by lysis of the host cells, which group together. Each gametocyte forms multiple gametes. The gametes fuse with another to form oocysts. The oocysts leave the host to be taken up by a new host.

Coccidians

In general, coccidians are parasites of vertebrates. Like gregarines, they are commonly parasites of the epithelial cells of the gut, but may infect other tissues.

The coccidian lifecycle involves merogony, gametogony, and sporogony. While similar to that of the gregarines it differs in zygote formation. Some trophozoites enlarge and become macrogamete, whereas others divide repeatedly to form microgametes (anisogamy). The microgametes are motile and must reach the macrogamete to fertilize it. The fertilized macrogamete forms a zygote that in its turn forms an oocyst that is normally released from the body. Syzygy, when it occurs, involves markedly anisogamous gametes. The lifecycle is typically haploid, with the only diploid stage occurring in the zygote, which is normally short-lived.

The main difference between the coccidians and the gregarines is in the gamonts. In the coccidia, these are small, intracellular, and without epimerites or mucrons. In the gregarines, these are large, extracellular, and possess epimerites or mucrons. A second difference between the coccidia and the gregarines also lies in the gamonts. In the coccidians, a single gamont becomes a macrogametocyte, whereas in the gregarines, the gamonts give rise to multiple gametocytes.

Haemosporidia

The Haemosporidia have more complex lifecycles that alternate between an arthropod and a vertebrate host. The trophozoite parasitises erythrocytes or other tissues in the vertebrate host. Microgametes and macrogametes are always found in the blood. The gametes are taken up by the insect vector during a blood meal. The microgametes migrate within the gut of the insect vector and fuse with the macrogametes. The fertilized macrogamete now becomes an ookinete, which penetrates the body of the vector. The ookinete then transforms into an oocyst and divides initially by meiosis and then by mitosis (haplontic lifecycle) to give rise to the sporozoites. The sporozoites escape from the oocyst and migrate within the body of the vector to the salivary glands where they are injected into the new vertebrate host when the insect vector feeds again.

Reproduction and Life Cycle of Apicomplexa

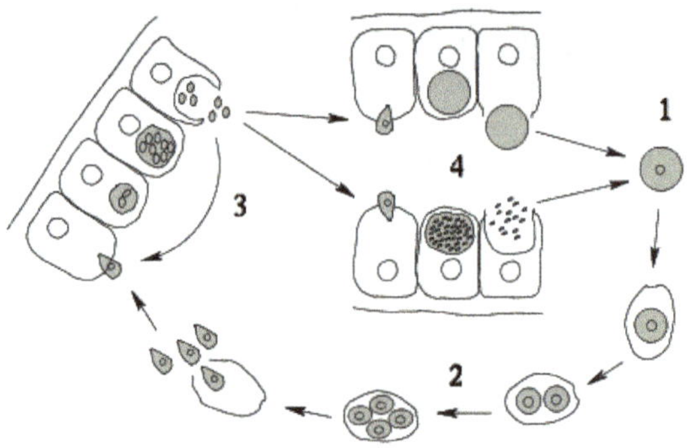

Generic lifecycle of an Apicomplexa: 1-zygote (cyst), 2-sporozoites, 3-merozoites, 4-gametocytes

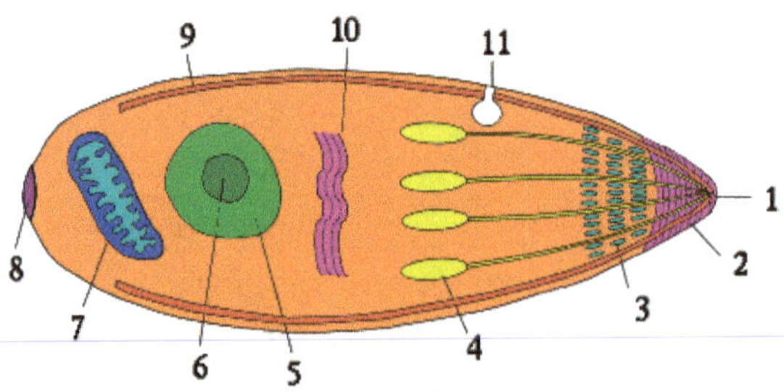

Apicomplexan structure: 1-polar ring, 2-conoid, 3-micronemes, 4-rhoptries, 5-nucleus, 6-nucleolus, 7-mitochondria, 8-posterior ring, 9-alveoli, 10-golgi apparatus, 11-micropore.

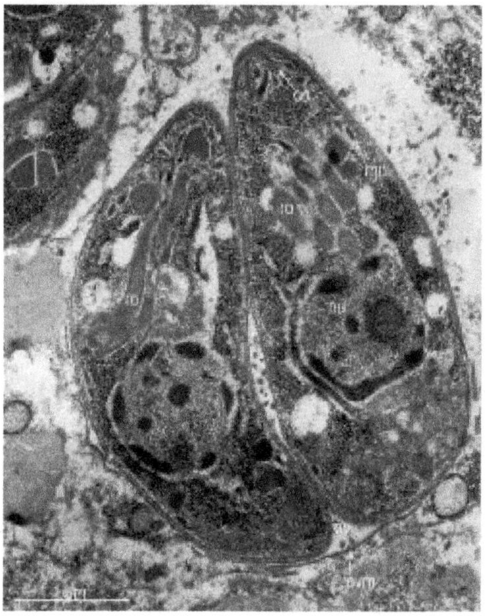

Two tachyzoites of *Toxoplasma gondii*, transmission electron microscopy

Most members have a complex lifecycle, involving both asexual and sexual reproduction. Typically, a host is infected via an active invasion by the parasites (similar to entosis), which divide to produce sporozoites that enter its cells. Eventually, the cells burst, releasing merozoites, which infect new cells. This may occur several times, until gamonts are produced, forming gametes that fuse to create new cysts. Many variations occur on this basic pattern, however, and many Apicomplexa have more than one host.

The apical complex includes vesicles called rhoptries and micronemes, which open at the anterior of the cell. These secrete enzymes that allow the parasite to enter other cells. The tip is surrounded by a band of microtubules, called the polar ring, and among the Conoidasida is also a funnel of tubulin proteins called the conoid. Over the rest of the cell, except for a diminished mouth called the micropore, the membrane is supported by vesicles called alveoli, forming a semirigid pellicle.

The presence of alveoli and other traits place the Apicomplexa among a group called the alveolates. Several related flagellates, such as *Perkinsus* and *Colpodella*, have structures similar to the polar ring and were formerly included here, but most appear to be closer relatives of the dinoflagellates. They are probably similar to the common ancestor of the two groups.

Another similarity is that many apicomplexan cells contain a single plastid, called the apicoplast, surrounded by either three or four membranes. Its functions are thought to include tasks such as lipid and heme biosynthesis, and it appears to be necessary for survival. In general, plastids are considered to have a common origin with the chloroplasts of dinoflagellates, and evidence points to an origin from red algae rather than green.

Genomics of Apicomplexa

Many of the apicomplexan parasites are important pathogens of human and domestic animals. In contrast to bacterial pathogens, these apicomplexan parasites are eukaryotic and share many metabolic pathways with their animal hosts. This makes therapeutic target development extremely difficult – a drug that harms an apicomplexan parasite is also likely to harm its human host. At present, no effective vaccines are available for most diseases caused by these parasites. Biomedical research on these parasites is challenging because it is often difficult, if not impossible, to maintain live parasite cultures in the laboratory and to genetically manipulate these organisms. In recent years, several of the apicomplexan species have been selected for genome sequencing. The availability of genome sequences provides a new opportunity for scientists to learn more about the evolution and biochemical capacity of these parasites. The predominant source of this genomic information is the EuPathDB family of websites, which currently provides specialised services for *Plasmodium* species (PlasmoDB), coccidians (ToxoDB), piroplasms (PiroplasmaDB), and *Cryptosporidium* species (CryptoDB). One possible target for drugs is the plastid, and in fact existing drugs such as tetracyclines, which are effective against apicomplexans, seem to operate against the plastid.

Taxonomy of Apicomplexa

Within the Apicomplexa are three suborders of parasites:

- suborder Adeleorina — eight genera
- suborder Haemosporina — all genera in this suborder
- suborder Eimeriorina — two genera (*Lankesterella* and *Schellackia*)

Within the Adelorina are species that infect invertebrates and others that infect vertebrates. The Eimeriorina — the largest suborder in this phylum — the lifecycle involves both sexual and asexual stages. The asexual stages reproduce by schizogony. The male gametocyte produces a large number of gametes and the zygote gives rise to an oocyst, which is the infective stage. The majority are monoxenous (infect one host only), but a few are heteroxenous (lifecycle involves two or more hosts).

The number of families in this later suborder is debated, with the number of families being between one and 20 depending on the authority and the number of genera being between 19 and 25.

Evolution of Apicomplexa

All members of this phylum are parasitic and evolved from a free-living ancestor. This lifestyle is presumed to have evolved at the time of the divergence of dinoflagellates and apicomplexans. Further evolution of this phylum has been estimated to have occurred about 800 million years ago. The oldest extant clade is thought to be the archigregarines.

Many Coccidiomorpha have an intermediate host, as well as a primary host, and the evolution of hosts proceeded in different ways and at different times in these groups. For some coccidiomorphs, the original host has become the intermediate host, whereas in others it has become the definitive host. In the genera *Aggregata*, *Atoxoplasma*, *Cystoisospora*, *Schellackia*, and *Toxoplasma*, the original is now definitive, whereas in *Akiba*, *Babesiosoma*, *Babesia*, *Haemogregarina*, *Haemoproteus*, *Hepatozoon*, *Karyolysus*, *Leucocytozoon*, *Plasmodium*, *Sarcocystis*, and *Theileria*, the original hosts are now intermediate.

Similar strategies to increase the likelihood of transmission have evolved in multiple genera. Polyenergid oocysts and tissue cysts are found in representatives of the orders Protococcidiorida and Eimeriida. Hypnozoites are found in *Karyolysus lacerate* and most species of *Plasmodium*; transovarial transmission of parasites occurs in lifecycles of *Karyolysus* and *Babesia*.

Horizontal gene transfer appears to have occurred early on in this phylum's evolution with the transfer of a histone H4 lysine 20 (H4K20) modifier, Set8, from an animal host to the ancestor of apicomplexans. A second gene — H3K36 methyltransferase (Ashr3 in plants) — may have also be horizontally transferred.

Taxonomy of Apicomplexa

This has rarely been studied at the subclass level. The Haemosporidia are related to the gregarines and the piroplasms and coccidians are sister groups. The Haemosporidia and the Piroplasma appear to be sister clades and are more closely related to the coccidians than to the gregarines.

Transposons appear to be rare in this phylum, but have been identified in the genera *Ascogregarina* and *Eimeria*.

HISTORY OF APICOMPLEXA TAXONOMY

The first Apicomplexa protozoan was seen by Antonie van Leeuwenhoek, who in 1674 saw probably oocysts of *Eimeria stiedae* in the gall bladder of a rabbit. The first species of the phylum to be described, *Gregarina ovata* in earwigs intestines, was named by Dufour in 1828. He thought that they were a peculiar group related to the trematodes, at that time included in Vermes. Since then, many more have been identified and named. During 1826–1850, 41 species and six genera of Apicomplexa were named. In 1951–1975, 1873 new species and 83 new genera were added.

The older taxon Sporozoa, included in Protozoa, was created by Leuckart in 1879 and adopted by Bütschli in 1880.Through history, it grouped with the current Apicomplexa many unrelated groups. For example, Kudo (1954) included in the Sporozoa species of the Ascetosporea (Rhizaria), Microsporidia (Fungi), Myxozoa (Animalia) and *Helicosporidium* (Chlorophyta), while Zierdt (1978) included the genus *Blastocystis* (Stramenopiles). Not all of these groups had spores, but all were parasitic. However, other parasitic or symbiotic unicellular organisms were included too in protozoan groups outside Sporozoa (Flagellata, Ciliophora and Sarcodina), if they had flagella (e.g., many Kinetoplastida, Retortamonadida, Diplomonadida, Trichomonadida, Hypermastigida), cilia (e.g., *Balantidium*) or pseudopods (e.g., *Entamoeba, Acanthamoeba, Naegleria*). If they had cell walls, they also could be included in plant kingdom between bacteria or yeasts.

Sporozoa is no longer regarded as biologically valid and its use is discouraged, although some authors still use it as a synonym for the Apicomplexa. More recently, other groups were excluded from Apicomplexa, e.g., *Perkinsus* and *Colpodella* (now in Protalveolata).

The field of classifying Apicomplexa is in flux and classification has changed throughout the years since it was formally named in 1970.

By 1987, a comprehensive survey of the phylum was completed: in all, 4516 species and 339 genera had been named. They consisted of:

- Class Conoidasida

- Subclass Gregarinasina *p.p.*
    - Order Eugregarinorida, with 1624 named species and 231 named genera
- Subclass Coccidiasina *p.p*
    - Order Eucoccidiorida *p.p*
        - Suborder Adeleorina *p.p*
            - Group Hemogregarines, with 399 species and four genera
        - Suborder Eimeriorina, with 1771 species and 43 genera

- Class Aconoidasida
    - Order Haemospororida, with 444 species and nine genera
    - Order Piroplasmorida, with 173 species and 20 genera
- Other minor groups omitted above, with 105 species and 32 genera

Although considerable revision of this phylum has been done (the order Haemosporidia now has 17 genera rather than 9), these numbers seems likely to be still approximately correct.

Jacques Euzéby (1988)

Jacques Euzéby in 1988 created a new class Haemosporidiasina by merging subclass Piroplasmasina and suborder Haemospororina.

- Subclass Gregarinasina (the gregarines)
- Subclass Coccidiasina
    - Suborder Adeleorina (the adeleorins)
    - Suborder Eimeriorina (the eimeriorins)
- Subclass Haemosporidiasina
    - Order Achromatorida
    - Order Chromatorida

The division into Achromatorida and Chromatorida, although proposed on morphological grounds, may have a biological basis, as the ability to store haemozoin appears to have evolved only once.

Roberts and Janovy (1996)

Roberts and Janovy in 1996 divided the phylum into the following subclasses and suborders (omitting classes and orders):

- Subclass Gregarinasina (the gregarines)
- Subclass Coccidiasina
  - Suborder Adeleorina (the adeleorins)
  - Suborder Eimeriorina (the eimeriorins)
  - Suborder Haemospororina (the haemospororins)
- Subclass Piroplasmasina (the piroplasms)

These form the following five taxonomic groups:

- The gregarines are, in general, one-host parasites of invertebrates.
- The adeleorins are one-host parasites of invertebrates or vertebrates, or two-host parasites that alternately infect haematophagous (blood-feeding) invertebrates and the blood of vertebrates.
- The eimeriorins are a diverse group that includes one host species of invertebrates, two-host species of invertebrates, one-host species of vertebrates and two-host species of vertebrates. The eimeriorins are frequently called the coccidia. This term is often used to include the adeleorins.
- Haemospororins, often known as the malaria parasites, are two-host Apicomplexa that parasitize blood-feeding dipteran flies and the blood of various tetrapod vertebrates.
- Piroplasms where all the species included are two-host parasites infecting ticks and vertebrates.

Perkins (2000)

This scheme is taken from Perkins et al. It is outdated as the Perkinsidae have since been recognised as a sister group to the dinoflagellates rather that the Apicomplexia. The remainder of the scheme appears to be valid:

- Class Aconoidasida

Conoid present only in the ookinete of some species

- Order Haemospororida

Macrogamete and microgamete develop separately. Syzygy does not occur. Ookinete has a conoid. Sporozoites have three walls. Heteroxenous: alternates between vertebrate host (in which merogony occurs) and invertebrate host (in which sporogony occurs). Usually blood parasites, transmitted by blood-sucking insects.

- Order Piroplasmorida
- Class Conoidasida
  - Subclass Gregarinasina
    - Order Archigregarinorida
    - Order Eugregarinorida
      - Suborder Adeleorina

- Suborder Eimeriorina
- Order Neogregarinorida
- Subclass Coccidiasina
- Order Agamococcidiorida
- Order Eucoccidiorida
- Order Ixorheorida
- Order Protococcidiorida
- Class Perkinsasida
- Order Perkinsorida
- Family Perkinsidae

The name Protospiromonadida has been proposed for the common ancestor of the Gregarinomorpha and Coccidiomorpha.

phyla

Animal phyla

	Protostome	Bilateria
	Deuterostome	
	Basal/disputed	
	Others (Radiata or Parazoa)	

Phylum	Meaning	Common name	Distinguishing characteristic	Species described
Acanthocephala	Thorny headed worms	Thorny-headed worms	Reversible spiny proboscis that bears many rows of hooked spines	approx. 1,100
Acoelomorpha	Without gut	Acoels	No mouth or alimentary canal (alimentary canal = digestive tract in digestive system)	approx. 350
Annelida	Little ring	Annelids	Multiple circular segment	17,000+ extant
Arthropoda	Jointed foot	Arthropods	Segmented bodies and jointed limbs, with Chitinexoskeleton	1,134,000+
Brachiopoda	Arm foot	Lamp shells	Lophophore and pedicle	300-500 extant
Bryozoa	Moss animals	Moss animals, sea mats	Lophophore, no pedicle, ciliated tentacles, anus outside ring of cilia	5,000 extant

Phylum	Meaning	Common name	Distinguishing characteristic	Species described
Chaetognatha	Longhair jaw	Arrow worms	Chitinous spines either side of head, fins	approx. 100 extant
Chordata	With a cord	Chordates	Hollow dorsal nerve cord, notochord, pharyngeal slits, endostyle, post-anal tail	approx. 100,000+
Cnidaria	Stinging nettle	Anemones / Jellyfish	Nematocysts (stinging cells)	approx. 11,000
Ctenophora	Comb bearer	Comb jellies	Eight "comb rows" of fused cilia	approx. 100 extant
Cycliophora	Wheel carrying	Symbion	Circular mouth surrounded by small cilia, sac-like bodies	3+
Echinodermata	Spiny skin	Echinoderms	Fivefold radial symmetry in living forms, mesodermal calcified spines	approx. 7,000 extant; approx. 13,000 extinct
Entoprocta	Inside anus	Goblet worm	Anus inside ring of cilia	approx. 150
Gastrotricha	Hair stomach	Hairybacks	Two terminal adhesive tubes	approx. 690
Gnathostomulida	Jaw orifice	Jaw worms		approx. 100
Hemichordata	Half cord	Acorn worms, pterobranchs	Stomochord in collar, pharyngeal slits	approx. 100 extant
Kinorhyncha	Motion snout	Mud dragons	Eleven segments, each with a dorsal plate	approx. 150
Loricifera	Corset bearer	Brush heads	Umbrella-like scales at each end	approx. 122
Micrognathozoa	Tiny jaw animals	—	Accordion-like extensible thorax	1
Mollusca	Soft	Mollusks / molluscs	Muscular foot and mantle round shell	112,000
Nematoda	Thread like	Round worms	Round cross section, keratin cuticle	25,000–1,000,000
Nematomorpha	Thread form	Horsehair worms		approx. 320
Nemertea	A sea nymph	Ribbon worms		approx. 1,200
Onychophora	Claw bearer	Velvet worms	Legs tipped by chitinous claws	approx. 200 extant
Orthonectida	Straight swim		Single layer of ciliated cells surrounding a mass of sex cells	approx. 20
Phoronida	Zeus's mistress	Horseshoe worms	U-shaped gut	11
Placozoa	Plate animals		Differentiated top and bottom surfaces, two ciliated cell layers, amoeboid fiber cells in between	1
Platyhelminthes	Flat worm	Flatworms		approx. 25,000
Porifera*	Pore bearer	Sponges	Perforated interior wall	5,000+ extant
Priapulida	Little Priapus	Penis worms		approx. 16
Rhombozoa	Lozenge animal	—	Single anteroposterior axial cell surrounded by ciliated cells	75
Rotifera	Wheel bearer	Rotifers	Anterior crown of cilia	approx. 2,000
Sipuncula	Small tube	Peanut worms	Mouth surrounded by invertible tentacles	144–320
Tardigrada	Slow step	Water bears	Four segmented body and head	1,000+
Xenacoelomorpha	Strange flatworm	—	Ciliated deuterostome	2
Total: 35				**2,000,000+**

Land Plant Phyla (divisions)

The ten Divisions into which the living embryophytes (land plants) are often placed are shown in the table below. To these may be added two algal Divisions, Chlorophyta and Charophyta, which are included with land plants in the clade Viridiplantae (see also current definitions of Plantae). The definition and classification of plants at this level varies from source to source and has changed progressively in recent years. Thus some sources place horsetails in division Arthrophyta and ferns in division Pteridophyta, while others place them both in Pteridophyta, as shown below. The division Pinophyta may be used for all gymnosperms (i.e. including cycads, ginkgos and gnetophytes), or for conifers alone as below.

Since the first publication of the APG system in 1998, which proposed a classification of angiosperms up to the level of orders, many sources have preferred to treat ranks higher than orders as informal clades. Where formal ranks have been provided, the traditional divisions listed below have been reduced to a very much lower level, e.g. subclasses.

Division	Meaning	Common name	Distinguishing characteristics
Anthocerotophyta	*Anthoceros*-like plants	hornworts	horn-shaped sporophytes, no vascular system
Bryophyta	*Bryum*-like plants, moss plants	mosses	persistent unbranched sporophytes, no vascular system
Marchantiophyta, Hepatophyta	*Marchantia*-like plants liver plants	liverworts	ephemeral unbranched sporophytes, no vascular system
Lycopodiophyta, Lycophyta	*Lycopodium*-like plants "wolf" plants	clubmosses & spikemosses	microphyll leaves, vascular system
Pteridophyta	*Pteris*-like plants, fern plants	ferns & horsetails	prothallus gametophytes, vascular system
Pinophyta, Coniferophyta	*Pinus*-like plants cone-bearing plants	conifers	cones containing seeds and wood composed of tracheids
Cycadophyta	*Cycas*-like plants, palm-like plants	cycads	seeds, crown of compound leaves
Ginkgophyta	*Ginkgo*-like plants	ginkgo, Maidenhair tree	seeds not protected by fruit (single living species)
Gnetophyta	*Gnetum*-like plants	gnetophytes	seeds and woody vascular system with vessels
Magnoliophyta	*Magnolia*-like plants	flowering plants, angiosperms	flowers and fruit, vascular system with vessels
Total: 10			

Fungal Divisions

- Chytridiomycota
- Blastocladiomycota
- Zygomycota

- Glomeromycota
- Ascomycota
- Basidiomycota
- Microsporidia
- Neocallimastigomycota

Protista Phyla (Divisions)

Group Description	Phylum	Meaning	Common name	Distinguishing characteristics	Example
Heterotrophs (no locomotor apparatus)	Rhizopoda	root-foot	Amoeba	Amoeboids have the ability to change their shape.	Amoeba
	Actinopoda	ray-foot	-------	long, thin axopodia	Radiolarians
	Foraminifera	hole bearers	Forams	Complex shells with one or more chambers	Forams
Photosynthetic protists	Dinoflagellata	whirling scourge	Dinoflagellates	Unicellular, have two dissimilar flagella	Red tides
	Euglenophyta	Good-eyed plant	Euglenids	Have a pellicle, which gives shape to the cell.	Euglena
	Chrysophyta	golden plant	golden algae		Diatoma
	Rhodophyta	rose plant	red algae	Cells do not have flagella or centrioles; use phycobiliproteins which gives red tint	Coralline Algae
	Phaeophyta	gray plant	brown algae	chloroplasts surrounded by four membranes - form differentiated tissues	Kelp
Heterotrophs (flagella)	Sarcomastigophora				Trypanosoma cruzi
	Ciliophora				Paramecium
Non-motile spore-formers	Apicomplexa				Plasmodium
Heterotrophs (restricted mobility)	Oomycota				Water Molds
	Acrasiomycota				Dictyostelium
	Myxomycota				Fuligo
Total: 14					

Bacterial Phyla/Divisions

Currently there are 29 phyla accepted by List of Prokaryotic names with Standing in Nomenclature (LPSN)

- Acidobacteria, phenotipically diverse and mostly uncultured
- Actinobacteria, High-G+C Gram positive species
- Aquificae, only 14 thermophilic genera, deep branching
- Bacteroidetes
- Caldiserica, formerly candidate division OP5, *Caldisericum exile* is the sole

representative

- Chlamydiae, only 6 genera
- Chlorobi, only 7 genera, green sulphur bacteria
- Chloroflexi, green non-sulphur bacteria
- Chrysiogenetes, only 3 genera (*Chrysiogenes arsenatis*, *Desulfurispira natronophila*, *Desulfurispirillum alkaliphilum*)
- Cyanobacteria, also known as the blue-green algae
- Deferribacteres
- Deinococcus-Thermus, *Deinococcus radiodurans* and *Thermus aquaticus* are "commonly known" species of this phyla
- Dictyoglomi
- Elusimicrobia, formerly candidate division Thermite Group 1
- Fibrobacteres
- Firmicutes, Low-G+C Gram positive species, such as the spore-formers Bacilli (aerobic) and Clostridia (anaerobic)
- Fusobacteria
- Gemmatimonadetes
- Lentisphaerae, formerly clade VadinBE97
- Nitrospira
- Planctomycetes
- Proteobacteria, the most known phyla, containing species such as *Escherichia coli* or *Pseudomonas aeruginosa*
- Spirochaetes, species include *Borrelia burgdorferi*, which causes Lyme disease
- Synergistetes
- Tenericutes, alternatively class Mollicutes in phylum Firmicutes (notable genus: *Mycoplasma*)
- Thermodesulfobacteria
- Thermomicrobia
- Thermotogae, deep branching
- Verrucomicrobia

Archaeal Phyla/Division/Kingdoms

- Crenarchaeota, Second most common archaeal phylum
- Euryarchaeota, most common archaeal phylum
- Korarchaeota
- Nanoarchaeota, ultra-small symbiotes, single known species
- Thaumarchaeota

TRICHOMONAS VAGINALIS

Trichomonas vaginalis is an anaerobic, flagellated protozoan parasite and the causative agent of trichomoniasis. It is the most common pathogenic protozoan infection of humans in industrialized countries. Infection rates between men and women are similar with women being symptomatic, while infections in men are usually asymptomatic. Transmission usually occurs via direct, skin-to-skin contact with an infected individual, most often through vaginal intercourse. The WHO has estimated that 160 million cases of infection are acquired annually worldwide. The estimates for North America alone are between 5 and 8 million new infections each year, with an estimated rate of asymptomatic cases as high as 50%. Usually treatment consists of metronidazole and tinidazole.

Clinical

Alfred Francois Donné (1801-1878) was the first to describe a procedure to diagnose trichomoniasis through "the microscopic observation of motile protozoa in vaginal or cervical secretions" in 1836. He published this in the article entitled, "Animalcules observés dans les matières purulentes et le produit des sécrétions des organes génitaux de l'homme et de la femme" in the journal, *Comptes rendus de l'Académie des sciences*. As a result, parasitologists often call the parasite, Tricomoniasis vaginalis Donné, in his name.

Mechanism of Infection

Trichomonas vaginalis, a parasitic protozoan, is the etiologic agent of trichomoniasis, and is a sexually transmitted infection. More than 160 million people worldwide are annually infected by this protozoan.

Symptoms

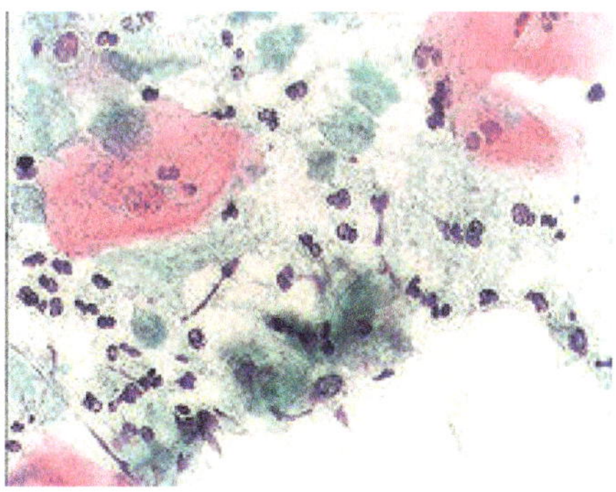

Pap smear, showing infestation by *Trichomonas vaginalis*. Papanicolaou stain, 400x

Trichomoniasis, a sexually transmitted infection of the urogenital tract, is a common cause of vaginitis in women, while men with this infection can display symptoms of urethritis. 'Frothy', greenish vaginal discharge with a 'musty' malodorous smell is characteristic.

Signs

Only 2% of women with the infection will have a "strawberry" cervix (*colpitis macularis*, an erythematous cervix with pinpoint areas of exudation) or vagina on examination. This is due to capillary dilation as a result of the inflammatory response.

Complications

Some of the complications of *T. vaginalis* in women include: preterm delivery, low birth weight, and increased mortality as well as predisposing to HIV infection, AIDS, and cervical cancer. *T. vaginalis* has also been reported in the urinary tract, fallopian tubes, and pelvis and can cause pneumonia, bronchitis, and oral lesions. Condoms are effective at reducing, but not wholly preventing, transmission.

Trichomonas vaginalis infection in males has been found to cause asymptomatic urethritis and prostatitis. It has been proposed that it may increase the risk of prostate cancer; however, evidence is insufficient to support this association as of 2014.

Diagnosis

Classically, with a cervical smear, infected women have a transparent "halo" around their superficial cell nucleus. It is unreliably detected by studying a genital discharge or with a cervical smear because of their low sensitivity. *T. vaginalis* was traditionally diagnosed via a wet mount, in which "corkscrew" motility was observed. Currently, the most common method of diagnosis is via overnight culture, with a sensitivity range of 75–95%. Newer methods, such as rapid antigen testing and transcription-mediated amplification, have even greater sensitivity, but are not in widespread use. The presence of *T. vaginalis* can also be diagnosed by PCR, using primers specific for GENBANK/L23861.

Treatment

Infection is treated and cured with metronidazole or tinidazole. The CDC recommends a one time dose of 2 grams of either metronidazole or tinidazole as the first-line treatment; the alternate treatment recommended is 500 milligrams of metronidazole, twice daily, for seven days if there is failure of the single-dose regimen. Medication should be prescribed to any sexual partner(s) as well because they may be asymptomatic carriers.

REFERENCES

1. Singleton, Paul (2006). Dictionary of Microbiology and Molecular Biology, 3rd Edition, revised. Chichester, UK: John Wiley & Sons. p. 32. ISBN 978-0-470-03545-0.
2. David J. Patterson. "Amoebae: Protists Which Move and Feed Using Pseudopodia". Tree of Life web project.
3. Flor-Parra, Ignacio; Bernal, Manuel; Zhurinsky, Jacob; Daga, Rafael R. (2013-12-17). "Cell migration and division in amoeboid-like fission yeast". Biology Open. 3 (1): 108–115. doi:10.1242/bio.20136783. ISSN 2046-6390. PMC 3892166Freely

accessible. PMID 24357230.

4. Friedl, P.; Borgmann, S.; Bröcker, E. B. (2001-10-01). "Amoeboid leukocyte crawling through extracellular matrix: lessons from the Dictyostelium paradigm of cell movement". Journal of Leukocyte Biology. 70 (4): 491–509. ISSN 0741-5400. PMID 11590185.
5. Marée, Athanasius FM, and Paulien Hogeweg. "How amoeboids self-organize into a fruiting body: multicellular coordination in Dictyostelium discoideum." Proceedings of the National Academy of Sciences 98.7 (2001): 3879–3883.
6. Mackerras, M. J., and Q. N. Ercole. "Observations on the action of paludrine on malarial parasites." Transactions of the Royal Society of Tropical Medicine and Hygiene 41.3 (1947): 365–376.
7. Jan Pawlowski: The twilight of Sarcodina: a molecular perspective on the polyphyletic origin of amoeboid protists. Protistology, Band 5, 2008, S. 281–302. (pdf, 570 kB)
8. Alberts Eds.; et al. (2007). Molecular Biology of the Cell 5th Edition. New York: Garland Science. p. 1037. ISBN 9780815341055.
9. Margulis, Lynn (2009). Kingdoms and Domains. Academic Press. pp. 206–7. ISBN 978-0-12-373621-5.
10. Ogden, C. G. (1980). An Atlas of Freshwater Testate Amoeba. Oxford, London, Glasgow: Oxford University Press, for British Museum (Natural History). pp. 1–5. ISBN 0198585020.
11. Alberts Eds.; et al. (2007). Molecular Biology of the Cell 5th Edition. New York: Garland Science. p. 663. ISBN 9780815341055.
12. Kudo, Richard Roksabro. "Protozoology." Protozoology 4th Edit (1954). p. 83
13. Thorp, James H. (2001). Ecology and Classification of North American Freshwater invertebrates. San Diego: Academic. p. 71. ISBN 0-12-690647-5.
14. Jeon, Kwang W. (1973). Biology of Amoeba. New York: Academic Press. p. 100.
15. Mylnikov, Alexander P.; Weber, Felix; Jürgens, Klaus; Wylezich, Claudia (2015-08-01). "Massisteria marina has a sister: Massisteria voersi sp. nov., a rare species isolated from coastal waters of the Baltic Sea". European Journal of Protistology. 51 (4): 299–310. doi:10.1016/j.ejop.2015.05.002. ISSN 1618-0429. PMID 26163290.
16. Gooday, A. J.; Aranda da Silva, A.; Pawlowski, J. (2011-12-01). "Xenophyophores (Rhizaria, Foraminifera) from the Nazaré Canyon (Portuguese margin, NE Atlantic)". Deep-Sea Research Part II: Topical Studies in Oceanography. The Geology, Geochemistry, and Biology of Submarine Canyons West of Portugal. 58 (23–24): 2401–2419. doi:10.1016/j.dsr2.2011.04.005.
17. Gooday, A. J.; Aranda da Silva, A.; Pawlowski, J. (2011-12-01). "Xenophyophores (Rhizaria, Foraminifera) from the Nazaré Canyon (Portuguese margin, NE Atlantic)". Deep-Sea Research Part II: Topical Studies in Oceanography. The Geology, Geochemistry, and Biology of Submarine Canyons West of Portugal. 58 (23–24): 2401–2419. doi:10.1016/j.dsr2.2011.04.005.

18. Friedl, Peter, Stefan Borgmann, and Eva-B. Bröcker. "Amoeboid leukocyte crawling through extracellular matrix: lessons from the Dictyostelium paradigm of cell movement." Journal of leukocyte biology 70.4 (2001): 491–509.
19. Nakagaki; et al. (2000). "Intelligence: Maze-solving by an amoeboid organism". Nature. 407 (6803): 470. doi:10.1038/35035159. PMID 11028990. Retrieved Sep 14, 2014.
20. Wehr, John D. (2003). Freshwater Algae of North America. San Diego and London: Academic Press. p. 353. ISBN 978-0-12-741550-5.
21. "Algae World: diatom sex and life cycles". Algae World. Royal Botanic Garden Edinburgh. Retrieved March 1, 2015.
22. Valle, L.G. (2014). "New species of Paramoebidium (trichomycetes, Mesomycetozoea) from the Mediterranean, with comments about the amoeboid cells in Amoebidiales". Mycologia. 106: 481–90. doi:10.3852/13-153. PMID 24895422.
23. Taylor, J. W. & Berbee, M. L. (2014). Fungi from PCR to Genomics: The Spreading Revolution in Evolutionary Biology. In: Systematics and Evolution. Springer Berlin Heidelberg. p. 52,
24. Corliss, J. O. (1987). Protistan phylogeny and eukaryogenesis. International Review of Cytology 100: 319–370, .
25. McAlpine, Daniel (1881). Biological atlas: a guide to the practical study of plants and animals. Edinburgh and London: W. & A. K. Johnston. p. 17.
26. Bory de Saint-Vincent, J. B. G. M. "Essai d'une classification des animaux microscopiques." Agasse, Paris (1826).p. 28
27. McGrath, Kimberley; Blachford, Stacey, eds. (2001). Gale Encyclopedia of Science Vol. 1: Aardvark-Catalyst (2nd ed.). Gale Group. ISBN 0-7876-4370-X. OCLC 46337140.
28. Ehrenberg, Christian Gottfried. Organisation, systematik und geographisches verhältniss der infusionsthierchen: Zwei vorträge, in der Akademie der wissenschaften zu Berlin gehalten in den jahren 1828 und 1830. Druckerei der Königlichen akademie der wissenschaften, 1832. p. 59
29. Dujardin, Felix (1841). Histoire Naturelle des Zoophytes Infusoires. Paris: Librarie Encyclopedique de Roret. p. 26.
30. Bütschli, Otto (1882). Klassen und Ordnungen des Thier-Reichs I. Abteilung: Sarkodina und Sporozoa. Paleontologische Entwicklung der Rhisopoda von C. Scwager. p. 1.
31. Adl, Sina M.; et al. (2012). "The Revised Classification of Eukaryotes". Journal of Eukaryotic Microbiology. 59: 429–93. doi:10.1111/j.1550-7408.2012.00644.x. PMC 3483872Freely accessible. PMID 23020233.
32. Park, J. S.; Simpson, A. G. B.; Brown, S.; Cho, B. C. (2009). "Ultrastructure and Molecular Phylogeny of two Heterolobosean Amoebae, Euplaesiobystra hypersalinica gen. Et sp. Nov. And Tulamoeba peronaphora gen. Et sp. Nov., Isolated from an Extremely Hypersaline Habitat". Protist. 160 (2): 265–283. doi:10.1016/j.protis.2008.10.002. PMID 19121603.
33. Ott, Donald W., Carla K. Oldham-Ott, Nataliya Rybalka, and Thomas Friedl. 2015. Xanthophyte, Eustigmatophyte, and Raphidophyte Algae. In: Wehr, J.D., Sheath, R.G., Kociolek, J.P. (Eds.) Freshwater Algae of North America: Ecology and Classification, 2nd edition. Academic Press, Amsterdam, pp. 483–534, .

34. Patterson, D.J., Simpson, A.G.B. & Rogerson, A., 2000. Amoebae of uncertain affinities. In: Lee, J.J., Leedale, G.F. & Bradbury, P. An Illustrated Guide to the Protozoa. Society of Protozoologists/Allen Press: Lawrence, Kansas, U.S.A, 2nd ed., vol. 2, p. 804-827, .

35. Khan NA, Siddiqui R (2015). "Is there evidence of sexual reproduction (meiosis) in Acanthamoeba?". Pathog Glob Health. 109 (4): 193–5. doi:10.1179/2047773215Y.0000000009. PMID 25800982.

36. Kelso AA, Say AF, Sharma D, Ledford LL, Turchick A, Saski CA, King AV, Attaway CC, Temesvari LA, Sehorn MG (2015). "Entamoeba histolytica Dmc1 Catalyzes Homologous DNA Pairing and Strand Exchange That Is Stimulated by Calcium and Hop2-Mnd1". PLoS ONE. 10 (9): e0139399. doi:10.1371/journal.pone.0139399. PMC 4589404Freely accessible. PMID 26422142.

37. Singh N, Bhattacharya A, Bhattacharya S (2013). "Homologous recombination occurs in Entamoeba and is enhanced during growth stress and stage conversion". PLoS ONE. 8 (9): e74465. doi:10.1371/journal.pone.0074465. PMC 3787063Freely accessible. PMID 24098652.

38. Flowers JM, Li SI, Stathos A, Saxer G, Ostrowski EA, Queller DC, Strassmann JE, Purugganan MD (2010). "Variation, sex, and social cooperation: molecular population genetics of the social amoeba Dictyostelium discoideum". PLoS Genet. 6 (7): e1001013. doi:10.1371/journal.pgen.1001013. PMC 2895654Freely accessible. PMID 20617172.

39. O'Day DH, Keszei A (2012). "Signalling and sex in the social amoebozoans". Biol Rev Camb Philos Soc. 87 (2): 313–29. doi:10.1111/j.1469-185X.2011.00200.x. PMID 21929567.

40. Lahr DJ, Parfrey LW, Mitchell EA, Katz LA, Lara E (2011). "The chastity of amoebae: re-evaluating evidence for sex in amoeboid organisms". Proc. Biol. Sci. 278 (1715): 2081–90. doi:10.1098/rspb.2011.0289. PMC 3107637Freely accessible. PMID 21429931.

CHAPTER 4

Helminths

Chapter Contents

- **Introduction**
- **Taxonomy**
- **Common Characteristics**
- **Detection in Medicine**

Helminth is a general term meaning worm. The helminths are invertebrates characterized by elongated, flat or round bodies. In medically oriented schemes the flatworms or platyhelminths (platy from the Greek root meaning "flat") include flukes and tapeworms. Roundworms are nematodes (nemato from the Greek root meaning "thread"). These groups are subdivided for convenience according to the host organ in which they reside, e.g., lung flukes, extraintestinal tapeworms, and intestinal roundworms. This chapter deals with the structure and development of the three major groups of helminths.

INTRODUCTION

Helminths , also commonly known as parasitic worms, are large multicellular organisms, which when mature can generally be seen with the naked eye. They are often referred to as intestinal worms even though not all helminths reside in the intestines; for example schistosomes are not intestinal worms, but rather reside in blood vessels.

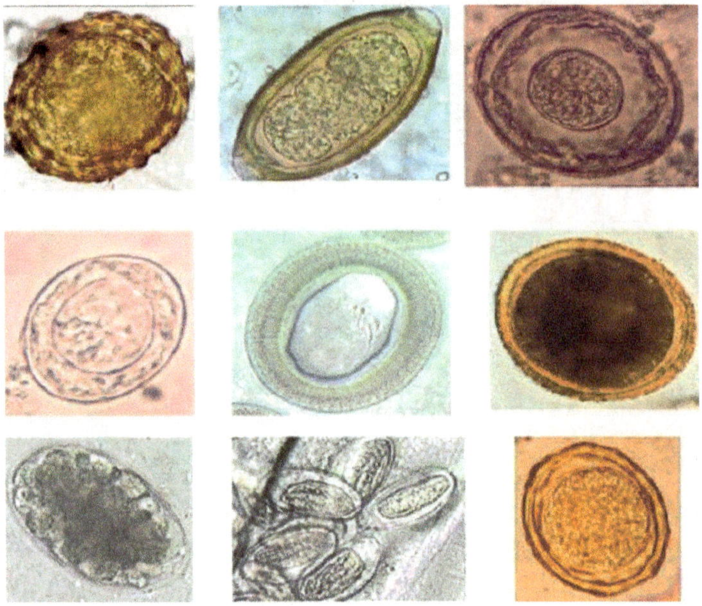

Helminth eggs of different helminth species, which are produced for reproduction of the worms.

There is no clear consensus on the taxonomy of helminths; it is more of a commonly used term to describe certain worms with superficial similarities. These are flatworms (platyhelminthes), namely cestodes (tapeworms) and trematodes (flukes), and roundworms or nemathelminths (nematodes) – both of these are parasitic worm types – and the annelida, which are not parasitic or at the most ectoparasites like the leeches.

Many, but not all, of the worms referred to as helminths belong to the group of intestinal parasites. An infection by a helminth is known as helminthiasis, soil-transmitted helminthiasis, helminth infection or intestinal worm infection. The same naming convention applies to all helminths whereby the ending "-asis" (or in veterinary science the ending "-osis") at the end of the name of the worm is added to signify the infection with that particular worm, for example *Ascaris* is the name of a particular helminth, and ascariasis is the name of the infectious disease caused by this helminth.

Helminths are worm-like organisms living in and feeding on living hosts, receiving nourishment and protection while disrupting their hosts' nutrient absorption, causing weakness and disease. Those that live inside the digestive tract are called intestinal parasites. They can live inside humans and other animals. In their adult form, helminths cannot multiply in humans. Helminths are able to survive in their mammalian hosts for many years due to their ability to manipulate the immune response by secreting immunomodulatory products. Helminth ova (or eggs) have a strong shell that protects the eggs against a range of environmental conditions.

Helminthology is the study of parasitic worms and their effects on their hosts. The word helminth comes from Greek *hélmins*, a kind of worm.

TAXONOMY

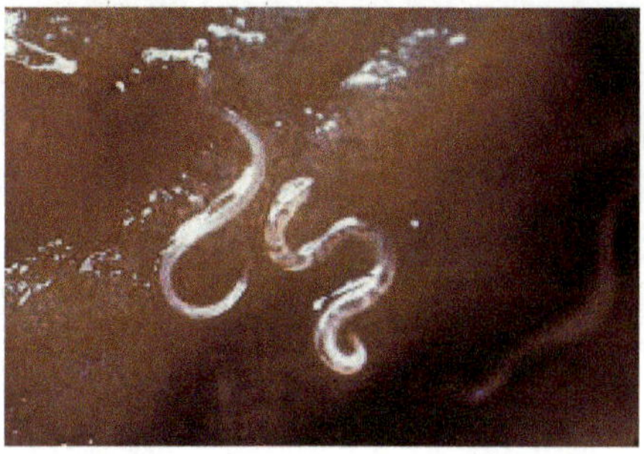

Hookworms attached to the intestinal mucosa

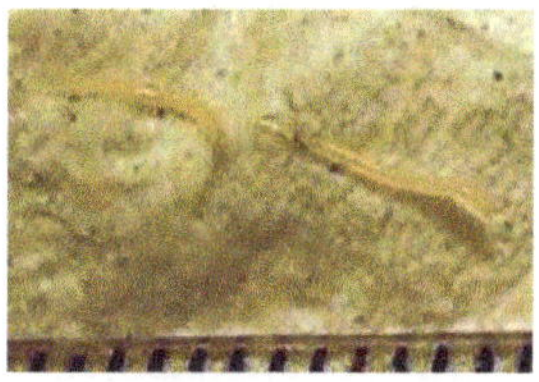

Two pinworms

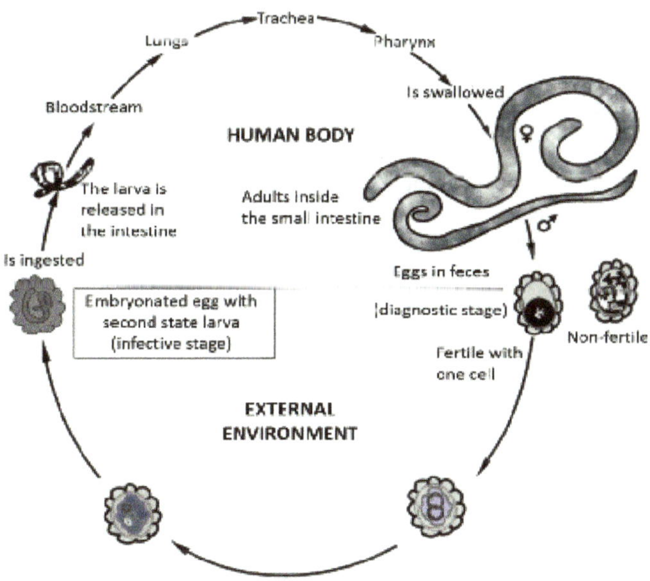

Ascaris lumbricoides **Life Cycle**, Nematode (Roundworm)

b

Image showing life cycle inside and outside of the human body of one fairly typical and well described helminth: Ascaris lumbricoides

There is no real consensus on the taxonomy (or groupings) of the helminths, particularly with the nematodes. The term "helminth" contains a number of phyla, many of which are completely unrelated. However, for practical considerations the term is still used nowadays to describe four groups with superficial similarities, the phyla Annelida, Platyhelminths, Nematoda and Acanthocephala.

There is in fact no helminth classification; it is an "artificial" term.

The most important helminths in the sanitation field are the human parasites, which is why most people relate the term helminth to them, where they are classified as nemathelminthes (nematodes) and platyhelminthes, depending on whether they possess a round or flat-shaped body respectively. The latter are further divided into cestodes and trematodes depending on whether or not they have a segmented body.

Ringworm (dermatophytosis) is actually caused by various fungi and not by a parasitic worm.

COMMON CHARACTERISTICS

Helminths are a group of evolutionary unrelated organisms which share a similar form. Helminths include members of the following taxa: monogeneans, cestodes (tapeworms), nematodes (roundworms), and trematodes (flukes). The number of different helminth species is vast: it is estimated to be around one million species. The nematodes are the most diverse of all the helminths with the highest number of species.

Characteristics that are common for all helminths include:

Life time:

- The life time of adult worms varies tremendously from one species to another but is generally in the range of 1 to 8 years (see following table). This life time of several years is a result of their ability to manipulate the immune response of their hosts by secreting immunomodulatory products.
- Helminths can be either hermaphrodites (i.e. can have both sexes), like tapeworms and the flukes (except the blood fluke which is not a hermaphrodite), or have their sexes differentiated, like the roundworms.

Eggs:

- All helminths produce eggs (also called ova) for reproduction.
- Helminth eggs have a strong shell that protects them against a range of environmental conditions. This shell consists of three layers: a lipoidal inner layer, a chitinous middle layer and outer proteinic layer.
- Generally thousands or even hundreds of thousands of eggs are produced each time the female worm deposits its eggs - a process called ovoposition. The following table shows a large variation in the amount of eggs produced by the different worms in one event; it varies in the range of 3,000 to 700,000.
- The frequency of egg deposition from an adult helminth is generally daily, or up to six times per day for some *Taenia* species.
- Adult trematodes lay smaller numbers of eggs compared to cestodes or nematodes. However, the egg develops into a miracidia from which thousands of *cercariae*, swimming larvae, develop. This means that one egg may produce thousands of adult worms.

- Helminth eggs remain viable for 1–2 months in crops and for many months in soil, fresh water and sewage, or even for several years in feces, fecal sludge (historically called night soil) and sewage sludge; a period that is much longer compared to other kind of microorganisms.

Larvae:

- Larvae hatch from these eggs (if the eggs are viable), inside or outside the host, depending on the type of helminth. Life cycles of the helminths differ in this and other specific aspects. Eggs that are no longer viable do not produce any larvae.
- The larvae maturing in the host take from about two weeks up to four months depending on the helminth species.

The following table shows the principal morphological and reproductive distinctions for three helminth groups:

Parasitic worms have been used as a medical treatment for various diseases, particularly those involving an overactive immune response. As humans have evolved with parasitic worms, proponents argue they are needed for a healthy immune system. Scientists are looking for a connection between the prevention and control of parasitic worms and the increase in allergies such as hay-fever in developed countries. Parasitic worms may be able to damp down the immune system of their host, making it easier for them to live in the intestine without coming under attack. This may be one mechanism for their proposed medicinal effect.

One study suggests a link between the rising rates of metabolic syndrome in the developed worlds and the largely successful efforts of Westerners to eliminate intestinal parasites. The work suggests eosinophils (a type of white blood cell) in fat tissue play an important role in preventing insulin resistance by secreting interleukin 4, which in turn switches macrophages into "alternative activation". Alternatively-activated macrophages are important to maintaining glucose homeostasis (i.e., blood sugar regulation). Helminth infection causes an increase in eosinophils. In the study, the authors fed rodents a high-fat diet to induce metabolic syndrome, and then injected them with helminths. Helminth infestation improved the rodents' metabolism.The authors concluded:

Although sparse in blood of persons in developed countries, eosinophils are often elevated in individuals in rural developing countries where intestinal parasitism is prevalent and metabolic syndrome rare. We speculate that eosinophils may have evolved to optimize metabolic homeostasis during chronic infections by ubiquitous intestinal parasites....

	Tapeworms (Cestodes)		Flukes (Trematodes)	Roundworms (Nematodes)			
Species (examples)	*Taenia solium*, *Taenia saginata*, *Hymenolepis* spp., *Echinoccocus granulosus*, *Multiceps multiceps*		*Schistosoma mansoni*, *Schistosoma japonicum*, *Fasciola hepatica*	*Ascaris*, *Onchocerca*, *Rhabditis*, *Trichuris*, *Necator americanus*, *Anchylostoma duodenale*			
Example diseases in humans	Tapeworm infection		Schistosomiasis, swimmer's itch	Ascariasis, dracunculiasis (guinea worm), elephantiasis, enterobiasis (pinworm), filariasis, hookworm infection (includes Necatoriasis and *Ancylostoma duodenale* infection), onchocerciasis, trichinosis, trichuriasis (whipworm)			
Shape	Segmented plane		Unsegmented plane	Cylindrical			
Body cavity	No		no	Present			
Body covering	Tegument		Tegument	Cuticle			
Digestive tube	No		Ends in cecum	Ends in anus			
Sex	Hermaphroditic		Hermaphroditic, except schistosomes which are dioecious	Dioecious			
Attachment organs	Sucker or bothridia, and rostellum with hooks		Oral sucker and ventral sucker or acetabulum	Lips, teeth, filariform extremities, and dentary plates			
Number of species	6000		Estimated > 15,000 and 9,000registered	800,000 to 1,000,000 estimated 25,000 registered			
Number of species known to infect humans	40		16	> 12,000			
Species	*Hymenolepis nana*	*Taenia solium* /*Taenia saginata*	*Fasciola hepatica*	*Ascaris lumbricoides*	Hookworm	*Trichuris trichiura*	*Toxocara*

Lifetime	Larvae formation		some days (eggs can survive for months)	9–15 days	18 days to several weeks	1–2 days	15–30 days	
	Larvae growth		After hatching the larvae move to develop into cysticercoid, which can survive for years in an animal	5–7 weeks as *cercariae* in snails and longer periods in wet environments as encysted *metacercariae*	10–14 days	5–10 days (after maturing can survive for weeks outside the host)	60–70 days (from hatching to mature state)	5–6 days
	Larvae maturing (in host)		2 months (form cysticercoid to adult)	3–4 months	2–3 months	2–8 weeks(can become dormant for months)		
	Adult worm	4–6 weeks	Several years	8–10 years	1–2 years	Several years	1 year	
Eggs laid per day		250,000 to 700,000		3,000 to 25,000	3,000 to 250,000			
Egg deposition	Frequency		up to 6 times a day		daily	daily	daily	
	Number of eggs per event		50,000-100,000		200,000to 250,000 or more	5,000-10,000	3,000-20,000	
Larvae per egg		1	1	300 *cercariae* (*Schistosoma*), 250,000 *metacercariae* (*Fasciola*)	1	1	1	1

Draft genomes for all categories of helminth have been sequenced in recent years and are available through the ParaSite sub-portal of WormBase.

DETECTION IN MEDICINE

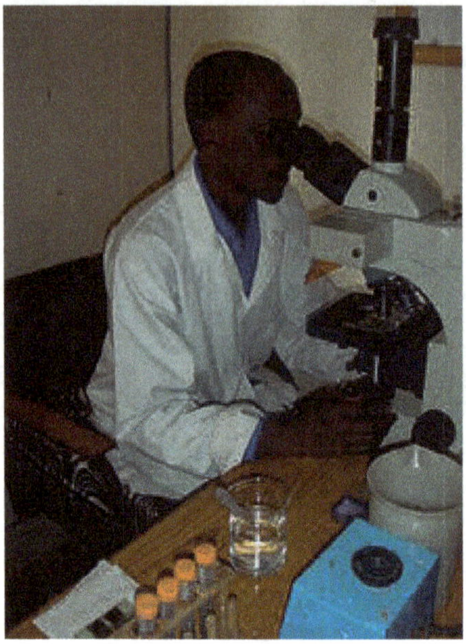

Analysing for helminth eggs in samples of feces from a dry toilet in Kenya

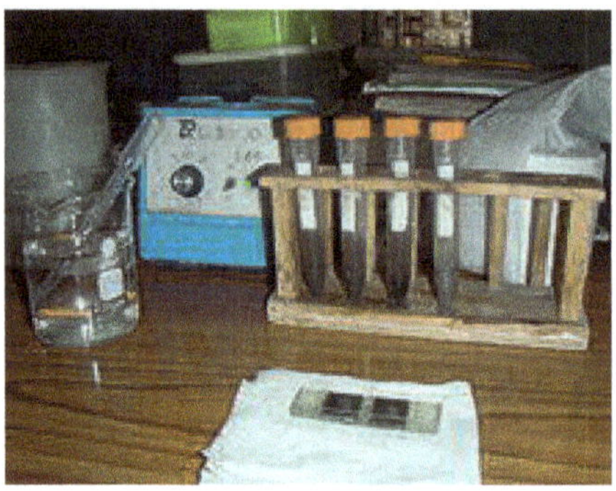

Processed helminth eggs samples from a dry toilet in Kenya

Eggs in the Environment

Eggs can reach the soil when polluted wastewater, sewage sludge or human excreta are used as fertilizer. Such soil is often characterized by moist and warm conditions. Therefore, the risk of using contaminated wastewater and sludge in agricultural fields is a real problem, especially in poor countries, where this practice is prevalent.Helminth eggs are regarded as the main biological health risk when applying sewage sludge, fecal sludge or fecal matter on agricultural soils. The eggs are the infective stage of the helminths' life cycle for causing the disease helminthiasis.

Helminth eggs are resistant to various environmental conditions due to the composition of the egg shell. Each helminth egg species has 3 to 4 layers with different physical and chemical characteristics: a) the 1 to 2 outer layers are formed of mucopolysaccharides and proteins, b) the middle layers consist of chitinous material and serve to give structure and mechanical resistance to the eggs, and c) the inner layer is composed of lipids and proteins and is useful to protect eggs from desiccation, strong acid and bases, oxidants and reductive agents as well as detergent and proteolytic compounds.

Due to this strong shell, helminth eggs or ova remain viable in soil, fresh water and sewage for many months. In feces, fecal sludge and sewage sludge they can even remain viable for several years. Helminth eggs of concern in wastewater used for irrigation have a size between 20 and 90 μm and a relative density of 1.06–1.23.It is very difficult to inactivate helminth eggs, unless temperature is increased above 40 °C or moisture is reduced to less than 5%.

Levels of Infectiousness

Helminth eggs contained in wastewater, sewage sludge or human excreta are not always infectious, i.e. able to cause the disease helminthiasis. Fertilized eggs and unfertilized eggs can exist side by side. Unfertilized eggs are identifiable under the microscope by their elongated shape. No larvae can hatch from these kinds of eggs. Therefore, unfertilized eggs do not pose a danger to human health.

In the case of *Ascaris lumbricoides* (giant roundworm), which has been considered the most resistant and common helminth type, fertilized eggs deposited in soil are resistant to desiccation but are, at this stage of development, very sensitive to environmental temperatures: The reproduction of a fertilized egg within the eggshell develops at an environmental soil temperature about 25 °C which is lower than the body temperature of the host (i.e., 37 °C for humans).

However, development of the larvae in the egg stops at temperatures below 15.5 °C, and eggs cannot survive temperatures much above 38 °C. If the temperature is around 25 °C, the infectiousness occurs after nearly 10 days of incubation.Finally, after 2 to 4 weeks in moist soil at optimal temperature and oxygen levels, the embryo develops into an infective larva, named "second-stage larva". This larva has the ability to get out of the egg, hatch in the small intestine and migrate to different organs. These infective larvae (or "infective eggs") may remain viable in soil for two years or longer.

Removal *Versus* Inactivation in Wastewater and Sludge Treatment

In order to physically remove (but not inactivate) helminth eggs from wastewater, processes that remove particles, such as sedimentation, filtration or coagulation-flocculation are employed. Therefore, waste stabilization ponds (lagoons), storage bassins, constructed wetlands, rapid filtration or upflow anaerobic sludge blanket (UASB) reactors can be used. These conventional wastewater treatment processes do not inactivate the helminth ova but only removes them from the wastewater and moves them to the sewage sludge.

Helminth ova cannot be inactivated with chlorine, UV light or ozone (in the latter case at least not with economical doses because >36 mg/L ozone are needed with 1 hour contact time).

Inactivation of helminth ova can be achieved in sewage sludge treatment where the temperature is increased over 40 °C or moisture is reduced to less than 5%. Best results can be obtained when both of these conditions are combined for an extended period of time. Details about the contact time under these conditions and other related environmental factors are generally not well-defined for every type of helminth egg species. Helminth eggs are considered highly resistant biological structures.

Indicator Organism

Helminth eggs (or ova) are a good indicator organism to assess the safety of sanitation and reuse systems because they are the most environmentally resistant pathogens of all pathogens (viruses, bacteria, protozoa and helminths) and can in extreme cases survive for several years in soil. Therefore, the presence or absence of viable helminth eggs ("viable helminth egg" means that a larva would be able to hatch from the egg) in a sample of dried fecal matter, compost or fecal sludge is often used as an indicator to assess the efficiency of diverse wastewater and sludge treatment processes in terms of pathogen removal. In particular, the number of viable Ascaris eggs is often taken as an indicator organism for all helminth eggs in treatment processes as they are very common in many parts of the world and relatively easy to identify under the microscope. However, the exact inactivation characteristics may vary for different types of helminth eggs.

Measurement Techniques

Environmental Samples

For the purpose of setting treatment standards and reuse legislation, it is important to be able to determine the amount of helminth eggs in an environmental sample with some accuracy. The detection of viable helminth eggs in samples of wastewater, sludge or fresh feces (as a diagnostic tool for the infection helminthiasis) is not straight forward. In fact, many laboratories in developing countries lack the right equipment or skilled staff required to do so. An important step in the analytical methods is usually the concentration of the eggs in the sample, especially in the case of wastewater samples. A concentration step may not be required in samples of dried feces, e.g. samples collected from urine-diverting dry toilets.

Human Stool Samples

For medical purposes, the exact number of helminth eggs is less important and therefore most diagnoses are made simply by identifying the appearance of the worm or eggs in feces. Due to the large quantity of eggs laid, physicians can diagnose using only one or two fecal smears. The Kato technique (also called the Kato-Katz technique) is a laboratory method for preparing human stool samples prior to searching for parasite eggs. Eggs per gram is a laboratory test that determines the number of eggs per gram of feces in patients suspected of having a parasitological infection, such as schistosomiasis.

Helminthic therapy

From Wikipedia, the free encyclopedia

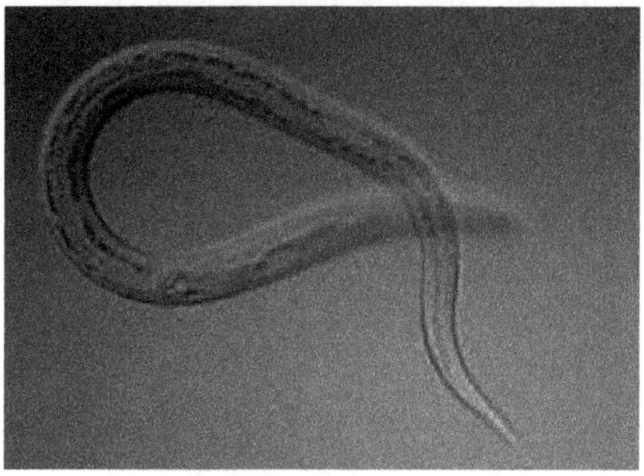

A *Necator americanus* larva. Invisible to the naked eye, 10 to 35 are applied to the skin in therapy, either in a single dose or in multiple smaller doses over the course of two or three months.

Helminthic therapy, an experimental type of immunotherapy, is the treatment of autoimmune diseases and immune disorders by means of deliberate infestation with a helminth or with the ova of a helminth. Helminths are parasitic worms such as hookworms, whipworms, and threadworms that have evolved to live within a host organism on which they rely for nutrients. These worms are members of two phyla; nematodes, which are primarily used in human helminthic therapy, and flat worms.

Helminthic therapy consists of the inoculation of the patient with specific parasitic intestinal nematodes (helminths). A number of such organisms are currently being investigated for their use as treatment including: *Trichuris suis* ova,commonly known as pig whipworm eggs; *Necator americanus*, commonly known as hookworms; *Trichuris trichiura* ova, commonly referred to as human whipworm eggs; *Hymenolepis diminuta*, commonly known as rat tapeworm, cysticerci, *Ascaris lumbricoides* commonly known as human giant roundworm; *Strongyloides stercoralis* commonly known as human roundworm; *Enterobius vermicularis* commonly known as threadworm or seatworm; and *Hymenolepis nana* also known as dwarf tapeworm.

Current research targets Crohn›s disease, ulcerative colitis, inflammatory bowel disease, multiple sclerosis, and asthma.

Helminthic infection has emerged as one possible explanation for the low incidence of autoimmune diseases and allergies in less developed countries, together with the significant and sustained increase in autoimmune diseases in industrialized countries.

Incidence of autoimmune diseases and parasitic infestation

While it is recognized that there is probably a genetic disposition in certain individuals for the development of autoimmune diseases, the rate of increase in incidence of autoimmune diseases is not a result of genetic changes in humans; the increased rate of autoimmune-related diseases in the industrialized world is occurring in too short a time to be explained in this way. There is evidence that one of the primary reasons for the increase in autoimmune diseases in industrialized nations is the significant change in environmental factors over the last century. Environmental factors include exposure to certain artificial chemicals from industrial processes, medicines, farming, and food preparation. It is posited that the absence of exposure to certain parasites, bacteria, and viruses is playing a significant role in the development of autoimmune diseases in the more sanitized and industrialized Western nations.

Lack of exposure to naturally occurring pathogens and parasites may result in an increased incidence of autoimmune diseases. Correlational data has shown the prevalence of helminthic infections to be greatest south of the equator where the rates of autoimmune diseases such as multiple sclerosis are low. This is consistent with the hygiene hypothesis which suggests that helminthic infections protect individuals from developing auto-immune diseases rather than being an agent responsible for inducing them. A complete explanation of how environmental factors play a role in autoimmune diseases has still not been proposed. Epidemiological studies such as the meta-analysis by Leonardi-Bee et al., however, have helped to establish the link between parasitic infestation and their protective role in autoimmune disease development.

Genetic research on the interleukin genes (IL genes) shows that helminths have been a major selective force on a subset of these human genes. In other words, helminths have shaped the evolution of at least parts of the human immune system, especially the genes responsible for Crohn›s disease, ulcerative colitis, and celiac disease; and provides further evidence that it is the absence of parasites, and in particular helminths, that has likely caused a substantial portion of the increase in incidence of diseases of immune dysregulation and inflammation in industrialized countries in the last century. A systematic approach was used to determine the relative pressure pathogens, such as helminths, viruses or bacteria exerted upon a selection of interleukin genes. Fumagalli et al. (2009) examined 52 globally dispersed human populations along with the diverse levels of pathogen richness, for >650,00 SNPs within 91 IL or IL receptor genes. Helminths were identified as a major selective pressure on a subset of IL genes. Through additional genome-wide association studies the subset of IL genes were associated with the human susceptibility to IBS and coeliac disease.

Hypotheses

Although the mechanism(s) of autoimmune disease development is not fully defined, there is broad agreement that the majority of autoimmune diseases are caused by inappropriate immunological responses to innocuous antigens, driven by a branch of the immune system known as the TH1 type immune response. Extra-cellular antigens primarily trigger the TH2 response, as observed with allergies, while intracellular antigens trigger a TH1 response. Th cells can be divided into subtypes based on the characteristic cytokines they secrete. Th2 immune responses result in the release of cytokines associated with inflammation reduction such as interleukin 4, interleukin 5 and interleukin 10. These cytokines are thought to improve the symptoms of many autoimmune disorders. Conversely, Th1 immune responses are characterized by the cytokines interferon gamma (IFNγ) and tumor necrosis factor alpha (TNFα), both of which are thought to increase inflammation and worsen the progression of autoimmune diseases and their symptoms. The relationship between these two types of immune response is a central theme of the biological basis of the hygiene hypothesis, which suggests that there is a regulatory action between the two types of response. However, the observation that allergies and autoimmune response are increasing at a similar rate in industrialized nations appears to undermine the hygiene hypothesis.

The hygiene hypothesis proposes that appropriate immune response is in part learned by exposure to microorganisms and parasites, and in part regulated by their presence. In industrialized nations, humans are exposed to somewhat lower levels of these organisms, potentially resulting in unbalanced immune systems. The development of vaccines, hygienic practices, and effective medical care have diminished or eliminated the prevalence and impact of many parasitic organisms, as well as bacterial and viral infections. This has been of obvious benefit with the effective eradication of many diseases that have plagued human beings. However, while many severe diseases have been eradicated, humans› exposure to benign and apparently beneficial parasites has also been reduced commensurately. The central thrust of the hypothesis is, therefore, that correct development of regulatory T cells in individuals may depend on exposure to organisms such as lactobacilli, various mycobacteria, and helminths. Lack of exposure to sufficient benign antigens, particularly during childhood, is sometimes suggested as a cause of the increase in autoimmune diseases and diseases for which chronic inflammation is a major component in the industrialized world. Two refinements to the hygiene hypothesis exist, the "old friends" hypothesis, and the "microbiome depletion theory".

The old friends hypothesis modifies the hygiene hypothesis by proposing that regulatory T cells can only become fully effective if they are stimulated by exposure to microorganisms and parasites that have low levels of pathogenicity and that have coexisted universally with human beings throughout our evolutionary history. This hypothesis has recently been given more credibility by a study demonstrating the impact of infectious organisms, and helminths in particular, upon genes responsible for the production of various cytokines, some involved in the regulation of inflammation, in particular those associated with the development of Crohn›s disease, ulcerative colitis, and celiac disease.

The microbiome depletion theory posits that the absence of an entire class of organisms from the human inner ecology is a profound evolutionary mismatch that destabilizes the immune system, resulting in disease. The microbiome is "depleted". The way to correct the dysregulation is to "reconstitute", or replenish, keystone species in healthy individuals prior to the development of human diseases of modern living. As keynote organisms, helminths are central to correcting immune dysregulation, and their replenishment may be a disease preventative. Biome depletion theory departs from a drug model approach, which remains the current focus of helminthic therapy as evidenced by numerous clinical trials now underway for existing disease states.

Proposed Mechanism of Action

Experimental data support the hypothesis that clinically induced helminthic infections have the ability to alleviate or mitigate immune responses. Most autoimmune disorders are believed to involve hyperactive Th1 or Th17 immune responses that are down regulated by the promotion of a Th2 response by helminths. Helminths secrete immunoregulatory molecules that promote the induction of regulatory T cells while inhibiting the function of antigen presenting cells and other T cells. As such, helminthic therapy attempts to restore homeostasis by shifting a hyperactive Th1 pro-inflammatory response to a Th2 response with reduced inflammation. Human and animal studies have provided evidence of decreased Th1 and Th17 immune responses with a shift to Th2 cytokine production resulting in significantly decreased levels of interleukin 12 and IFNy with simultaneous increases in the regulatory T cells, interleukin 4, interleukin 5 and interleukin 10 of test subjects. These observations indicate that helminth therapy can provide protection against autoimmune disease not only through prevention, since helminths can be present before autoimmune disease develops, but also after autoimmune responses are initiated. Furthermore, responses of type-two T helper cells rarely kill the parasitic worms. Rather, the Th2 response limits the infection by reducing the viability and reproductive capacity of the parasite.

Given the down regulation of Th1 and Th17 immune responses with helminthic therapy, immune responses to other pathogens and allergens may be suppressed. Consequently, unmonitored and uncontrolled helminthic infections may be associated with suppressed immunity to the viruses and bacteria that normally trigger Th1 and Th17 immune responses required for protection against them leading to illness or disease.

Immunity

Evidence in support of the idea that helminthic infections reduce the severity of autoimmune diseases is primarily derived from animal models. Studies conducted on mice and rat models of colitis, muscular sclerosis, type 1 diabetes, and asthma have shown helminth-infected subjects to display protection from the disease. While helminths are often considered a homogenous group, considerable differences exist between species and the utilization of species in clinical research varies between human and animal trials. As such, caution must be exercised when interpreting the results from animal models.

Helminthic therapy is currently being studied as a treatment for several (non-viral) autoimmune diseases in humans including celiac disease, Crohn›s disease, multiple sclerosis, ulcerative colitis, and atherosclerosis. It is currently unknown which clinical dose or species of helminth is the most effective method of treatment. Hookworms have been linked to reduced risk of developing asthma, while *Ascaris lumbricoides* (roundworm infection) was associated with an *increased* risk of asthma. Similarly, *Hymenolepis nana*, *Trichoris trichiura*, *Ascaris lumbricoides*, *Strongyloides stercolaris*, *Enterobius vermicularis*, and *Trichuris suis* ova have all been found to lower the number of symptom exacerbations, reduce the number of symptom relapses, and decrease the number of new or enlarging brain lesions in patients with multiple sclerosis at doses ranging from 1,180 to 9,340 eggs per gram.

Trichuris suis ova has been used in most cases to treat autoimmune disorders because it is thought to be non-pathogenic in humans and therefore has been rendered as safe. The use of *Trichuris suis* ova has been granted by the USA Food and Drug Administration as an investigational medicinal product (IMP). While in the UK, the hookworm *Necator americanus* has been granted an IMP license by the Medicines and Healthcare Regulatory Authority. This hookworm is likely to be relatively safe, but can cause some gastrointestinal complications.

The general ideal characteristics for a therapeutic helminth are as follows:

- Little or no pathogenic potential
- Does not multiply in the host
- Cannot be directly spread to close contacts
- Produces a self-limited colonization in humans
- Produces an asymptomatic colonization in humans
- Does not alter behaviour in patients with depressed immunity
- Is not affected by most commonly used medications
- Can be eradicated with an anti-helminthic drug
- Can be isolated free of other potential pathogens
- Can be isolated or produced in large numbers
- Can be made stable for transport and storage
- Easy to administer

Potential Side Effects

Helminths are extremely successful parasites capable of establishing long-lasting infections within a host. During this time, helminths compete with the host organism's cells for nutrient resources and thus possess the potential to cause harm. While the majority of clinically infected individuals are asymptomatic, helminthic therapy does carry a number of potential side effects that can be alleviated through the use of anti-helminthic medications. The most common clinical symptoms of helminthic therapy include;

- Fatigue
- Malnutrition
- Gastrointestinal discomfort
- Anemia
- Fever
- Abdominal pain
- Weight loss
- Anorexia
- Diarrhea
- General malaise

Diseases of Affluence

Diseases of affluence is a term sometimes given to selected diseases and other health conditions which are commonly thought to be a result of increasing wealth in a society. Psychologists' research is probing why affluent people enjoy better health. Epidemiological studies have confirmed the relationship between income, education and occupation on the one hand and health outcomes on the other. Studies have found that relative risk of death increased significantly as rank decreased. The message is simple: the lower a person›s socioeconomic status, the greater their risk of both physical and psychological health problems.

Also referred to as the "Western disease" paradigm, these diseases are in contrast to so-called "diseases of poverty", which largely result from and contribute to human impoverishment. The modern diet and sedentary lifestyle is argued to be the blame for current levels of obesity, cardiovascular disease, high blood pressure, type 2 diabetes, osteoporosis, colorectal cancer, acne, gout, depression, and diseases related to vitamin and mineral deficiencies. These diseases of affluence have vastly increased in prevalence since the end of World War II.

Examples of diseases of affluence include mostly chronic non-communicable diseases (NCDs) and other physical health conditions for which personal lifestyles and societal conditions associated with economic development are believed to be an important risk factor — such as type 2 diabetes, asthma, coronary heart disease, cerebrovascular disease, peripheral vascular disease, obesity, hypertension, cancer, alcoholism, gout, and some types of allergy.

They may also be considered to include depression and other mental health conditions associated with increased social isolation and lower levels of psychological well being observed in many developed countries. Many of these conditions are interrelated, for example obesity is thought to be a partial cause of many other illnesses.

In contrast, the diseases of poverty tend to be largely infectious diseases, or the result of poor living conditions. These include tuberculosis, asthma, and intestinal diseases. Increasingly, research is finding that diseases thought to be diseases of affluence also appear in large part in the poor. These diseases include obesity and cardiovascular disease and, coupled with infectious diseases, these further increase global health inequalities.

Diseases of affluence are predicted to become more prevalent in developing countries as diseases of poverty decline, longevity increases, and lifestyles change. In 2008, nearly 80% of deaths due to NCDs — including heart disease, strokes, chronic lung diseases, cancers and diabetes — occurred in low- and middle-income countries.

Causes

Factors associated with the increase of these conditions and illnesses ironically appear to be things that are a direct result of technological advances. They include:

- Less strenuous physical exercise, often through increased use of motor vehicles
- Irregular exercise as a result of office jobs involving no physical labor.
- Easy accessibility in society to large amounts of low-cost food (relative to the much-lower caloric food availability in a subsistence economy)
    - More food generally, with much less physical exertion expended to obtain a moderate amount of food
    - More high fat and high sugar foods in the diet are common in the affluent developed economies of the late-twentieth century
    - Higher consumption of meat and dairy products
    - Higher consumption of refined flours and products made of such, like white bread or white noodles

- More foods which are processed, cooked, and commercially provided (rather than seasonal, fresh foods prepared locally at time of eating)

- Prolonged periods of little activity
- Greater use of alcohol and tobacco
- Longer life-spans
    - Reduced exposure to infectious agents throughout life (this can result in a more idle and inexperienced immune system [as compared to an individual that experienced relatively frequent exposure to certain pathogens in their time of life])

Parasitic worms (helminths)

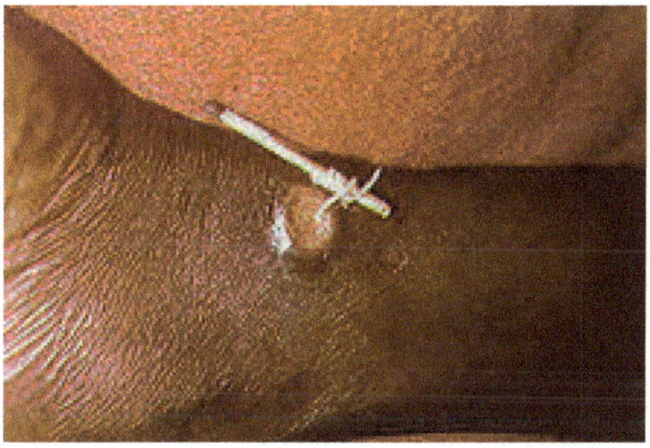

Guinea worm (Dracunculus) wrapped around a match stick

Hookworm

Hookworm infection, also known as hookworm disease, is an infection by a parasitic bloodsucking roundworm. Hookworm infections include ancylostomiasis and necatoriasis. These worms live in the small intestine which may be that of a bird or mammal such as a dog, cat, or human. Hookworm infection in pregnancy can cause poor growth, premature birth and a low birth weight of the baby. Hookworms in children can cause intellectual and growth problems. Two species of hookworms commonly infect humans: *Ancylostoma duodenale* and *Necator americanus*. *A. duodenale* is the more common type in the Middle East, North Africa, India and (formerly) in southern Europe, while *N. americanus* is the more common type in the Americas, Sub-Saharan Africa, Southeast Asia, China, and Indonesia. *A. tubaeforme* infects cats, *A. caninum* infects dogs and *A. braziliense* and *Uncinaria stenocephala* infect both cats and dogs. Hookworms are much smaller than the giant roundworms *Ascaris lumbricoides*. The most significant risk of hookworm infection is anemia, secondary to loss of iron (and protein) in the gut. The worms suck blood and damage the mucosa. However, the blood loss in the stools is not visibly apparent. Hookworm infection affects over half a billion people globally. It is a leading cause of health problems in mothers and children in developing countries of the tropics and subtropics. In developed countries, hookworm infection is rarely fatal, but anemia can be significant in a heavily infected individual. Hookworm infection is a soil-transmitted helminthiasis and therefore classified as a neglected tropical disease. Ancylostomiasis is the disease caused when *Ancylostoma duodenale* hookworms, present in large numbers, produce an iron deficiency anemia by sucking blood from the host's intestinal walls.

Tapeworm

Cestoda (Cestoidea) is a class of parasitic flatworms of the phylum Platyhelminthes. Biologists informally refer to them as cestodes. The best-known species are commonly called **tapeworms**. All cestodes are parasitic and their life histories vary, but typically they live in the digestive tracts of vertebrates as adults, and often in the bodies of other species of animals as juveniles. Over a thousand species have been described, and all vertebrate species may be parasitised by at least one species of tapeworm.

Humans are subject to infection by several species of tapeworms if they eat undercooked meat such as pork (*Taenia solium*), beef (*T. saginata*), and fish (*Diphyllobothrium* spp.), or if they live in, or eat food prepared in, conditions of poor hygiene (*Hymenolepis* or *Echinococcus* species).

T. saginata, the beef tapeworm, can grow up to 20 m (65 ft); the largest species, the whale tapeworm *Polygonoporus giganticus*, can grow to over 30 m (100 ft).Species using small vertebrates as hosts, though, tend to be small. For example, vole and lemming tapeworms are only 13–240 mm (0.51–9.45 in) in length, and those parasitizing shrews only 0.8–60 mm (0.031–2.362 in).

Tapeworm parasites of vertebrates have a long history: recognizable clusters of cestode eggs, one with a developing larva, have been discovered in fossil feces (coprolites) of a shark dating to the mid- to late Permian, some 270 million years ago.

Whipworm

The **human whipworm (*Trichuris trichiura or Trichocephalus trichiuris*)** is a round worm (a type of helminth) that causes trichuriasis (a type of helminthiasis which is one of the neglected tropical diseases) when it infects a human large intestine. It is commonly known as the *whipworm* **which refers to the shape of the worm; it looks like a whip with wider "handles" at the posterior end.**

Parasitic flukes

- *Schistosoma* - causes Schistosomiasis
- *Gnathostoma* - causes Gnathostomiasis
- *Paragonimus* - causes Paragonimiasis
- *Fasciola hepatica* - causes Fascioliasis
- *Trichobilharzia regenti* - causes Swimmer's itch

Ectoparasites

- *Sarcoptes scabiei* - causes scabies
- *Pediculus humanus capitis* - causes headlice
- *Phthirus pubis* - causes pubic lice
- *Human botfly maggots* - causes Myiasis
- Chigoe flea *Tunga penetrans* - causes Tungiasis
- Ticks (*Ixodoidea*)

REFERENCES

1. Ezzati M, Vander Hoorn S, Lawes CM, et al. (May 2005). "Rethinking the "diseases of affluence" paradigm: global patterns of nutritional risks in relation to economic development". PLoS Med. 2 *(5): e133. doi:10.1371/journal.pmed.0020133. PMC 1088287. PMID 15916467.*
2. Wood LE (October 2006). "Obesity, waist–hip ratio and hunter–gatherers". BJOG: an International Journal of Obstetrics & Gynaecology. 113 *(10): 1110–16. doi:10.1111/j.1471-0528.2006.01070.x. PMID 16972857.*
3. Kopp, Wolfgang (May 2006). "The atherogenic potential of dietary carbohydrate". Preventive Medicine. 42 *(5): 336–42. doi:10.1016/j.ypmed.2006.02.003. PMID 16540158.*
4. Tekol, Yalcin (April 2008). "Maternal and infantile dietary salt exposure may cause hypertension later in life". Birth Defects Research Part B: Developmental and Reproductive Toxicology. 83 *(2): 77–79. doi:10.1002/bdrb.20149. PMID 18330898.*
5. Dedoussis GV, Kaliora AC, Panagiotakos DB (Spring 2007). "Genes, Diet and Type 2 Diabetes Mellitus: A Review". Review of Diabetic Studies. 4 *(1): 13–24. doi:10.1900/RDS.2007.4.13. PMC 1892523. PMID 17565412.*
6. Sebastian A, Frassetto LA, Sellmeyer DE, Merriam RL, Morris RC Jr (1 December 2002). "Estimation of the net acid load of the diet of ancestral preagricultural Homo sapiens and their hominid ancestors". The American Journal of Clinical Nutrition. 76 *(6): 1308–16. PMID 12450898.*
7. Leach, Jeff D. (January 2007). "Evolutionary perspective on dietary intake of fibre and colorectal cancer". European Journal of Clinical Nutrition. 61 *(1): 140–42. doi:10.1038/sj.ejcn.1602486. PMID 16855539.*
8. Keri, Jonette E; Nijhawan, Rajiv (August 2008). "Diet and acne". Expert Review of Dermatology. 3 *(4): 437–40. doi:10.1586/17469872.3.4.437.*
9. Chen LX, Schumacher HR (October 2008). "Gout: an evidence-based review". J Clin Rheumatol. 14 *(5 Suppl): S55–62. doi:10.1097/RHU.0b013e3181896921. PMID 18830092.*
10. Cunnane, Stephen C. (1 August 2005). "Origins and evolution of the Western diet: implications of iodine and seafood intakes for the human brain". The American Journal of Clinical Nutrition. 82 *(2): 483; author reply 483–4. PMID 16087997.*

11. Von Hertzen LC, Haahtela T (February 2004). "Asthma and atopy — the price of affluence?". *Allergy.* 59 *(2): 124–37. doi:10.1046/j.1398-9995.2003.00433.x. PMID 14763924.*

12. Luthar SS (2003). "The culture of affluence: psychological costs of material wealth". Child Dev. 74 *(6): 1581–93. doi:10.1046/j.1467-8624.2003.00625.x. PMC 1950124. PMID 14669883.*

13. Hamilton C. (15 October 2004). "Diseases of affluence and other paradoxes". The Australian Financial Review.

14. Singh AR, Singh SA (January 2008). "Diseases of poverty and lifestyle, well-being and human development". Mens Sana Monogr. 6 *(1): 187–225. doi:10.4103/0973-1229.40567. PMC 3190550* PMID 22013359.

15. World Health Organization. New WHO report: deaths from noncommunicable diseases on the rise, with developing world hit hardest. Geneva, 27 April 2011.

16. Boseley, Sarah (2004-12-31). "15-Year Study Links Fast Food To Obesity". The Guardian. London. Retrieved 2010-05-01.

17. Lo CT, Ayele Y, Birrie H. Helminth and snail survey in Harerge region of Ethiopia with special reference to Schistosomiasis. Ethiop Med J 1989;27:73-83.

18. McMillan B, Kelly A, Walkar JC. Prevalence of Hymenolepis diminuta infection in man in the New Guinea Highlands. Trop Geogr Med 1971;23:390-2.

19. Mercado R, Arias B. Infections by Taenia sp and other intestinal cestodos in patients of consultorios hospitals and the public sector north of Santiago de Chile (1985–1995). Bol Chil Parasitol 1995:50:80-3.

20. Tena D, Pırez Simón M, Gimeno C, Pırez Pomata MT, Illescas S, Amondarain I, et al. Human infection with Hymenolepis diminuta : Case report from Spain. J Clin Microbiol 1998;36:2375-6.

21. Marangi M, Zechini B, Fileti A, Quaranta G, Aceti A. Hymenolepis diminuta infection in a child living in the urban area of Rome, Italy. J Clin Microbiol 2003;41:3994-5.

22. Kan SK, Kok RT, Marto S, Thomas I , Teo WW. The first report in Hymenolepis diminuta infection in Sabah, Malaysia. Trans R Soc Trop Med Hyg 1981;75:609.

23. "CDC - DPDx - Hymenolepiasis (Life Cycles)". cdc.gov. Center for Disease Control. Hymenolepis diminuta. Retrieved 2016-04-15.

24. Pappas, P. W., and A. J. Barley. 1999. Beetle-to-beetle transmission and dispersal of Hymenolepis diminuta (Cestoda) eggs via the feces of Tenebrio molitor. J. Parasitol. 85:384-385.

25. Watwe S, Dardi CK. Hymenolepis diminuta in a child from rural area. Indian Journal of Pathology & Microbiology 2008; 51(1): 149-150.

26. Cohen IP. A case report of Hymenolepis diminuta in a child in St James Parish, Jamaica. J La State Med Soc 1989;141: 23-4.

27. Sheiman IM, Shkutin MF, Terenina NB, Gustafsson MK. A behavioral study of the beetle Tenebrio molitor infected with cysticercoids of the rat tapeworm Hymenolepis diminuta. Naturwissenschaften. 2006 Jun;93(6):305-8. Epub 2006 Mar 23.

28. Parker W, Perkins SE, Harker M, Muehlenbein MP. A prescription for clinical immunology: the pills are available and ready for testing. A review. Curr Med Res Opin. 2012 Jul;28(7):1193-202. Epub 2012 Jun 12.

29. Finlay, Conor; Walsh, Kevin; Mills, Kingston (2014). "Induction of regulatory cells by helminth parasites: exploitation for the treatment of inflammatory diseases". Immunological Reviews. 259: 206–230. doi:10.1111/imr.12164.

30. «Ovamed". Retrieved 2013-09-27.

31. Fleming, J; Isaak, A; Lee, J; Luzzio, C; Carrithers, M; Cook, T; Field, A; Boland, J; Fabry, Z (2011). "Probiotic helminth administration in relapsing–remitting multiple sclerosis: a phase 1 study". Multiple Sclerosis Journal. 17 *(6): 743–754.* doi:10.1177/1352458511398054.

32. «Helminthic therapy or worm therapy using human hookworm or whipworm.". Retrieved 2009-05-22.

33. [i] Correale, Jorge; Farez, Mauricio (2007). "Association Between Parasite Infection and Immune Responses in Multiple Sclerosis". Annals of Neurology. 61: 97–108. doi:10.1002/ana.21067. PMID 17230481.

34. Correale, Jorge; Farez, Mauricio (2011). "The impact of parasite infections on the course of multiple sclerosis". Journal of Neuroimmunology. 233: 6–11. doi:10.1016/j.jneuroim.2011.01.002.

35. Leonardi-Bee, J.; Pritchard, D.; Britton, J. (2006). "Asthma and current intestinal parasite infection: systematic review and meta-analysis". American Journal of Respiratory and Critical Care Medicine. 174 *(5): 514–523.* doi:10.1164/rccm.200603-331OC. PMID 16778161.

36. P Zaccone; * Z Fehervari; * J M Phillips; D W Dunne; A Cooke (2006). "Parasitic worms and inflammatory diseases". Parasite Immunol. 28 *(10): 515–523. doi:10.1111/j.1365-3024.2006.00879.x. PMC 1618732.* PMID 16965287.

37. Pugliatti M, Sotgiu S, Rosati G (July 2002). "The worldwide prevalence of multiple sclerosis" (PDF). Clin Neurol Neurosurg. 104 *(3): 182–191.* doi:10.1016/S0303-8467(02)00036-7. PMID 12127652. Retrieved 4 March 2011.

38. Weinstock JV, Summers R, Elliott DE (2004). "Helminths and harmony". Gut. 53 *(1): 7–9. doi:10.1136/gut.53.1.7. PMC 1773927. PMID 14684567.*

39. Fumagalli, Matteo; Pozzoli, Uberto; Cagliani, Rachele; Comi, Giacomo P; Riva, Stefania; Clerici, Mario; Bresolin, Nereo; Sironi, Manuela (June 8, 2009). "Parasites represent a major selective force for interleukin genes and shape the genetic predisposition to autoimmune conditions". The Journal of Experimental Medicine. 206 *(6): 1395–1405. doi:10.1084/jem.20082779. PMC 2715056* PMID 19468064. Retrieved January 20, 2015.

40. David E. Elliott; Robert W. Summers; Joel V. Weinstock. (2005). "Helminths and the Modulation of Mucosal Inflammation". Current Opinion in Gastroenterology. 21 *(2): 51–58. PMID 15687885.*

41. Mohan C. (2006). "Environment versus genetics in autoimmunity: a geneticist›s perspective". Lupus. 15 *(11): 791–793.* doi:10.1177/0961203306070005. PMID 17153852.

42. Libbey, Jane; Cusick, Matthew; Fujinami, Robert (2014). "Role of pathogens in multiple sclerosis". International reviews of immunology. 22: 266–283.

43. World Health Organization. "Intestinal Worms". Retrieved 8 February 2015.

44. Strachan D P. (2006). "Hay fever, hygiene, and household size". BMJ. 299 *(6710): 1259–1260. doi:10.1136/bmj.299.6710.1259. PMC 1838109. PMID 2513902.*

45. Correale, Jorge (2014). "Helminth/Parasite Treatment of Multiple Sclerosis". Current Treatment Options in Neurology. 16: 1–12. doi:10.1007/s11940-014-0296-3.

46. Fumagalli M, Pozzoli U, Cagliani R, et al. (June 2009). "Parasites represent a major selective force for interleukin genes and shape the genetic predisposition to autoimmune conditions". The Journal of Experimental Medicine. 206 *(6): 1395–408. doi:10.1084/jem.20082779. PMC 2715056. PMID 19468064.*

47. Oreja-Guevara, Celia; Ramos-Cejudo, Jaime; Aroeira, Luiz; Chamorro, Beatriz; Diez-Tejedor, Exuperio (2012). "TH1/TH2 Cytokine profile in relapsing-remitting multiple sclerosis patients treated with Glatiramer acetate or Natalizumab". BioMed Central Neurology. 12: 1–6.

48. Hadley C (2004). "Should auld acquaintance be forgot...". *EMBO Rep. 5 (12): 1122–4. doi:10.1038/sj.embor.7400308. PMC 1299202. PMID 15577925.*

49. Parker W, Ollerton J. "Evolutionary biology and anthropology suggest biome reconstitution as a necessary approach toward dealing with immune disorders". Evol Med Public Health. 2013 *(1): 89–103. doi:10.1093/emph/eot008.*

50. Parker W, Perkins SE, Harker M, Muehlenbein MP (Jul 2012). "A prescription for clinical immunology: the pills are available and ready for testing. A review". Curr Med Res Opin. 28 *(7): 1193–202. doi:10.1185/03007995.2012.695731.*

51. Elliott, David; Summers, Robert; Weinstock, Joel (2007). "Helminths as governors of immune-mediated inflammation". International Journal for Parasitology. 37: 457–464. doi:10.1016/j.ijpara.2006.12.009. PMID 17313951.

52. McKay, D (2006). "The beneficial helminth parasite?". *Parasitology.* 132: 1–12. doi:10.1017/s003118200500884x.

53. Experimental hookworm infection and gluten microchallenge promote tolerance in celiac disease". Journal of Allergy and Clinical Immunology. 135: 508–516.e5. doi:10.1016/j.jaci.2014.07.022.

54. «Inoculating Celiac Disease Patients With the Human Hookworm Necator Americanus: Evaluating Immunity and Gluten-Sensitivity - Full Text View - ClinicalTrials.gov". Retrieved 2009-05-22.

55. Hunter MM, McKay DM (2004). "Review article: helminths as therapeutic agents for inflammatory bowel disease". Aliment. Pharmacol. Ther. 19 *(2): 167–77. doi:10.1111/j.0269-2813.2004.01803.x. PMID 14723608.*

56. Croese J, O›neil J, Masson J, Cooke S, Melrose W, Pritchard D, Speare R (2006). "A proof of concept study establishing Necator americanus in Crohn›s patients and reservoir donors". Gut. 55 *(1): 136–137. doi:10.1136/gut.2005.079129. PMC 1856386. PMID 16344586.*

57. Summers RW, Elliott DE, Urban JF, Thompson R, Weinstock JV (2005). "Trichuris suis therapy in Crohn›s disease". Gut. 54 *(1): 87–90. doi:10.1136/gut.2004.041749. PMC 1774382. PMID 15591509.*

58. Summers RW, Elliott DE, Qadir K, Urban JF, Thompson R, Weinstock JV (2003). "Trichuris suis seems to be safe and possibly effective in the treatment of inflammatory bowel disease". Am. J. Gastroenterol. 98 *(9): 2034–41. doi:10.1111/j.1572-*

0241.2003.07660.x. PMID 14499784.

59. Correale J, Farez M (2007). “Association between parasite infection and immune responses in multiple sclerosis”. Annals of Neurology. 61 *(2): 97–108. doi:10.1002/ana.21067. PMID 17230481.*

60. Summers RW, Elliott DE, Urban JF, Thompson RA, Weinstock JV (2005). “Trichuris suis therapy for active ulcerative colitis: a randomized controlled trial”. Gastroenterology. 128 *(4): 825–32. doi:10.1053/j.gastro.2005.01.005. PMID 15825065.*

61. Magen E, Bychkov V, Ginovker A, Kashuba E.Chronic Opisthorchis felineus infection attenuates atherosclerosis - An autopsy study.Int J Parasitol. 2013 Jun 19. pii: S0020-7519(13)00153-7. doi:

62. Elliott, David; Summers, Robert W; Weinstock, Joel V (2007). “Helminths as governors of immune-mediated inflammation”. International Journal for Parasitology. 37: 457–464. doi:10.1016/j.ijpara.2006.12.009. PMID 17313951.

63. Elliott, David; Weinstock, Joel V (2009). “Helminthic therapy: using worms to treat immune-mediated disease”. Advanced Experimental Medical Biology. 666: 157–66. doi:10.1007/978-1-4419-1601-3_12. PMID 20054982.

64. Pritchard, D,I. (2011). “Worm therapy: for or against?”. *Journal of Helminthology.* 85 *(03): 225–227.* doi:10.1017/S0022149X11000204. PMID 21729383.

CHAPTER 5

Veterinary Parasitology

Chapter Contents

INTRODUCTION

Veterinary parasitology is the study of animal parasites, especially relationships between parasites and animal hosts. Parasites of domestic animals, (livestock and pet animals), as well as wildlife animals are considered. Veterinary parasitologists study the genesis and development of parasitoses in animal hosts, as well as the taxonomy and systematics of parasites, including the morphology, life cycles, and living needs of parasites in the environment and in animal hosts. Using a variety of research methods, they diagnose, treat, and prevent animal parasitoses. Data obtained from parasitological research in animals helps in veterinary practice and improves animal breeding. The major goal of veterinary parasitology is to protect animals and improve their health, but because a number of animal parasites are transmitted to humans, veterinary parasitology is also important for public health.

DIAGNOSTIC METHODS

Various methods are used to identify parasites in animals, using feces, blood, and tissue samples from the host animal.

Coprological

Coprological examinations involve examining the feces of animals to identify and count parasite eggs. Some common methods include fecal flotation and sedimentation to separate eggs from fecal matter. Others include the McMaster method, which uses a special two-chamber slide that allows parasite eggs to be more clearly visible and easily counted. It is most commonly used to monitor parasites in horses and other grazing and livestock animals. The Baermann method is similar but requires more specialized equipment and more time and is typically used to diagnose lungworm and threadworm.

Haematological

Haematological examinations involve examining the blood of animals to determine the presence of parasites. Blood parasites tend to inhabit the erythrocytes or white blood cells and are most likely to be detected during the acute phase of infection. Veterinary parasitologists use blood smears, which involve placing a drop of blood onto a slide and spreading it over the surface in a thin film in order to examine it under a microscope. The blood is stained with a dye in order for the cells to be easily distinguished.

Histopathological

Histopathological examinations involve examining tissue samples from animals. A small slice of the organ suspected of being infected by parasites is mounted on a slide, stained, and examined under a microscope.

Though not technically considered a histopathological technique, skin scraping – which involves taking a small sample of the epidermal cells of a dog, cat, or other household pet – is commonly used to detect the presence of mites.

Immunological

Immunological examinations, such as indirect immunofluorescence, ELISA, Immunoblotting (Western blot), and Complement fixation test are methods of identifying different kinds of parasites by detecting the presence of their antigens on or within the parasite itself. These diagnostic methods are used in conjunction with coprological examinations for more specific identification of different parasite species in fecal samples.

Molecular biological

Molecular biological methods involve studying the DNA of the parasite in order to identify it. PCR and RFLP are used to detect and amplify parasite DNA found in the feces, blood, or tissue of the host. These techniques are very sensitive, which is useful for diagnosing parasites even when they are present in very low numbers; they are also useful for identifying parasites not only in large animal hosts but smaller insect vectors.

DIVISIONS OF VETERINARY PARASITOLOGY

Veterinary Protozoology

Protozoology is the study of protozoa, the "animal-like" (i.e., motile and heterotrophic) protists.

This term has become dated as understanding of the evolutionary relationships of the eukaryotes has improved. For example, the Society of Protozoloogists, founded in 1947, was renamed International Society of Protistologists in 2005. However, the term persists in some cases (e.g., the Polish journal *Acta Protozoologica*).

- focused on veterinary important protozoans

Examples of protozoan parasites:

- *Trypanosoma brucei*
- *Trypanosoma equiperdum*
- *Leishmania donovani*
- *Leishmania infantum*
- *Giardia duodenalis*
- *Trichomonas gallinae*
- *Tritrichomonas foetus*
- *Histomonas meleagridis*
- *Cryptosporidium parvum*
- *Balantidium coli*
- *Eimeria acervulina*
- *Eimeria tenella*
- *Isospora canis*
- *Toxoplasma gondii*
- *Neospora caninum*
- *Hammondia hammondi*
- *Besnoitia besnoiti*
- *Babesia divergens*

Veterinary Helminthology

- focused on veterinary important helminth parasites

Examples of helminth parasites:

- *Ancylostoma duodenale*
- *Ascaris suum*
- *Dicrocoelium dendriticum*
- *Dictyocaulus bovis*
- *Dipylidium caninum*
- *Echinococcus granulosus*

- *Fasciola hepatica*
- *Fascioloides magna*
- *Habronema muscae*
- *Habronema majus*
- *Haemonchus contortus*
- *Metastrongylus*
- *Muellerius capillaris*
- *Ostertagia ostertagi*
- *Paragonimus westermani*
- *Schistosoma bovis*
- *Strongyloides canis*
- *Strongylus vulgaris*
- *Syngamus trachea*
- *Taenia pisiformis*
- *Taenia saginata*
- *Taenia solium*
- *Toxocara canis*
- *Trichinella spiralis*
- *Trichobilharzia regenti*
- *Trichostrongylus axei*
- *Trichuris suis*

Veterinary Entomology (Arachnoentomology)

Entomology is the scientific study of insects, a branch of zoology. In the past the term "insect" was more vague, and historically the definition of entomology included the study of terrestrial animals in other arthropod groups or other phyla, such as arachnids, myriapods, earthworms, land snails, and slugs. This wider meaning may still be encountered in informal use.

Like several of the other fields that are categorized within zoology, entomology is a taxon-based category; any form of scientific study in which there is a focus on insect-related inquiries is, by definition, entomology. Entomology therefore overlaps with a cross-section of topics as diverse as molecular genetics, behavior, biomechanics, biochemistry, systematics, physiology, developmental biology, ecology, morphology, paleontology

At some 1.3 million described species, insects account for more than two-thirds of all known organisms, date back some 400 million years, and have many kinds of interactions with humans and other forms of life on earth.

- focused on veterinary important Arachnids, Insects, and Crustaceans

Examples of arachnid, insect, and crustacean parasites:

- *Sarcoptes equi*

- *Psoroptes ovis*
- *Ixodes ricinus*
- *Dermacentor marginatus*
- *Caligus clemensi*
- *Caligus cuneifer*
- *Caligus elongatus*
- *Caligus rogercresseyi*
- *Cimex colombarius.*
- *Cimex lectularius*
- *Culex pipiens*
- *Culicoides imicola*
- *Demodex bovis*
- *Gasterophilus intestinalis*
- *Haematobia irritans*
- *Hypoderma bovis*
- *Knemidocoptes mutans*
- *Lepeophtheirus salmonis (sea louse)*
- *Lucilia sericata*
- *Musca domestica*
- *Nosema apis*
- *Notoedres cati*
- *Oestrus ovis*
- *Otodectes cynotis*
- *Phlebotomus*
- *Pulex irritans*
- *Rhipicephalus sanguineus*
- *Sarcophaga carnaria*
- *Tabanus atratus*
- *Triatoma*
- *Ctenocephalides canis*
- *Ctenocephalides felis*

REFERENCES

1. Jurášek, V., Dubinský, P., 1993. Veterinárna parazitológia. Príroda a.s., Bratislava, 382 pp.

2. Kaufmann, J., 1996. Parasitic infections of domestic animals: a diagnostic manual. Birkhauser, Berlin, 423 pp.

3. Elsheikha, HM; Khan, NA (editor) (2011). Essentials of Veterinary Parasitology. Caister Academic Press. ISBN 978-1-904455-79-0.

4. Leland S. Shapiro; Patricia Mandel (22 May 2009). Pathology & Parasitology for Veterinary Technicians. Cengage Learning. pp. 237–239. ISBN 978-1-4354-3855-2.

5. A. Zajac; Gary A. Conboy; American Association of Veterinary Parasitologists (24 March 2006). Veterinary clinical parasitology. Wiley-Blackwell. p. 162. ISBN 978-0-8138-1734-7.

6. John E. Hyde (1993). Protocols in molecular parasitology. Humana Press. pp. 213–214. ISBN 978-0-89603-239-2.

CHAPTER 6

Human Parasitology

Chapter Contents

- **Introduction**
- **Terminology**
- **List of Parasites of Humans**
- **Treatment**
- **Humans**

Parasitic diseases are illnesses caused by infestation (infection) with parasites such as protozoa (one-celled animals), worms, or insects. These diseases are widespread in Africa, southern Asia, and Central and South America, especially among children. They include malaria and schistosomiasis, the world's most common serious infectious diseases.

INTRODUCTION

A parasitic disease, also known as parasitosis, is an infectious disease caused or transmitted by a parasite. Many parasites do not cause diseases. Parasitic diseases can affect practically all living organisms, including plants and mammals. The study of parasitic diseases is called parasitology.

Some parasites like *Toxoplasma gondii* and *Plasmodium* spp. can cause disease directly, but other organisms can cause disease by the toxins that they produce.

TERMINOLOGY

Although organisms such as bacteria function as parasites, the usage of the term "parasitic disease" is usually more restricted. The three main types of organisms causing these conditions are protozoa (causing protozoan infection), helminths (helminthiasis), and ectoparasites. Protozoa and helminths are usually endoparasites (usually living inside the body of the host), while ectoparasites usually live on the surface of the host. Occasionally the definition of "parasitic disease" is restricted to diseases due to endoparasites.

SIGNS AND SYMPTOMS

Symptoms of parasites may not always be obvious. However, such symptoms may mimic anemia or a hormone deficiency.Some of the symptoms caused by several worm infestation can include itching affecting the anus or the vaginal area, abdominal pain, weight loss, increased appetite, bowel obstructions, diarrhea, and vomiting eventually leading to dehydration, sleeping problems, worms present in the vomit or stools, anemia, aching muscles or joints, general malaise, allergies, fatigue, nervousness. Symptoms may also be confused with pneumonia or food poisoning.

The effects caused by parasitic diseases range from mild discomfort to death. The nematode parasites *Necator americanus* and *Ancylostoma duodenale* cause human hookworm infection, which leads to anaemia and protein malnutrition. This infection affects approximately 740 million people in the developing countries, including children and adults, of the tropics specifically in poor rural areas located in sub-Saharan Africa, Latin America, South-East Asia and China. Chronic hookworm in children leads to impaired physical and intellectual development, school performance and attendance are reduced. Pregnant women affected by a hookworm infection can also develop aneamia, which results in negative outcomes both for the mother and the infant. Some of them are: low birth weight, impaired milk production, as well as increased risk of death for the mother and the baby.

CAUSES

Mammals can get parasites from contaminated food or water, bug bites, or sexual contact. Ingestion of contaminated water can produce Giardia infections.

Parasites normally enter the body through the skin or mouth. Close contact with pets can lead to parasite infestation as dogs and cats are host to many parasites.

Other risks that can lead people to acquire parasites are walking barefeet, inadequate disposal of feces, lack of hygiene, close contact with someone carrying specific parasites, and eating undercooked or exotic foods.

Parasites can also be transferred to their host by the bite of an insect vector, i.e. mosquito, bed bug.

LIST OF PARASITES OF HUMANS

Endoparasites

Protozoan Organisms

Common name of organism or disease	Latin name (sorted)	Body parts affected	Diagnostic specimen	Prevalence	Source/ Transmission (Reservoir/ Vector)
Granulomatous amoebic encephalitis and *Acanthamoeba* keratitis (eye infection)	*Acanthamoeba* spp.	eye, brain, skin	culture	worldwide	contact lenses cleaned with tap water, open wounds
Granulomatous amoebic encephalitis (skin infection)	*Balamuthia mandrillaris*	brain, skin	culture	worldwide	open wounds
Babesiosis	*Babesia B. divergens*, *B. bigemina*, *B. equi*, *B. microfti*, *B. duncani*	red blood cells	Giemsa-stained thin blood smear	New York, Martha's Vineyard, Nantucket (different species have worldwide distribution)	tick bites, e.g. *Ixodes scapularis*
Balantidiasis	*Balantidium coli*	intestinal mucosa, may become invasive in some patients	stool (diarrhea=ciliated trophozoite; solid stool=large cyst with horseshoe shaped nucleus)		ingestion of cyst, zoonotic infection acquired from pigs (feces)
Blastocystosis	*Blastocystis* spp.	intestinal	direct microscopy of stool (PCR, anti body)	• worldwide: one of the most common human parasites • United States: infected ~23% of the population during year 2000 • Developing regions: infects 40–100% of the total populations	eating food contaminated with feces from an infected human or animal
Cryptosporidiosis	*Cryptosporidium* spp.	intestines	stool	widespread	ingestion of oocyst (sporulated), some species are zoonotic (e.g. bovine fecal contamination)
Cyclosporiasis	*Cyclospora cayetanensis*	intestines	stool	United States	ingestion of oocyst thru contaminated food

Common name of organism or disease	Latin name (sorted)	Body parts affected	Diagnostic specimen	Prevalence	Source/ Transmission (Reservoir/ Vector)
Dientamoebiasis	*Dientamoeba fragilis*	intestines	stool	up to 10% in industrialized countries	ingesting water or food contaminated with feces
Amoebiasis	*Entamoeba histolytica*	Intestines (mainly Large, can go to extraintestinal sites)	stool (fresh diarrheic stools have amoeba, solid stool has cyst)	areas with poor sanitation, high population density and tropical regions	fecal-oral transmission of cyst, not amoeba
Giardiasis	*Giardia lamblia*	lumen of the small intestine	stool	widespread	ingestion of cysts in fecal contaminated water or food, can be zoonotic (deer, beavers)
Isosporiasis	*Isospora belli*	epithelial cells of small intestines	stool	worldwide – less common than *Toxoplasma* or *Cryptosporidium*	fecal oral route – ingestion of sporulated oocyst
Leishmaniasis	*Leishmania* spp.	cutaneous, mucocutaneous, or visceral	visual identification of lesion or microscopic stain with Leishman's or Giemsa's stain	Visceral leishmaniasis – Worldwide; Cutaneous leishmaniasis – Old World; Mucocutaneous leishmaniasis – New World	*Phlebotomus*, *Lutzomyia* – bite of several species of phlebotomine sandflies
Primary amoebic meningoencephalitis (PAM)	*Naegleria fowleri*	brain and skin	culture	rare but deadly	Nasal insufflation of contaminated warm fresh water, poorly chlorinated swimming pools, hot springs, soil
Malaria	*Plasmodium falciparum* (80% of cases), *Plasmodium vivax*, *Plasmodium ovale curtisi*, *Plasmodium ovale wallikeri*, *Plasmodium malariae*, *Plasmodium knowlesi*	red blood cells, liver	Blood film	tropical – 250 million cases/year	Anopheles mosquito, bites at night
Rhinosporidiosis	*Rhinosporidium seeberi*	nose, nasopharynx	biopsy	India and Sri Lanka	nasal mucosa came into contact with infected material through bathing in common ponds

Common name of organism or disease	Latin name (sorted)	Body parts affected	Diagnostic specimen	Prevalence	Source/ Transmission (Reservoir/ Vector)
Sarcocystosis	*Sarcocystis bovihominis,Sarcocystis suihominis*	intestine, muscle	muscle biopsy	widespread	ingestion of uncooked/ undercooked beef/pork with *Sarcocystis* sarcocysts
Toxoplasmosis (Acute and Latent)	*Toxoplasma gondii*	eyes, brain, heart, liver	blood and PCR	worldwide: one of the most common human parasites; estimated to infect between 30–50% of the global population.	ingestion of uncooked/ undercooked pork/lamb/goat with *Toxoplasma* bradyzoites, ingestion of raw milk with Toxoplasma tachyzoites, ingestion of contaminated water food or soil with oocysts in cat feces that is more than one day old
Trichomoniasis	*Trichomonas vaginalis*	female urogenital tract (males asymptomatic)	microscopic examination of genital swab	7.4 million Americans	sexually transmitted infection – only trophozoite form (no cyst)
Sleeping sickness	*Trypanosoma brucei*	blood lymph and central nervous systems	microscopic examination of chancre fluid, lymph node aspirates, blood, bone marrow	50,000 to 70,000 people	tsetse fly, day biting fly of the genus Glossina
Chagas disease	*Trypanosoma cruzi*	colon, esophagus, heart, nerves, muscle and blood	Giemsa stain – blood	Mexico, Central America, South America – 16-18 million	*Triatoma*/ Reduviidae – "Kissing bug" Insect Vector, feeds at night

Helminths Organisms (worms)

Helminth organisms (also called helminths or intestinal worms) include:

Tapeworms

Common name of organism or disease	Latin name (sorted)	Body parts affected	Diagnostic specimen	Prevalence	Transmission/Vector
Tapeworm – Tapeworm infection	*Cestoda, Taenia multiceps*	intestine	stool	rare	
Diphyllobothriasis – tapeworm	*Diphyllobothrium latum*	intestines, blood	stool (microscope)	Europe, Japan, Uganda, Peru, Chile	ingestion of raw fresh water fish
Echinococcosis – tapeworm	*Echinococcus granulosus, Echinococcus multilocularis, E. vogeli, E. oligarthrus*	liver, lungs, kidney, spleen	imaging of hydatid cysts in the liver, lungs, kidney and spleen	Mediterranean countries	as intermediate host, ingestion of material contaminated by feces from a carnivore; as definite host, ingestion of uncooked meat (offal) from a herbivore
Hymenolepiasis	*Hymenolepis nana, Hymenolepis diminuta*				ingestion of material contaminated by flour beetles, meal worms, cockroaches
Beef tapeworm	*Taenia saginata*	Intestines	stool	worldwide distribution	ingestion of undercooked beef
Cysticercosis-Pork tapeworm	*Taenia solium*	Brain, muscle, Eye (Cysts in conjuntiva/ anterior chamber/ sub-retinal space)	stool, blood	Asia, Africa, South America, Southern Europe, North America.	ingestion of undercooked pork
Bertielliasis	*Bertiella mucronata, Bertiella studeri*	Intestines	Stool	Rare	Contact with non human primates
Sparganosis	*Spirometra erinaceieuropaei*				ingestion of material contaminated with infected dog or cat faeces (humans: dead-end host)

Flukes

Common name of organism or disease	Latin name (sorted)	Body parts affected	Diagnostic specimen	Prevalence	Transmission/ Vector
Clonorchiasis	*Clonorchis sinensis*; *Clonorchis viverrini*	gall bladder ducts and inflammation of liver			ingestion of under prepared fresh water fish
Lancet liver fluke	*Dicrocoelium dendriticum*	gall bladder		rare	ingestion of ants
Liver fluke – Fasciolosis	*Fasciola hepatica*, *Fasciola gigantica*	liver, gall bladder	stool	*Fasciola hepatica* in Europe, Africa, Australia, the Americas and Oceania; *Fasciola gigantica* only in Africa and Asia, 2.4 million people infected by both species	freshwater snails
Fasciolopsiasis – intestinal fluke	*Fasciolopsis buski*	intestines	stool or vomitus (microscope)	East Asia – 10 million people	ingestion of infested water plants or water (intermediate host:amphibic snails)
Gnathostomiasis	*Gnathostoma spinigerum*, *Gnathostoma hispidum*	subcutaneous tissues (under the skin)	physical examination	rare – Southeast Asia	ingestion of raw or undercooked meat (e.g., freshwater fish, chicken, snails, frogs, pigs) or contaminated water
Metagonimiasis – intestinal fluke	*Metagonimus yokogawai*		stool	Siberia, Manchuria, Balkan states, Israel, Spain	ingestion of undercooked or salted fish
Metorchiasis	*Metorchis conjunctus*			Canada, USA, Greenland	ingestion of raw fish
Chinese Liver Fluke	*Opisthorchis viverrini*, *Opisthorchis felineus*, *Clonorchis sinensis*	bile duct		1.5 million people in Russia	consuming infected raw, slightly salted or frozen fish

Common name of organism or disease	Latin name (sorted)	Body parts affected	Diagnostic specimen	Prevalence	Transmission/ Vector
Paragonimiasis, Lung Fluke	*Paragonimus westermani*; *Paragonimus africanus*; *Paragonimus caliensis*; *Paragonimus kellicotti*; *Paragonimus skrjabini*; *Paragonimus uterobilateralis*	lungs	sputum, feces	East Asia	ingestion of raw or undercooked freshwater crabs crayfishes or other crustaceans
Schistosomiasis – bilharzia, bilharziosis or snail fever (all types)	*Schistosoma* sp.			Africa, Caribbean, eastern South America, east Asia, Middle East – 200 million people	skin exposure to water contaminated with infected fresh water snails
intestinal schistosomiasis	*Schistosoma mansoni* and *Schistosoma intercalatum*	intestine, liver, spleen, lungs, skin,rarely infects the brain	stool	Africa, Caribbean, South America, Asia, Middle East – 83 million people	skin exposure to water contaminated with infected *Biomphalaria* fresh water snails
urinary schistosomiasis	*Schistosoma haematobium*	kidney, bladder, ureters, lungs, skin	urine	Africa, Middle East	skin exposure to water contaminated with infected *Bulinus* sp. snails
Schistosomiasis by *Schistosoma japonicum*	*Schistosoma japonicum*	intestine, liver, spleen, lungs, skin	stool	China, East Asia, Philippines	skin exposure to water contaminated with infected Oncomelania sp. snails
Asian intestinal schistosomiasis	*Schistosoma mekongi* -			South East Asia	skin exposure to water contaminated with infected *Neotricula aperta* – fresh water snails
	Echinostoma echinatum	small intestine		Far East	ingestion of raw fish, mollusks, snails
Swimmer's itch	*Trichobilharzia regenti*, Schistosomatidae				skin exposure to contaminated water (snails and vertebrates)

Roundworms

Common name of organism or disease	Latin name (sorted)	Body parts affected	Diagnostic specimen	Prevalence	Transmission/ Vector
Ancylostomiasis/ Hookworm	*Ancylostoma duodenale*, Necator americanus	lungs, small intestine, blood	stool	common in tropical, warm, moist climates	penetration of skin by L3 larva
Angiostrongyliasis	*Angiostrongylus costaricensis*	intestine	stool		ingestion of infected faeces or infected slugs
Anisakiasis	*Anisakis*	allergic reaction	biopsy	incidental host	ingestion of raw fish, squid, cuttlefish, octopus
Roundworm – Parasitic pneumonia	*Ascaris* sp. *Ascaris lumbricoides*	Intestines, liver, appendix, pancreas, lungs, Löffler's syndrome	stool	common in tropical and subtropical regions	
Roundworm – Baylisascariasis	*Baylisascaris procyonis*	Intestines, liver, lungs, brain, eye		rare: North America	stool from raccoons
Roundworm-lymphatic filariasis	*Brugia malayi*, *Brugia timori*	lymph nodes	blood samples	tropical regions of Asia	Arthropods
Dioctophyme renalis infection	*Dioctophyme renale*	kidneys (typically the right)	Urine	Rare	Ingestion of undercooked or raw freshwater fish

Common name of organism or disease	**Latin name (sorted)**	**Body parts affected**	**Diagnostic specimen**	**Prevalence**	**Transmission/ Vector**
Guinea worm – Dracunculiasis	*Dracunculus medinensis*	subcutaneous tissues, muscle	skin blister/ulcer	South Sudan (eradication ongoing)	
Pinworm – Enterobiasis	*Enterobius vermicularis, Enterobius gregorii*	intestines, anus	stool; tape test around anus	widespread; temperate regions	
Halicephalobiasis	*Halicephalobus gingivalis*	brain			soil contaminated wounds
Loa loa filariasis, Calabar swellings	*Loa loa filaria*	Connective tissue, lungs, eye	blood (Giemsa, haematoxylin, eosin stain)	rain forest of West Africa – 12-13 million people	Tabanidae – horse fly, bites in the day
Mansonelliasis, Filariasis	*Mansonella streptocerca*	subcutaneous layer of skin			insect
River blindness, Onchocerciasis	*Onchocerca volvulus*	skin, eye, tissue	bloodless skin snip	Africa, Yemen, Central and South America near cool, fast flowing rivers	Simulium/Black fly, bite during the day
Strongyloidiasis – Parasitic pneumonia	*Strongyloides stercoralis*	Intestines, lungs, skin (Larva currens)	stool, blood		skin penetration
Thelaziasis	*Thelazia californiensis, Thelazia callipaeda*	Eyes	ocular examination	Asia, Europe	*Amiota (Phortica) variegata, Phortica okadai*

Common name of organism or disease	Latin name (sorted)	Body parts affected	Diagnostic specimen	Prevalence	Transmission/ Vector
Toxocariasis	*Toxocara canis, Toxocara cati*	liver, brain, eyes (Toxocara canis – Visceral larva migrans, Ocular larva migrans)	blood, ocular examination	worldwide distribution	pica, unwashed food contamined with Toxocara eggs, undercooked livers of chicken
Trichinosis	*Trichinella spiralis, Trichinella britovi, Trichinella nelsoni, Trichinella nativa*	muscle, periorbital region, small intestine	blood	more common in developing countries due to improved feeding practices in developed countries.	ingestion of undercooked pork
Whipworm	*Trichuris trichiura, Trichuris vulpis*	large intestine, anus	stool (eggs)	common worldwide	accidental ingestion of eggs in dry goods such as beans, rice, and various grains or soil contaminated with human feces
ElephantiasisLymphatic filariasis	*Wuchereria bancrofti*	lymphatic system	thick blood smears stained with hematoxylin.	Tropical and subtropical	mosquito, bites at night

Other Organisms

Common name of organism or disease	**Latin name (sorted)**	**Body parts affected**	**Diagnostic specimen**	**Prevalence**	**Transmission/ Vector**
Acanthocephaliasis	Archiacanthocephala, *Moniliformis moniliformis*	Gastrointestinal tract, peritoneum, eye	Faeces, parasite itself	worldwide	ingestion of intermediate hosts
Halzoun Syndrome	*Linguatula serrata*	nasopharynx	physical examination	Mid East	ingestion of raw or undercooked lymph nodes (e.g., meat from infected camels and buffalos)
Myiasis	Oestroidea, Calliphoridae, Sarcophagidae	dead or living tissue			
Screwworm, Cochliomyia	*Cochliomyia hominivorax* (family Calliphoridae)	skin and wounds	visual	North America (eradicated), Central America, North Africa	direct contact with fly
Chigoe flea	*Tunga penetrans*	Subcutaneous tissue	physical examination	Central and South America	
Bedbug	Cimicidae: *Cimex lectularius*	skin	visual	Worldwide	sharing of clothing and bedding
Human Botfly	*Dermatobia hominis*	Subcutaneous tissue	physical examination	Central and South America	Mosquitoes and biting flies

Ectoparasites

Common name of organism or disease	**Latin name (sorted)**	**Body parts affected**	**Diagnostic specimen**	**Prevalence**	**Transmission/ Vector**
Head louse – Pediculosis	*Pediculus humanus*	hair follicles	visual identification under magnification	Common worldwide	head-to-head contact

Common name of organism or disease	Latin name (sorted)	Body parts affected	Diagnostic specimen	Prevalence	Transmission/ Vector
Body louse – Pediculosis	*Pediculus humanus corporis*		visual identification under magnification (Vagabond's disease)	Worldwide	skin-to-skin contact such as sexual activity and via sharing clothing or bedding
Crab louse – Pediculosis	*Pthirus pubis*	pubic area, eyelashes	visual identification under magnification	Worldwide	skin-to-skin contact such as sexual activity and via sharing clothing or bedding
Demodex – Demodicosis	*Demodex folliculorum/ brevis/canis*	eyebrow, eyelashes	Microscopy of eyelash or eyebrow hair follicle	Pandemic, worldwide	prolonged skin-to-skin contact
Scabies	*Sarcoptes scabiei*	skin	microscopy of surface scrapings	Worldwide	skin-to-skin contact such as sexual activity and via sharing clothing or bedding
"Chiggers" (Trombiculidae) – Trombiculosis	Arachnida: Trombiculidae	skin	visual identification under magnification, microscopy	worldwide (mesic habitats)	High grass, weeds
Flea, Siphonaptera	*Pulex irritans*	skin	visual identification under magnification	Worldwide	environment
Tick	Arachnida: Ixodidae and Argasidae	skin	visual	Worldwide	High grass, leaf litter, weeds

TREATMENT

Parasitic infections can usually be treated with antiparasitic drugs.

Albendazole and mebendazole have been the treatments administered to entire populations to control hookworm infection. However, it is a costly option and both children and adults become reinfected within a few months after deparasitation occurs raising concerns because the treatment has to repeatedly be administered and drug resistance may occur.

Another medication administered to kill worm infections has been pyrantel pamoate. For some parasitic diseases, there is no treatment and, in the case of serious symptoms, medication intended to kill the parasite is administered, whereas, in other cases, symptom relief options are used. Recent papers have also proposed the use of viruses to treat infections caused by protozoa.

HUMANS

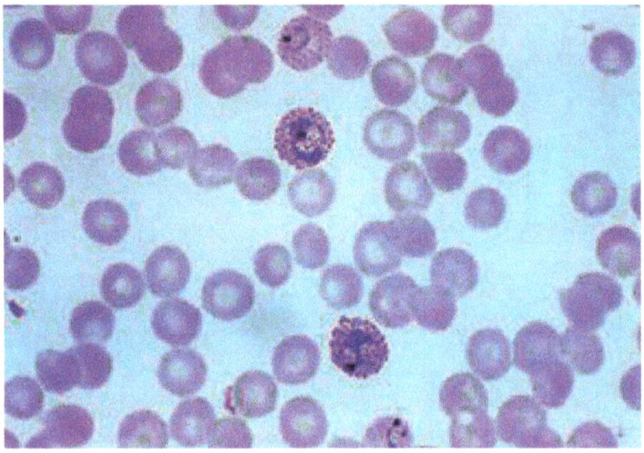

Trophozoites of the *Plasmodium vivax* parasite among human red blood cells

The species of *Plasmodium* that infect humans include:

- *Plasmodium falciparum* (the cause of malignant tertian malaria)
- *Plasmodium vivax* (the most frequent cause of benign tertian malaria)
- *Plasmodium ovale* (the other, less frequent, cause of benign tertian malaria)
- *Plasmodium malariae* (the cause of benign quartan malaria)
- *Plasmodium knowlesi* (the cause of severe quotidian malaria in South East Asia since 1965)

P. falciparum, *P. vivax*, *P. ovale*, and *P. malariae* together account for nearly all human infections with *Plasmodium* species, with *P. falciparum* accounting for the overwhelming majority of malaria deaths. An increasing number of cases of severe malaria in Southeast Asia have been attributed to *P. knowlesi*.

With the use of the polymerase chain reaction additional species have been identified in humans, although whether these species can regularly infect humans is not known. An experimental infection of a human volunteer with *Plasmodium eylesi* and *Plasmodium cynomolgi* has been reported, although the infection was not able to be transferred to another susceptible host, suggesting the parasites may not be able to productively infect humans. A possible infection with *Plasmodium tenue* has also been reported, however doubts have been raised as to the validity of this diagnosis. Other species which have been reportedly isolated from humans include *Plasmodium brasilianum*, *Plasmodium inui*, *Plasmodium rhodiani*, *Plasmodium schweitzi*, *Plasmodium semiovale*, and *Plasmodium simium*.

In addition to humans, *P. vivax* can infect chimpanzees and orangutans. In these hosts, infection tends to not cause severe disease, but may persist for some time.

P. ovale can be transmitted to chimpanzees, and is found in Africa, the Philippines and New Guinea.

REFERENCES

1. Boorom KF, Smith H, Nimri L, Viscogliosi E, Spanakos G, Parkar U, Li LH, Zhou XN, Ok UZ, Leelayoova S, Jones MS (2008). "Oh my aching gut: irritable bowel syndrome, Blastocystis, and asymptomatic infection". Parasit Vectors. 1 (1): 40. doi:10.1186/1756-3305-1-40. PMC 2627840Freely accessible. PMID 18937874.
2. Roberts T, Stark D, Harkness J, Ellis J (May 2014). "Update on the pathogenic potential and treatment options for Blastocystis sp". Gut Pathog. 6: 17. doi:10.1186/1757-4749-6-17. PMC 4039988Freely accessible. PMID 24883113.
3. "Seasonal prevalence of intestinal parasites in the United States during 2000" (PDF). Am. J. Trop. Med. Hyg. 66 (6): 799–803. PMID 12224595. Retrieved 3 January 2016.
4. El Safadi D, Gaayeb L, Meloni D, Cian A, Poirier P, Wawrzyniak I, Delbac F, Dabboussi F, Delhaes L, Seck M, Hamze M, Riveau G, Viscogliosi E (March 2014).
5. Cogo PE, Scaglia M, Gatti S, Rossetti F, Alaggio R, Laverda AM, et al. Fatal Naegleria fowleri Meningoencephalitis, Italy Emerging Infectious Diseases [serial on the Internet]. 2004 Oct; accessed Jan 2009
6. Bennett, Nicholas John State University of New York Upstate Medical University Domachowske, Joseph; Khan, Asad A Louisiana State University Health Science Center; King, John W; Cross, J Thomas Naegleria eMedicine; accessed Jan 2009
7. Flegr J, Prandota J, Sovičková M, Israili ZH (March 2014). "Toxoplasmosis--a global threat. Correlation of latent toxoplasmosis with specific disease burden in a set of 88 countries". PLoS ONE. 9 (3): e90203. doi:10.1371/journal.pone.0090203.
8. Pappas, G; Roussos, N; Falagas, ME (October 2009). "Toxoplasmosis snapshots: global status of Toxoplasma gondii seroprevalence and implications for pregnancy and congenital toxoplasmosis.". International Journal for Parasitology. 39 (12): 1385–94. doi:10.1016/j.ijpara.2009.04.003. PMID 19433092.
9. Yılmaza, Hasan; Gödekmerdan, Ahmet Human fasciolosis in Van province, Turkey doi:10.1016/j.actatropica.2004.04.009

CHAPTER 7

Neglected Parasites

Chapter Contents

INTRODUCTION

Structural parasitology is the study of the structures of proteins of parasites. It applies the techniques of structural biology (such as X-ray crystallography or NMR) to determine the 3-D structures of protein molecules involved in a parasitic relationship. One goal is to distinguish the workings of functional pathways in these organisms in comparison to humans. More importantly, it is hoped that structures of parasite proteins will lead to faster discovery of drugs for diseases neglected by pharmaceutical companies.

This is a challenging field because parasite proteins are often more difficult to express using a heterologous system. The challenge is particularly great for proteins from eukaryotic parasites.

Parasites of interest include Plasmodium, Trypanosoma, Leishmania, Giardia, Entamoeba, Cryptosporidium, Helminth and Toxoplasma, many of which are agents for Neglected Diseases are:

NEGLECTED TROPICAL DISEASES

Neglected tropical diseases (NTDs) are a diverse group of tropical infections which are especially common in low-income populations in developing regions of Africa, Asia, and the

Americas. They are caused by a variety of pathogens such as viruses, bacteria, protozoa and helminths. These diseases are contrasted with the big three diseases (HIV/AIDS, tuberculosis, and malaria), which generally receive greater treatment and research funding. In sub-Saharan Africa, the impact of these diseases as a group is comparable to malaria and tuberculosis. NTD co-infection can also make HIV/AIDS and tuberculosis more deadly. In some cases, the treatments are relatively inexpensive. For example, the treatment for schistosomiasis is US$0.20 per child per year.Nevertheless, control of neglected diseases is estimated to require funding of between US$2 billion to US$3 billion over the next five to seven years. Some pharmaceutical companies have committed to donating all the drug therapies required, and mass drug administration (for example mass deworming) has been successfully accomplished in several countries. However, preventative measures are often more accessible in the developed world, but not universally available in poorer areas. Within developed countries, neglected tropical diseases affect the very poorest in society. In the United States, there are up to 1.46 million families in poverty, with 2.8 million children living on less than two dollars a day. In countries such as these, the burdens of neglected tropical diseases are often overshadowed by other public health issues. However, many of the same issues put populations at risk in developed as developing nations. For example, from poverty stem problems such as lack of adequate housing, thus exposing individuals to the vectors of these diseases. Seventeen neglected tropical diseases are prioritized by WHO, though other organizations define NTDs differently. These diseases are common in 149 countries, affecting more than 1.4 billion people (including more than 500 million children) and costing developing economies billions of dollars every year. They resulted in 142,000 deaths in 2013—down from 204,000 deaths in 1990.Of these 17, two were targeted for eradication (dracunculiasis (guinea-worm disease) by 2015 and yaws by 2020), and four for elimination (blinding trachoma, human African trypanosomiasis, leprosy and lymphatic filariasis by 2020).

List of Diseases

There is some debate among the WHO, CDC, and infectious disease experts over which diseases are classified as neglected tropical diseases. Feasey, a researcher in neglected tropical diseases, notes 13 neglected tropical diseases: ascariasis, Buruli ulcer, Chagas disease, dracunculiasis, hookworm infection, human African trypanosomiasis, Leishmaniasis, leprosy, lymphatic filariasis, onchocerciasis, schistosomiasis, trachoma, and trichuriasis. Fenwick recognizes 12 "core" neglected tropical diseases: ascariasis, Buruli ulcer, Chagas disease, dracunculiasis, human African trypanosomiasis, Leishmaniasis, leprosy, lymphatic filariasis, onchocerciasis, schistosomiasis, trachoma, and trichuriasis.

These diseases result from four different classes of causative pathogens: (i) protozoa (for Chagas disease, human African trypanosomiasis, leishmaniases); (ii) bacteria (for Buruli ulcer, leprosy, trachoma, yaws), (iii) helminths or metazoan worms (for cysticercosis/taeniasis, dracunculiasis, echinococcosis, foodborne trematodiases, lymphatic filariasis, onchocerciasis, schistosomiasis, soil-transmitted helminthiasis); and (iv) viruses (dengue and chikungunya, rabies). The World Health Organization recognizes the seventeen diseases below as neglected tropical diseases.

<table>
<tr><th>WHO/CDC</th><th>PLOS
Major NTDs</th><th>Others</th></tr>
<tr><td>Buruli Ulcer
Chagas disease
Dengue & Chikungunya*
Dracunculiasis
Echinococcosis
Yaws
Fascioliasis
African trypanosomiasis
Leishmaniasis
Leprosy
Lymphatic filariasis
Onchocerciasis
Rabies
Schistosomiasis
Soil-transmitted helminthiasis
Cysticercosis
Trachoma</td><td>Protozoan infections:
• Amebiasis
• Balantidiasis
• Chagas Disease
• Giardiasis
• Human African Trypanosomiasis
• Leishmaniasis
Helminth infections:
• Taeniasis-Cysticercosis
• Dracunculiasis
• Echinococcosis
• Food-borne Trematodiases
• Loiasis
• Lymphatic Filariasis
• Onchocerciasis
• Schistosomiasis
• Soil-transmitted Helminthiases: Ascariasis
• Hookworm Diseases: Trichuriasis, Strongyloidiasis
• Toxocariasis and other Larva Migrans
Viral infections:
• Dengue
• Japanese encephalitis
• Jungle yellow fever
• Other arboviral infections
• Rabies
• Rift Valley fever
• Viral hemorrhagic fevers
Bacterial infections:
• Bartonella
• Bovine Tuberculosis in Humans
• Buruli Ulcer
• Cholera
• Enteric pathogens, Shigella, Salmonella, E. coli
• Leprosy
• Leptospirosis
• Relapsing Fever
• Trachoma
• Treponematoses: Bejel, Pinta, Syphilis, Yaws
Fungal infections:
• Mycetoma
• Paracoccidiomycosis
Ectoparasitic infections:
• Scabies
• Myiasis</td><td>Podoconiosis</td></tr>
<tr><td>* Only WHO</td><td></td><td></td></tr>
</table>

Buruli ulcer

Buruli ulcer is caused by the bacterium *Mycobacterium ulcerans*. It is related to the family of organisms that cause tuberculosis and leprosy, but *Mycobacterium ulcerans* produces a toxin, mycolactone, that destroys tissue. The prevalence of Buruli ulcer is unknown. The risk of mortality is low, although secondary infections can be lethal. Morbidity takes the form of deformity, disability, and skin lesions, which can be prevented through early treatment and treated with antibiotics and surgery. It is found in Africa, Asia, and Latin America.

Chagas Disease

Chagas disease is also known as American trypanosomiasis. There are approximately 15 million people infected with Chagas disease. The chance of morbidity is higher for immuno-compromised individuals, children, and elderly, but very low if treated early. Chagas disease does not kill victims rapidly, instead causing years of debilitating chronic symptoms. It is caused by a vector-borne protozoa and spread by contact with *Trypanosoma cruzi* infected feces of the triatomine (assassin) bug. The protozoan can enter the body via the bug›s bite, skin breaks, or mucous membranes. Infection can result from eating infected food and coming into contact with contaminated bodily fluids. There are two phases of Chagas disease. The acute phase is usually asymptomatic. The first symptoms are usually skin chancres, unilateral purplish orbital oedema, local lymphoadenopathies, and fever accompanied by a variety of other symptoms depending on infection site.The chronic phase occurs in 30 percent of total infections and can take three forms, which are asymptomatic (most prevalent), cardiac, and digestive lesions.

Chagas disease can be prevented by avoiding insect bites through insecticide spraying, home improvement, bed nets, hygienic food, medical care, laboratory practices, and testing. It can be treated etiologically or with drugs, although the drugs used to treat Chagas disease have severe side effects It can be diagnosed through a serological test, although the test is not very accurate.

Dengue and chikungunya fever

There are 50–100 million dengue virus infections annually. Dengue fever is usually not fatal, but infection with one of four serotypes can increase later susceptibility to other serotypes, resulting in a potentially fatal disease called severe dengue.Dengue fever is caused by a flavivirus, and is spread mostly by the bite of the *A. Aegypti* mosquito. No treatment for either dengue or severe dengue exists beyond palliative care. The symptoms are high fever and flu-like symptoms. It is found in Asia, Latin America, and Northern Australia.

Chikungunya is an arboviral disease transmitted by *A. albopictus* and *A. aegypti* mosquitoes. The virus was first isolated form an outbreak in Tanzania in 1952. Chikungunya virus is a member of the genus Alphavirus and family Togaviridae. The word chikungunya is from the Makonde which means "that which bends up," and this refers to the effect of the debilitating joint pain on the patient. The symptoms can be confused with dengue and include fever, rash, joint pain, and swelling. The disease mainly occurs in Africa and Asia.

Dracunculiasis

Dracunculiasis is also known as Guinea-worm disease. There were 126 cases of dracunculiasis in 2014, a decrease from 542 cases in 2012, and a substantial decrease from 3,500,000 cases in 1986. It is not fatal, but can cause months of inactivity. It is caused by drinking water contaminated by water fleas infected with guinea-worm larvae. Approximately one year after infection, a painful blister forms and one or more worm emerges. Worms can be up to one meter long.

It is usually treated by World Health Organization volunteers who clean and bandage wounds caused by worms and return daily to pull the worm out a few more inches. Dracunculiasis is preventable by water filtration, immediate case identification to prevent spread of disease, health education, and treating ponds with larvicide. An eradication program has been able to reduce prevalence. As of 2014, the four endemic countries are Chad, Ethiopia, Mali, and South Sudan.

Echinococcosis

The rates of echinococcosis is higher in rural areas, and there are more than one million people infected currently.Untreated alveolar echinococcosis is fatal. It is caused by ingesting parasites in animal feces. There are two versions of the disease: cystic and alveolar. Both versions involve an asymptomatic incubation period of several years. In the cystic version, liver cysts cause abdominal pain, nausea and vomiting while cysts in the lungs cause chronic cough, chest pain, and shortness of breath. In alveolar echinococcosis, a primary cyst develops, usually in the liver, in addition to weight loss, abdominal pain, general feeling of ill health, and signs of liver failure.

Surgery and drugs can both be used to treat echinococcosis. It can be prevented by deworming dogs, sanitation, proper disposal of animal feces, health education, and livestock vaccination. Cystic echinococcosis is found in the eastern portion of the Mediterranean region, northern Africa, southern and eastern Europe, the southern portion of South America, and central Asia. Alveolar echinococcosis is found in western and northern China, Russia, Europe, and northern North America. It can be diagnosed through imaging techniques and serological tests.

Endemic Treponematoses (Yaws)

There are limited data available on the prevalence of yaws, although it primarily affects children. The mortality risk is very low, but the disease causes disfigurement and disability if untreated. The most common symptom is skin lesions. It is a chronic bacterial infection, transmitted by skin contact, and caused by treponemes. It is treated with antibiotics and can be prevented through improved hygiene and sanitation. Yaws is most prevalent in the warm, moist, tropical regions of the Americas, Africa, Asia, and the Pacific.

Foodborne Trematodiases

The foodborne trematode infections include clonorchiasis, opisthorchiasis, fascioliasis, and paragonimiasis. These infections are all zoonotic, primarily affecting domestic or wild animals, but also transmitted to humans. They are acquired by eating food, such as raw fish, contaminated with the larval stages of the parasites. At least 40 million people are thought to be infected.

Human African Trypanosomiasis

African trypanosomiasis is also known as African sleeping sickness. There are fewer than 10,000 cases currently. Human African trypanosomiasis is vector-borne, and spread through the bite of the tsetse fly. The most common symptoms are fever, headache, lymphadenopathy, nocturnal sleeping pattern, personality changes, cognitive decline, and coma. The disease is always fatal if untreated.

The current forms of treatment are highly toxic and ineffective as resistance is spreading. It is diagnosed through an inexpensive serological test.

Leishmaniasis

The three forms of leishmaniasis are visceral (Kala-azar), cutaneous, and mucocutaneous. There are an estimated 12 million people infected. It is fatal if untreated and 20,000 deaths from visceral leishmaniasis occur annually. It is a vector-borne disease that is caused by the bite of sandflies. At least 90 percent of visceral leishmaniasis occurs in Bangladesh, Brazil, Ethiopia, India, South Sudan, and Sudan. Cutaneous leishmaniasis occurs in Afghanistan, Algeria, Brazil, Colombia, Iran, Pakistan, Peru, Saudi Arabia, and Syria. Around 90 percent of mucocutaneous leishmaniasis occurs in Bolivia, Brazil, and Peru.

The only method of prevention is a vaccine that is under development and prevention of sandfly bites. Diagnosis can by made by identifying clinical signs, serological tests, or parasitological tests. Leishmaniasis can be treated with expensive medications.

Leprosy

There were 189,018 known cases of leprosy in March 2013, and 232,857 new cases were diagnosed in 2012. It is found in Angola, Brazil, Central African Republic, Democratic Republic of the Congo, India, Madagascar, Mozambique, Nepal, Tanzania. There are one to two million individuals currently disabled or disfigured due to past or present leprosy. It is caused by bacteria and transmitted through droplets from the mouth and nose of infected individuals. Leprosy causes disfigurement and physical disabilities if untreated. It is curable if treated early.

Treatment requires multidrug therapy. The BCG vaccine has some preventative effect against leprosy. Leprosy has a 5–20 year incubation period, and the symptoms are damage to the skin, nerves, eyes, and limbs.

Lymphatic filariasis

Lymphatic filariasis is also known as elephantiasis. There are approximately 120 million individuals infected and 40 million with deformities. Approximately two-thirds of cases are in Southwest Asia and one-third in Africa. Lymphatic filariasis is rarely fatal. Lymphatic filariasis has lifelong implications, such as lymphoedema of the limbs, genital disease, and painful recurrent attacks. Most people are asymptomatic, but have lymphatic damage. Up to of 40 percent of infected individuals have kidney damage. It is a vector-borne disease, caused by nematode worms that are transmitted by mosquitoes.

It can be treated with cost-effective antihelminthic treatments, and washing skin can slow or even reverse damage. It is diagnosed with a finger-prick blood test.

Onchocerciasis

Onchocerciasis is also known as "river blindness". There are 37 million people infected and prevalence is higher in rural areas. Over 99 percent of cases are in Sub-Saharan Africa. It causes blindness, skin rashes, lesions, intense itching, and skin depigmentation. It is a vector-borne disease, caused by filarial worm infected blackflies.

It can be treated with ivermectin. It can be prevented by insecticide spraying or preventative dosing with ivermectin. The symptoms are generally itching and skin lesions.

Rabies

There are two forms of rabies: furious and paralytic. There are 60,000 deaths from rabies annually. It is mostly found in Asia and Africa. There is a higher prevalence in rural areas and it disproportionately affects children. Rabies is usually fatal after symptoms develop. It is caused by a lyssavirus transmitted through wounds or bites from infected animals. The first symptoms are fever and pain near the infection site which occur after a one to three month incubation period. Furious (more common type) rabies causes hyperactivity, hydrophobia, aerophobia, and death by cardio-respiratory arrest occurs within days. Paralytic rabies causes a slow progression from paralysis to coma to death.

It can be prevented in dogs by vaccination, and cleaning and disinfecting bite wounds (post-exposure prophylaxis).Rabies is undiagnosable before symptoms develop. It can be detected through tissue testing after symptoms develop.

Schistosomiasis

There are over 200 million cases of schistosomiasis. Approximately 85 percent of cases are in sub-Saharan Africa. The disease can be fatal by causing bladder cancer and hematemesis. *Schistosoma* species have a complex life cycle that alternates between humans and freshwater snails. Infection occurs when skin comes into contact with contaminated freshwater in which the snail that carry the parasite are living. Symptoms for schistosomiasis not caused by the worms but by the body's reaction the eggs. The eggs that do not pass out of the body can become lodged in the intestine or bladder, causing inflammation or scarring. Children who are repeatedly infected can develop anemia, malnutrition and learning difficulties. The symptoms are usually haematuria, bladder obstruction, renal failure, bladder cancer, periportal fibrosis, bladder fibrosis, liver fibrosis, portal hypertension, cervical lesions, ascites, and varies.

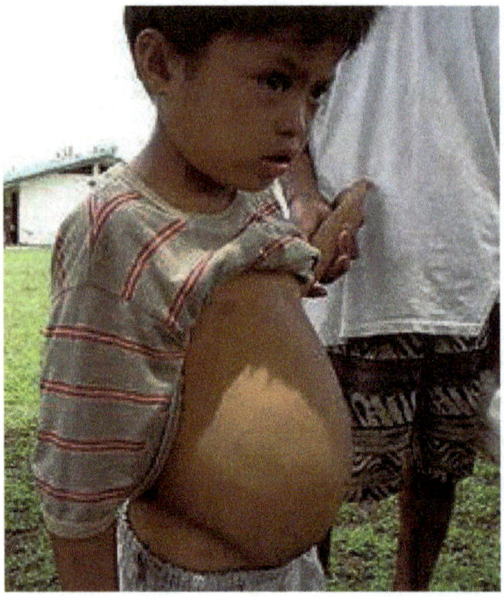

11-year-old boy with ascites and portal hypertension due to schistosomiasis (Agusan del Sur, Philippines)

Inexpensive praziquantel can be used to treat individuals with schistosomiasis, but cannot prevent reinfection. The cost of prevention is US$0.32 per child per year.Mass deworming treatment with praziquantel, better access to safe water, sanitation, health education can all be used to prevent schistosomiasis. Vaccines are under development. It can be diagnosed through a serological test, but it often produces false negatives.

Soil-transmitted Helminthiasis

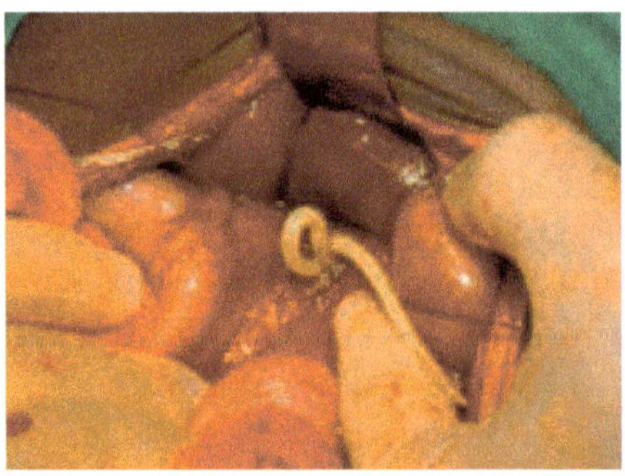

Adult ascaris worms being removed from the bile duct of a patient in South Africa

The three major worm species responsible for soil-transmitted helminthiasis are Ascaris (roundworms), Trichuris (whipworm), the hookworms *Necator americanus* and *Ancylostoma duodenale*, and *Strongyloides stercoralis*. There are 1.5 billion currently infected. Soil-transmitted heminthiasis occurs in sub-Saharan Africa, the Americas, China, and east Asia. The mortality risk is very low. The most common symptoms are anemia, stunted growth, intestinal problems, lack of energy, and compromised physical and cognitive development. Infected children often fall behind in schooling. The severity of symptoms depends on the number of worms in the body.

Parasitic worms are generally transmitted via exposure to infected human feces and soil which are spread in the environment, for example, due to open defecation. The most common treatment is medicine. It can be prevented through hygienically prepared food and clean water, improved sanitation, periodic deworming, and health education. The World Health Organisation recommends mass deworming without prior diagnosis.

Taeniasis/cysticercosis

Cysticercosis is a tapeworm larvae infection, while taeniasis is infection with adult tapeworms . Both are found in Asia, Africa, Latin America, particularly on farms in which pigs are exposed to human excrement.

Cysticercosis is the most common preventable cause of epilepsy in the developing world. Cysticercosis occurs after ingestion of contaminated food, water, or soil. Cysts and lesions can cause headaches, blindness, seizures, hydrocephalus, meningitis, and dementia. Neurocystocercosis, or the parasitic infection of the nervous system, can be fatal. Taeniasis is not fatal. It is usually contracted after eating undercooked contaminated pork. Taeniasis has mild symptoms, including abdominal pain, nausea, diarrhea, or constipation.

Drugs are used to treat both diseases. Infection can be prevented through stricter meat-inspection standards, livestock confinement, improved hygiene and sanitation, health education, safe meat preparation, and identifying and treating human and pig carriers.

Trachoma

There are 21.4 million people infected with trachoma, of whom 2.2 million are partially blind and 1.2 million are blind. It is found in Africa, Asia, Central and South America, Middle East, and Australia. The disease disproportionately affects women and children. The mortality risk is very low, although multiple re-infections eventually lead to blindness. The symptoms are internally scarred eyelids, followed by eyelids turning inward. Trachoma is caused by a micro-organism that spreads through eye discharges (on hands, cloth, etc.) and by “eye-seeking flies”.

It is treated with antibiotics. The only known prevention method is interpersonal hygiene.

Health Impact

Deworming treatment

Deworming treatments in those who are infected are correlated with healthy weight gain since worms are often partially responsible for malnutrition. Whether or not mass deworming campaigns improve long term outcomes is unclear. This included a lack of definite proof of sustained health benefits with respect to nutritional status, haemoglobin in blood and levels of school attendance or performance. To achieve health gains in the longer term, improvements in sanitation and hygiene behaviors are also required, together with deworming treatments.

Coinfection

Coinfection is a major concern with neglected tropical diseases, making NTDs more damaging than their mortality rates might portray. Because the factors that support neglected tropical diseases (poverty, inadequate healthcare, inadequate sanitation practices etc) support all NTDs, they are often found in overlapping distributions. Helminth infections, as the most common infection of humans, are often found to be in multi-infection systems. For example, in Brazil, low socioeconomic status contributes to overcrowded housing. In these same areas, connection by *Necator americanus* and *Schistosoma mansoni* is common. The impact of each worm separate weakens the immune system of those infected, making infection from the other easier and more severe. For this reason, coinfection carries a higher risk of mortality. NTDs may also play a role in infection with other diseases, such as malaria, HIV/AIDS, and tuberculosis. The ability of helminths to manipulate the immune system may create a physiological environment that could exacerbate the progression of HIV/AIDS. Some evidence from Senegal, Malawi, and Thailand has shown that helminth infections raise the risk of malarial infection.

Integration of Treatment

Inclusion of NTDs into initiatives for malaria, HIV/AIDS, and tuberculosis, as well as integration of NTD treatment programs, may have advantages given the strong link between these diseases and NTDs. Some neglected tropical diseases share common vectors (sandflies, black flies, and mosquitos). Both medicinal and vector control efforts may be combined.

A four-drug rapid-impact package has been proposed for widespread proliferation. Administration may be made more efficient by targeting multiple diseases at once, rather than separating treatment and adding work to community workers. This package is estimated to cost US$0.40 per patient. When compared to stand-alone treatment, the savings are estimated to be 26–47%. While more research must be done in order to understand how NTDs and other diseases interact in both the vector and the human stages, safety assessments have so far produced positive results.

Many neglected tropical diseases and other prevalent diseases share common vectors, creating another opportunity for treatment and control integration. One such example of this is malaria and lymphatic filariasis. Both diseases are transmitted by the same or related mosquito vectors. Vector control, through the distribution of insecticide treated nets, reduces the human contact with a wide variety of disease vectors. Integrated vector control may also alleviate pressure on mass drug administration, especially with respect to rapidly evolving drug resistance. Combining vector control and mass drug administration deemphasizes both, making each less susceptible to resistance evolution.

Economic Impact

The low cost of treatment for NTDs can be attributed to the large scale of the programs, free provision of drugs by pharmaceutical companies, delivery modes of drugs, and the un-paid volunteers who distribute the drugs. The economic burden of NTDs is undervalued and therefore the corresponding economic impact and cost-effectiveness of decreased prevalence of NTDs is underestimated. The investment return on measures to control neglected tropical diseases is estimated to be between 14–30 percent, depending on the disease and region. The long term benefits of deworming include a decrease in school absenteeism by 25 percent, and an increase in adult earnings by 20 percent.

The cost of treatment of some of these diseases, however, such as Buruli ulcer, can amount to over twice the yearly income of an average household in the lowest income quartile, while for the highest income quartile, the burden is slightly less than the average household income. These enormous financial costs often cause deferral of treatment and financial ruin, but there is inequality between the wealthy and poor in terms of economic burden. These diseases also cost the government in terms of health care and lost worker productivity through morbidity and shortened life spans. In Kenya, for example, deworming is estimated to increase average adult income by 40 percent, which is a benefit-to-cost ratio of 100. Each untreated case of Trachoma is estimated to cost US$118 in lost productivity. Each case of schistosomiasis causes a loss of 45.4 days of work per year. Most of the diseases cost the economies of various developing countries millions of dollars. Large scale prevention campaigns are predicted to increase agricultural output and education levels.

Social Impact

Social Stigma

Several NTDs, such as leprosy, cause severe deformities that result in social stigma. Stigma is considered to be the 'hidden burden' of neglected tropical diseases, and is not accounted for in measures such as DALYs. Other NTDs that carry heavy social stigma include onchocerciasis, lymphatic filariasis, plague, Buruli ulcer, leishmaniasis, and Chagas disease.Lymphatic filariasis, for example, causes severe deformities that can result in denial of marriage and inability to work.Studies in Ghana and Sri Lanka have demonstrated that support groups for patients with lymphatic filariasis can increase participants' self-esteem, quality of life, and social relations through social support and providing practical advice on how to manage their illness. The social effects of neglected tropical diseases have been shown to affect men and women in different ways. Men are socially stigmatized in a way that detrimentally affects their economic prospects. Women are more likely to be affected in the areas of marriage and family.

Effect on Mental Health

A 2012 review found that infection with a neglect tropical disease predisposes individuals to poor mental health. This is partially due to the social stigma that surround NTDs, but is also likely caused by the subsequent lack of access to health and social services. Overall, being a member of the infected community was found to cut individuals off from multiple aspects of society via civic rights, educational opportunities, and employment. The authors suggest that more research be directed into the psychological aspects of neglected tropical diseases in order to fully untangle their co-effects.

Gender

The impact of NTDs is tied to gender in some situations. NTDs disproportionately affect females. This is especially true in the cases of schistosomiasis, dengue, hookworm, and Chagas disease. There is also the added risk of hookworm infection during pregnancy and the potential to transfer diseases such as Chagas during pregnancy. A study in Uganda found that women were more easily able to obtain treatment because they had fewer occupational responsibilities than men and were more trusting of treatment, but ignorance of the effects of medicines on pregnant women prevented adequate care. The paper concludes that gender should be considered when designing treatment programs. Additionally, women often bear a heavier social stigma in relation to the pressure to marry.

School Attendance

Deworming treatment is correlated with increased school attendance, which has long lasting impacts. Schools are a focal point in the fight against neglected tropical diseases, as they are often used as centers for the distribution of treatment. One study of such a school found that boys were enrolled in primary school for more years than boys who were in schools that did not offer such programs. Girls in the same study were about a quarter more likely to attend secondary school if they received past treatment. Both groups went on to participate in more skilled sectors of the labor market. The economic growth generated from school programs such as this may balance out the actual expenses of the program.

Reasons for Neglect

This group of diseases has been overlooked because they mainly affect the poorest countries of the developing world and because of recent emphasis on decreasing the prevalence of HIV/AIDS, tuberculosis, and malaria. Far more resources are given to the "big three" diseases (HIV/AIDS, malaria, and tuberculosis) because of their higher mortality and public awareness rates. Neglected tropical diseases do not have a prominent cultural figure to champion the cause.

The importance of neglected tropical diseases has been underestimated since many are asymptomatic and have long incubation periods. The connection between a death and a neglected tropical disease that has been latent for a long period of time is not often realized. Areas of high endemicity are often in geographically isolated areas, making treatment and prevention much more difficult.

Stigma

Additionally, neglected tropical diseases are often associated with some kind of social stigma, making their treatment more complex. Public health research has only recently begun to focus on stigma as a component of the issue. From the 1960s onward, approximately one citation a year related to social stigma. In 2006, there were 458. Disease control is greatly affected by this stigma, as it decreases help-seeking and treatment adherence. Disease control programs, starting as early as the 1980s, have begun to integrate stigma mitigation into their offerings. In India, the leprosy program prioritized the message that “leprosy is curable, not hereditary” in order to inspire optimism in highly affected communities. The goal was to make leprosy a disease “like any other,” so as to reduce stigma. Supplementally, the medical resources available in the area were optimized in order to fulfill the curable promise made.

Economic Incentives

One reason for neglect for these disease is that they are not commercial and consequently patents and profit play no role in stimulating innovation. Like all non-commercial areas, these diseases are the responsibility of governments and philanthropy (including industry philanthropy). Currently, the pharmaceutical industry views research and development as highly risky. For this reason, resources are not often put into the field of NTDs (as diseases of the poor) and new chemical products are often expensive. A review of public and private initiatives found that of the 1393 new chemical products that were marketed in the period of 1975 and 1999, just 16 related to tropical diseases and tuberculosis. The same review additionally found that there was a 13-fold greater chance of a drug entering the marking being for central-nervous-system disorders and cancer than an NTD.

Due to lack of incentive in the pharmaceutical industry, successful NTD treatment programs have often relied on the donation format. The Mectizan Donation Program has donated over 1800 million tablets of ivermectin. While often developed countries will rely on government-run and private partnerships to fund such projects, developing nations frequently have significantly lower per head per annum spending on these diseases.

Developed Nations

In developed nations, neglected tropical disease also pose a threat to human health. In the United States alone, there are at least 12 million people suffering from these neglected parasitic infections. They make up a hidden disease burden among the poorest of wealthy societies. In developed nations, lack of knowledge in the healthcare industry and few conclusive diagnostic tests perpetuate the neglect of this group of diseases.

In the United States, high rates of parasitic infection can be found to be distributed along geographic, racial, and socio-economic lines. Within the African-American community, there may be up to 2.8 million cases of toxocariasis. Rates of toxocariasis, trichomoniasis, and other neglected infections occur in the United States at the same rate as Nigeria. Within the Hispanic community, neglected infections are concentrated near the US-Mexico border. Vector-born illnesses are especially high, with some rates approaching those of Latin America. Chagas disease was found in the US as early as the 1970s.However, in the developed world, diseases that are associated with poverty are often not addressed as comprehensively as they should be. This may be due to lack of economic incentives and public policy failings. Here, a lack of awareness prevents effective policy generation and leaves health care services unequipped to address the issue. Additionally, there is little effort put into taking and maintaining large data sets on neglected disease in the United States and other developed nations. The first summit on the issue was held by the Adler Institute on Social Exclusion in the United States in 2009.

In Europe, a similar trend is seen. Neglected tropical diseases are concentrated in eastern and southern Europe, where poverty levels are the highest. The most prevalent diseases in this region are ascariasis, trichuriasis, zoonotic helminth infections, and visceral leishmaniasis. Migration paths to Europe, most notably to Spain, have brought diseases to Europe as well. As many as 6,000 cases of Chagas disease have been introduced via this method. In response to a growing awareness to the burden on these populations, the European Centre for Disease Prevention and Control has laid out ten public health guidelines. They cover a variety of topics, from health education and promotion to community partnerships and the development of a minority healthcare workforce.

Prevention

Prevention and eradication are important because "of the appalling stigma, disfigurement, blindness and disabilities caused by NTDs." The possibility of eliminating or eradicating dracunculiasis, leprosy, lymphatic filariasis, onchocerciasis, trachoma, sleeping sickness, visceral leishmaniasis, and canine rabies within the next ten years was the principal aim of the London Declaration on Neglected Tropical Diseases, which is a collaborative effort involving the WHO, the World Bank, the Bill & Melinda Gates Foundation, the world›s 13 leading pharmaceutical companies, and government representatives from US, UK, United Arab Emirate, Bangladesh, Brazil, Mozambique and Tanzania. It was launched in January 2012.

While the current era has had a noticeable uptick in biological research in to neglected tropical diseases, prevention may be supplemented by social and development outreach. Spiegal and his coauthors advocated for this to take the form of "social offset." Social offset entails the delegation of some of the funding for biotechnological research to social programs. The attempts to alleviate some of the surrounding factors (such as poverty, poor sanitation, overcrowding, poor healthcare etc) that greatly exacerbate the conditions brought on by neglected tropical diseases. Projects such as these also strengthen the goal of sustained eliminations, rather than quickly addressing symptoms.

Policy Initiatives

There are many prevention and eradication campaigns funded for example by the World

Health Organization, US Agency for International Development, Bill and Melinda Gates Foundation, UK Department for International Development.

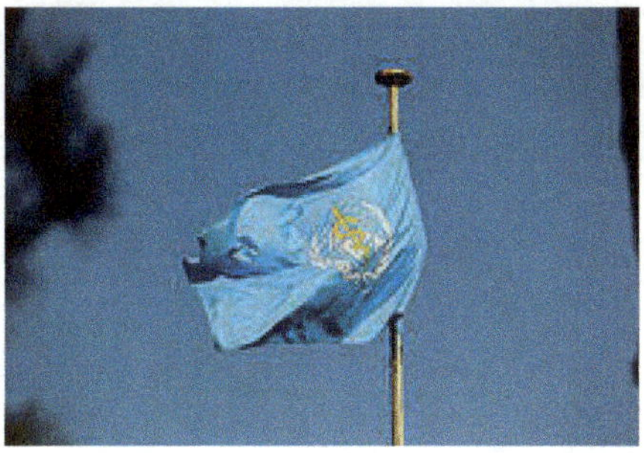

Flag of the World Health Organization (WHO)

WHO Roadmap of 2012

WHO published in 2012 the NTD "roadmap" which contains milestones for 2015 and 2020 and which specifies targets for eradication, elimination, and intensified control of the different NTDs. For example:

- NTDs planned to be eradicated: dracunculiasis (by the year 2015), endemic treponematoses (yaws) (by 2020)
- NTDs planned to be eliminated globally by 2020: blinding trachoma, leprosy, human African trypanosomiasis, lymphatic filariasis
- NTDs planned to be eliminated in certain regions: rabies (by 2015 in Latin America, by 2020 in Southeast Asia and western Pacific regions), chagas disease (transmission through blood transfusion by 2015, intra-domiciliary transmission by 2020 in the region of the Americas), visceral leishmaniasis (by 2020 in the Indian subcontinent), oncocerciasis (by 2015 in Latin America), schistosomiasis (by 2015 in eastern Mediterranean region, Caribbean, Indonesia and the Mekong River basin, by 2020 in the region of the Americas and western Pacific region)
- NTDs planned to be eliminated in certain countries: human African trypanosomiasis (by 2015 in 80 percent of areas in which it occurs), oncocerciasis (by 2015 in Yemen, by 2020 in selected countries in Africa), schistosomiasis (by 2020 in selected countries in Africa)
- Intensified control with specific targets for the years 2015 and 2020 are provided for these NTDs: dengue, buruli ulcer, cutaneous leishmaniasis, taeniasis/cysticercosis and echinococcosis/hydatidosis, foodborne tremadode infections, soil-transmitted helmintheases

Others

The U.S. Food and Drug Administration priority review voucher is an incentive for companies to invest in new drugs and vaccines for tropical diseases. A provision of the Food and Drug Administration Amendments Act (HR 3580) awards a transferable "priority review voucher" to any company that obtains approval for a treatment for one of the listed diseases. The voucher can later be used to accelerate review of an unrelated drug. This program is for all tropical diseases and includes medicines for malaria and tuberculosis. The first voucher given was for Coartem, a malaria treatment. It does not use or define the term "neglected" though most of the diseases listed are often included on lists of neglected diseases.

The prize was proposed by Duke University faculty Henry Grabowski, Jeffrey Moe, and David Ridley in their 2006 *Health Affairs* paper: "Developing Drugs for Developing Countries." In 2007 United States Senators Sam Brownback (R-KS) and Sherrod Brown (D-OH) sponsored an amendment to the Food and Drug Administration Amendments Act of 2007. President George W. Bush signed the bill in September 2007.

Integration with WASH Programs

Water, sanitation, and hygiene (WASH) interventions are essential in preventing many NTDs, for example soil-transmitted helminthiasis. Mass drug administrations alone will not protect people from re-infection. A more holistic and integrated approach to NTDs and WASH efforts will benefit both sectors along with the communities they are aiming to serve. This is especially true in areas that are endemic with more than one NTD.

In August 2015 the World Health Organization unveiled a global strategy and action plan to integrate WASH with other public health interventions in order to accelerate elimination of NTDs. The plan aims to intensify control or eliminate certain NTDs in specific regions by 2020 and refers to the NTD "roadmap" milestones from 2012 that include for example eradication of dracunculiasis by 2015 and of yaws by 2020, elimination of trachoma and lymphatic filariasis as public health problems by 2020, intensified control of dengue, schistosomiasis and soil-transmitted helminthiases.

A closer collaboration between WASH and NTD programmes can lead to synergies. They can be achieved through collaborative planning, delivery and evaluation of programmes, strengthening and sharing of evidence, and using monitoring tools to improve the equity of health services.

Reasons why WASH plays an important role in NTD prevention and patient care include:

- NTDs affect more than one billion people in 149 countries. They occur mainly in regions with a lack of basic sanitation. About 2.4 billion people worldwide do not have adequate sanitation facilities. 663 million do not have access to improved drinking water sources.
- One leading cause of preventable blindness is trachoma. The bacterial infection is transmitted through contact with eye-seeking flies, fingers, and fomites. Prevention components are facial cleanliness which requires water for face washing and environmental improvement which includes safe disposal of excreta to reduce fly populations.
- Improved sanitation prevents soil-transmitted helminthiases. It impedes fecal pathogens such as intestinal worm eggs from contaminating the environment

and infecting people through contaminated food, water, dirty hands, and direct skin contact with the soil.

- Improved sanitation and water management can contribute to reduce proliferation of mosquitoes that transmit diseases, such as lymphatic filariasis, dengue and chikungunya. Breeding of the *Culex* mosquito which transmits filarial parasites is facilitated through poorly constructed latrines. Breeding of the *Aedes aegypti* and *Aedes albopictus* mosquitoes which transmit dengue and chikungunya can be prevented through safe storage of water.
- Feces and urine which contain worm eggs can contaminate surface water and lead to transmission of schistosomiasis. This can be prevented through improved sanitation. Not only human but also animal (cow, buffalo) urine or feces can transmit some schistosome species. Therefore, it is important to protect freshwater from animals and animal waste.
- Treatment of many NTDs require clean water and hygienic condition for healthcare facilities and households. For guinea worm, Buruli ulcer, or cutaneous leishmaniasis, wound management is needed to speed up healing and reduce disability. Lymphatic filariasis causes chronic disabilities. People who suffer from this disease need to maintain rigorous personal hygiene with water and soap to prevent secondary infections.
- NTDs that lead to permanent disabilities make tasks such as carrying water long distances or accessing toilets difficult. However, people affected by these diseases often face stigma and can be excluded from accessing water and sanitation facilities. This increases their risk of poverty and severe illness. Clean water and soap are essential for these groups to maintain personal hygiene and dignity. Therefore, additional efforts to reduce stigma and exclusion are needed. In this manner, WASH can improve quality of life of people affected by NTDs.
- In a meta-analysis safe water was associated with significantly reduced odds of *Schistosoma* infection, and adequate sanitation was associated with significantly lower odds of infection with both *S. mansoni* and *S. haematobium*.
- A systematic review and meta-analysis showed that better hygiene in children is associated with lower odds of trachoma. Access to sanitation was associated with 15 percent lower odds of active trachoma and 33 percent lower odds of *C. trachomatis* infection of the eyes.
- Another systematic review and meta-analysis found a correlation between WASH access and practices and lower odds of soil-transmitted helminthiasis infections by 33 to 77 percent. Persons who washed their hands after defecating were less than half as likely to be infected as those who did not. Traditionally, preventive chemotherapy is used as a measure of control, although this measure does not stop the transmission cycle and cannot prevent reinfection. In contrast, improved sanitation can.

Pharmaceutical Market

Biotechnology companies in the developing world have targeted neglected tropical diseases due to need to improve global health.

Mass drug administration is considered a possible method for eradication, especially for lymphatic filariasis, onchocerciasis, and trachoma, although drug resistance is a potential problem. According to Fenwick, Pfizer donated 70 million doses of drugs in 2011 to eliminate trachoma through the International Trachoma Initiative. Merck has helped The African Programme for the Control of Onchocerciasis (APOC) and Oncho Elimination Programme for the Americas to greatly diminished the impact of Onchocerciasis by donating ivermectin. Merck KGaA pledged to give 200 million tablets of praziquantel over 10 years, the only cure for schistosomiasis. GlaxoSmithKline has donated two billion tablets of medicine for lymphatic filariasis and pledged 400 million deworming tablets per year for five years in 2010. Johnson & Johnson has pledged 200 million deworming tablets per year. Novartis has pledged leprosy treatment, EISAI pledged two billion tablets to help treat lymphatic filariasis.

NGO Initiatives

There are currently only two donor-funded non-governmental organizations that focus exclusively on NTDs: the Schistosomiasis Control Initiative and Deworm the World. Despite under-funding, many neglected diseases are cost-effective to treat and prevent. The cost of treating a child for infection of soil transmitted helminths and schistosomes (some of the main causes of neglected diseases), is less than US$0.50 per year, when administered as part of school-based mass deworming by Deworm the World. This programme is recommended by Giving What We Can and the Copenhagen Consensus Centre as one of the most efficient and cost-effective solutions. The efforts of Schistosomiasis Control Initiative to combat neglected diseases include the use of rapid impact packages: supplying schools with packages including four or five drugs, and training teachers in how to administer them.

Public-private Initiatives

An alternative model to the profit-driven drug development emerged in the years 2000 to provide an answer to the needs of these neglected patients. Product development partnerships (PDPs) aim at implementing and accelerating the research and development (R&D) of safe and effective health tools (diagnostics, vaccines, drugs) to notably combat diseases that are neglected. Drugs for Neglected Diseases *initiative* (DNDi) is one of these PDPs that has already developed new treatments for NTDs

The Sabin Vaccine Institute, founded in 1993, works to address the issues of vaccine-preventable diseases as well as NTDs. They run three main programs, Sabin Vaccine Development, Global Network for Neglected Tropical Diseases, and Vaccine Advocacy and Education. Their product development partnership affiliates them with the Texas Children›s Hospital as well as the Baylor College of Medicine. Their major campaign, End7, aims to end seven of the most common NTDs (elephantiasis, river blindness, snail fever, trachoma, roundworm, whipworm and hookworm) by 2020. Through End7, college campuses undertake fundraising and educational initiatives for the broader goals of the campaign.

WIPO Re:Search was established in 2011 by the World Intellectual Property Organization in collaboration with BIO Ventures for Global Health (BVGH) and with the active participation of leading pharmaceutical companies and other private and public sector research organizations. It allows organizations to share their intellectual property, compounds, expertise, facilities and know-how royalty-free with qualified researchers worldwide working on new solutions for NTDs, malaria and tuberculosis.

In 2013, the Government of Japan, five Japanese pharmaceutical companies, the Bill and Melinda Gates Foundation, and the UNDP established a new public-private partnership, Global Health Innovative Technology Fund. They pledged over US$100 million to the fund over five years, to be awarded as grants to R&D partnerships across sectors in Japan and elsewhere, working to develop new drugs and vaccines for 17 neglected diseases, in addition to HIV, malaria and tuberculosis.Affordability of the resulting drugs and vaccines is one of the key criteria for grant awards.

Others

An open-access journal dedicated to neglected tropical diseases called *PLOS Neglected Tropical Diseases* first began publication in 2007.

One of the first large-scale initiatives to address NTDs came from a collaboration between Kenneth Warren and the Rockefeller Foundation. Ken Warren is regarded as one of the founding figures in neglected tropical disease research. The Great Neglected Tropical Diseases Network was a consortium of scientists from all over the world, hand picked by Ken Warren, working to expand the research base in neglected diseases. Many of the scientists that he recruited had not been involved in NTD research before. The network ran from 1978 to 1988. Warren›s vision was to establish units within biological labs across the world, dedicated to R&D. By forming a critical mass of scientists in NTD research, he hoped to attract new students into the field. The interdisciplinary group met annually to update the community on research progress. Much of the work done by this group focused on the understanding of the mechanisms behind infection. At these informally structured meetings, research partnerships were formed. Warren himself encouraged these partnerships, especially if they bridged the divide between developed and developing nations. Through the Great Neglected Tropical Disease Network, a great number of scientists were brought into the field of parasitology.

Epidemiology

The six most common NTDs include soil-transmitted helminths (STHs)—specifically roundworm (*Ascaris lumbricoides*), whipworm (*Trichuris trichiura*) and hookworms (*Necator americanus* and *Ancylostoma duodenale*)—schistosomiasis, trachoma, and lymphatic filariasis (LF). These diseases affect one-sixth of the world's population with 90 percent of the disease burden occurring in sub-Saharan Africa.

Information on the frequency of neglected tropical diseases is of low quality. It is currently difficult to summarize all of the information on this family of diseases. One effort to do so is the Global Burden of Disease framework. It aims to create a standardized method of measurement. The principle components of the approach involve 1) the measuring of premature mortality as well as disability, 2) the standardized usage of DALYs (disability-adjusted life years), and 3) wide spread inclusion of diseases and injury causes with the estimation of missing data. However, the DALY has been criticized as a 'systematic undervaluation' of disease burden. King asserts that the DALY emphasizes the individual too much, while ignoring the effects of the ecology of the disease. In order for the measure to become more valid, it may gave to take the context of poverty more into account. King also emphasizes that DALYs may not capture the non-linear effects of poverty on cost-utility analysis of disease control.

Many academic labs around the world study structural parasitology. Two groups in particular have contributed many parasite structures: the SGPP (Structural Genomnics of Pathogenic Protozoa) and the SGC (Structural Genomics Consortium).

REFERENCES

1. Hotez PJ (November 2013). "NTDs V.2.0: "blue marble health"—neglected tropical disease control and elimination in a shifting health policy landscape". PLoS Negl Trop Dis. 7 (11): e2570. doi:10.1371/journal.pntd.0002570. PMC 3836998Freely accessible. PMID 24278496.
2. Hotez PJ, Kamath A (2009). Cappello, Michael, ed. "Neglected Tropical Diseases in Sub-Saharan Africa: Review of Their Prevalence, Distribution, and Disease Burden". PLoS Negl Trop Dis. 3 (8): e412. doi:10.1371/journal.pntd.0000412. PMC 2727001Freely accessible. PMID 19707588.
3. Mike Shanahan (31 January 2006). "Beat neglected diseases to fight HIV, TB and malaria". SciDev.Net.
4. "Making the Case to Fight Schistosomiasis". National Public Radio. Retrieved 2008-12-01.
5. Hotez PJ (January 2010). "How To Cure 1 Billion People? — Defeat Neglected Tropical diseases". Scientific America. 302 (1): 90–4, 96. doi:10.1038/scientificamerican0110-90. PMID 20063641.
6. Reddy M, Gill SS, Kalkar SR, Wu W, Anderson PJ, Rochon PA (October 2007). "Oral drug therapy for multiple neglected tropical diseases: a systematic review". JAMA. 298 (16): 1911–24. doi:10.1001/jama.298.16.1911. PMID 17954542.
7. Hotez, Peter (2009-11-01). "Neglected Diseases Amid Wealth In The United States And Europe". Health Affairs. 28 (6): 1720–1725. doi:10.1377/hlthaff.28.6.1720. ISSN 0278-2715.
8. Hotez, Peter (2012). "Fighting neglected tropical diseases in the southern United States". BMJ. Houston, Texas.
9. GBD 2013 Mortality and Causes of Death, Collaborators (17 December 2014). "Global, regional, and national age-sex specific all-cause and cause-specific mortality for 240 causes of death, 1990-2013: a systematic analysis for the Global Burden of Disease Study 2013.". Lancet. 385 (9963): 117–71. doi:10.1016/S0140-6736(14)61682-2. PMC 4340604Freely accessible. PMID 25530442.

10. Feasey N, Wansbrough-Jones M, Mabey DC, Solomon AW (2010). "Neglected tropical diseases". Br. Med. Bull. 93 (1): 179–200. doi:10.1093/bmb/ldp046. PMID 20007668.

11. Fenwick A (March 2012). "The global burden of neglected tropical diseases". Public Health. 126 (3): 233–6. doi:10.1016/j.puhe.2011.11.015. PMID 22325616.

12. "PLOS Neglected Tropical Diseases". journals.plos.org. Retrieved 2016-10-30.

13. Korevaar, D. A.; Visser, B. J. (2012-06-01). "Podoconiosis, a neglected tropical disease". The Netherlands Journal of Medicine. 70 (5): 210–214. ISSN 1872-9061. PMID 22744921.

14. Pialoux, Gilles; Gaüzère, Bernard-Alex; Jauréguiberry, Stéphane; Strobel, Michel (2007-05-01). "Chikungunya, an epidemic arbovirosis". The Lancet. Infectious Diseases. 7 (5): 319–327. doi:10.1016/S1473-3099(07)70107-X. ISSN 1473-3099. PMID 17448935.

15. "Dracunculiasis eradication — global surveillance summary, 2009" (PDF). Wkly. Epidemiol. Rec. World Health Organization. 85 (19): 166–76. May 2010. PMID 20449943.

16. Mohammed KA, Hail HJ, Gabrielli AF, et al. (2008). Utzinger J, ed. "Triple Co-Administration of Ivermectin, Albendazole and Praziquantel in Zanzibar: A Safety Study". PLoS Negl Trop Dis. 2 (1): e171. doi:10.1371/journal.pntd.0000171. PMC 2217668Freely accessible. PMID 18235853. open access publication - free to read

17. "Schistosomiasis-Disease". CDC, Division of Parasitic Diseases. Retrieved "Signs, symptoms and treatment of taeniasis/cysticercosis". Retrieved 13 March 2014.

18. Taylor-Robinson, DC; Maayan, N; Soares-Weiser, K; Donegan, S; Garner, P (14 November 2012). "Deworming drugs for soil-transmitted intestinal worms in children: effects on nutritional indicators, haemoglobin and school performance.". The Cochrane database of systematic reviews. 11: CD000371. doi:10.1002/14651858.CD000371.pub5. PMID 23152203.

19. Lindoso, Jos A.L.; Lima, Ana C.S.; Cunha, Mirella A.; Gomes, Claudia M.C. (2015-08-23). "Diagnosing Neglected Tropical Diseases in HIV Coinfection". Human Parasitic Diseases. 2015 (7): 11. doi:10.4137/HPD.S19569. replacement character in |first= at position 4 (help)

20. Singer, Merrill; Bulled, Nicola (2012-11-01). "Interlocked Infections: The Health Burdens of Syndemics of Neglected Tropical Diseases". Annals of Anthropological Practice. 36 (2): 328–345. doi:10.1111/napa.12007. ISSN 2153-9588.

21. Brady, Molly A.; Hooper, Pamela J.; Ottesen, Eric A. "Projected benefits from integrating NTD programs in sub-Saharan Africa". Trends in Parasitology. 22 (7): 285–291. doi:10.1016/j.pt.2006.05.007.

22. van den Berg, Henk; Kelly-Hope, Louise A.; Lindsay, Steve W. (2013-01-01). "Malaria and lymphatic filariasis: the case for integrated vector management". The Lancet. Infectious Diseases. 13 (1): 89–94. doi:10.1016/S1473-3099(12)70148-2. ISSN 1474-4457. PMID 23084831.

23. Conteh L, Engels T, Molyneux DH (January 2010). "Socioeconomic aspects of neglected tropical diseases". Lancet. 375 (9710): 239–47. doi:10.1016/S0140-6736(09)61422-7. PMID 20109925.
24. Molyneux DH (2004). ""Neglected" diseases but unrecognised successes—challenges and opportunities for infectious disease control". Lancet. 364 (9431): 380–3. doi:10.1016/S0140-6736(04)16728-7. PMID 15276399.
25. Weiss MG (2008). "Stigma and the social burden of neglected tropical diseases". PLoS Negl Trop Dis. 2 (5): e237. doi:10.1371/journal.pntd.0000237. PMC 2359851Freely accessible. PMID 18478049. open access publication - free to read
26. Litt, Elizabeth; Baker, Margaret C.; Molyneux, David (2012-05-01). "Neglected tropical diseases and mental health: a perspective on comorbidity". Trends in Parasitology. 28 (5): 195–201. doi:10.1016/j.pt.2012.03.001. ISSN 1471-5007. PMID 22475459.
27. Rilkoff H, Tukahebwa EM, Fleming FM, Leslie J, Cole DC (2013). "Exploring gender dimensions of treatment programmes for neglected tropical diseases in Uganda". PLoS Negl Trop Dis. 7 (7): e2312. doi:10.1371/journal.pntd.0002312. PMC 3708858Freely accessible. PMID 23875047. open access publication - free to read
28. Hotez, Peter; Ottesen, Eric; Fenwick, Alan; Molyneux, David (2006-01-01). "The neglected tropical diseases: the ancient afflictions of stigma and poverty and the prospects for their control and elimination". Advances in Experimental Medicine and Biology. 582: 23–33. doi:10.1007/0-387-33026-7_3. ISSN 0065-2598. PMID 16802616.
29. Payne, Lara; Fitchett, Joseph R. (2010-09-01). "Bringing neglected tropical diseases into the spotlight". Trends in Parasitology. 26 (9): 421–423. doi:10.1016/j.pt.2010.06.002. ISSN 1471-5007. PMID 20591739.
30. Weiss, Mitchell G. (2008-01-01). "Stigma and the social burden of neglected tropical diseases". PLoS neglected tropical diseases. 2 (5): e237. doi:10.1371/journal.pntd.0000237. ISSN 1935-2735. PMC 2359851Freely accessible. PMID 18478049.
31. http://www.ft.com/intl/cms/s/0/07bfe8f2-5e05-11e4-bc04-00144feabdc0.html#axzz3MMnaQdHZ
32. Trouiller, Patrice; Olliaro, Piero; Torreele, Els; Orbinski, James; Laing, Richard; Ford, Nathan (2002-06-22). "Drug development for neglected diseases: a deficient market and a public-health policy failure". Lancet (London, England). 359 (9324): 2188–2194. doi:10.1016/S0140-6736(02)09096-7. ISSN 0140-6736. PMID 12090998.
33. Colatrella, B. (2008-09-01). "The Mectizan Donation Program: 20 years of successful collaboration - a retrospective". Annals of Tropical Medicine and Parasitology. 102 Suppl 1: 7–11. doi:10.1179/136485908X337418. ISSN 0003-4983. PMID 18718147.
34. Hotez, Peter J. (2014-09-04). "Neglected Parasitic Infections and Poverty in the United States". PLOS Negl Trop Dis. 8 (9): e3012. doi:10.1371/journal.

pntd.0003012. ISSN 1935-2735. PMC 4154650Freely accessible. PMID 25188455.

35. World Health Organization (WHO) (2015): Water Sanitation and Hygiene for accelerating and sustaining progress on Neglected Tropical Diseases. A global strategy 2015 - 2020. Geneva, Switzerland, p. 26
36. Kirchhoff, Louis V. (1993-08-26). "American Trypanosomiasis (Chagas› Disease) – A Tropical Disease Now in the United States". New England Journal of Medicine. 329 (9): 639–644. doi:10.1056/NEJM199308263290909. ISSN 0028-4793. PMID 8341339.
37. Spiegel, Jerry M.; Dharamsi, Shafik; Wasan, Kishor M.; Yassi, Annalee; Singer, Burton; Hotez, Peter J.; Hanson, Christy; Bundy, Donald A. P. (2010-05-18). "Which New Approaches to Tackling Neglected Tropical Diseases Show Promise?". PLOS Medicine. 7 (5): e1000255. doi:10.1371/journal.pmed.1000255. ISSN 1549-1676. PMC 2872649Freely accessible. PMID 20502599.
38. World Health Organization (WHO) (2012). Accelerating work to overcome the global impact of Neglected Tropical Diseases. A roadmap for implementation. Geneva, Switzerland.
39. "FDA Approves Coartem Tablets to Treat Malaria". USFDA. Retrieved 11 December 2009.
40. Ridley DB, Grabowski HG, Moe JL (2006). "Developing drugs for developing countries". Health Aff (Millwood). 25 (2): 313–24. doi:10.1377/hlthaff.25.2.313. PMID 16522573.
41. Johnston, E. A.; Teague, Jordan; Graham, Jay P. (2015-06-11). "Challenges and opportunities associated with neglected tropical disease and water, sanitation and hygiene intersectoral integration programs". BMC Public Health. 15 (1): 547. doi:10.1186/s12889-015-1838-7. ISSN 1471-2458. PMID 26062691.
42. "WHO strengthens focus on water, sanitation, and hygiene to accelerate elimination of neglected tropical diseases". World Health Organization (WHO). 27 August 2015. Retrieved 14 September 2015.
43. "Collaboration between WASH and NTD". World Health Organization (WHO). Retrieved 14 September 2015.
44. "NTDs and access to water and sanitation are major global challenges". World Health Organization (WHO). Retrieved 14 September 2015.
45. "Facial cleanliness and environmental improvement are key to eliminating trachoma". World Health Organization (WHO). Retrieved 14 September 2015.
46. "Sanitation prevents soil transmitted helminth infections". World Health Organization (WHO). Retrieved 14 September 2015.
47. "Breeding sites for mosquitoes are reduced through improved sanitation and water management". World Health Organization (WHO). Retrieved 14 September 2015.
48. "Protecting freshwater from contamination reduces schistosomiasis". World Health Organization (WHO). Retrieved 14 September 2015.
49. "Safe water is essential to treat and care for NTDs". World Health Organization (WHO). Retrieved 14 September 2015.

50. "WASH improves the quality of life for people affected by NTDs". World Health Organization (WHO). Retrieved 14 September 2015.
51. Grimes, Jack E.T.; Croll, David; Harrison, Wendy E.; Utzinger, Jürg; Freeman, Matthew C.; Templeton, Michael R. (4 December 2014). "The Relationship between Water, Sanitation and Schistosomiasis: A Systematic Review and Meta-analysis". PLOS Neglected Tropical Diseases. 8: e3296. doi:10.1371/journal.pntd.0003296. Retrieved 16 September 2015.
52. Stocks, Meredith E. (25 February 2014). "Effect of Water, Sanitation, and Hygiene on the Prevention of Trachoma: A Systematic Review and Meta-Analysis". PLOS Medicine. 11: e1001605. doi:10.1371/journal.pmed.1001605. Retrieved 16 September 2015.
53. Strunz, Eric C. (24 March 2014). "Water, Sanitation, Hygiene, and Soil-Transmitted Helminth Infection: A Systematic Review and Meta-Analysis". PLOS Medicine. 11: e1001620. doi:10.1371/journal.pmed.1001620. Retrieved 16 September 2015.
54. Campbell, Suzy J. (10 April 2014). "Water, Sanitation, and Hygiene (WASH): A Critical Component for Sustainable Soil-Transmitted Helminth and Schistosomiasis Control". PLOS Neglected Tropical Diseases. 8: e2651. doi:10.1371/journal.pntd.0002651. Retrieved 16 September 2015.
55. Frew SE, Liu VY, Singer PA (2009). "A business plan to help the ‹global South› in its fight against neglected diseases" (PDF). Health Aff (Millwood). 28 (6): 1760–73. doi:10.1377/hlthaff.28.6.1760. PMID 19887417.
56. Keenan JD, Hotez PJ, Amza A, et al. (2013). "Elimination and eradication of neglected tropical diseases with mass drug administrations: a survey of experts". PLoS Negl Trop Dis. 7 (12): e2562. doi:10.1371/journal.pntd.0002562. PMC 3855072Freely accessible. PMID 24340111.
57. Burns, Melinda (3 October 2010). "Lifesaving Drug Praziquantel Too Expensive for Africa". Pacific Standard. The Miller-McCune Center for Research, Media and Public Policy. Retrieved 8 December 2015.
58. 5.7. Croft SL. Public-private partnership: from there to here. Trans R Soc Trop Med Hyg 2005; 99(suppl 1):S9-14.
59. "An Innovative Approach to R&D for Neglected Patients: Ten Years of Experience and Lessons Learned by DNDi". DNDi. January 2014
60. Ramamoorthi, R; Graef, KM; Dent, J (December 2014). "WIPO Re:Search: Accelerating anthelmintic development through cross-sector partnerships.". International journal for parasitology. Drugs and drug resistance. 4 (3): 220–5. doi:10.1016/j.ijpddr.2014.09.002. PMID 25516832.
61. Japan in pioneering partnership to fund global health research", by Andrew Jack, Financial Times, May 30, 2013
62. "An Audience with ... Tachi Yamada", by Asher Mullard, Nature magazine, September 2013, Volume 12, p.658
63. "Joining the Fight Against Neglected Diseases", Science magazine, June 7,

2013, Volume 340, p.1148

64. Keating, Conrad (2014-12-16). “Ken Warren and the Rockefeller Foundation›s Great Neglected Diseases Network, 1978–1988: The Transformation of Tropical and Global Medicine”. Molecular Medicine. 20 (Suppl 1): S24–S30. doi:10.2119/molmed.2014.00221. ISSN 1076-1551. PMC 4374516Freely accessible. PMID 25549230.
65. Mathers, Colin D.; Ezzati, Majid; Lopez, Alan D. (2007-11-07). “Measuring the Burden of Neglected Tropical Diseases: The Global Burden of Disease Framework”. PLoS Neglected Tropical Diseases. 1 (2): e114. doi:10.1371/journal.pntd.0000114. ISSN 1935-2727. PMC 2100367Freely accessible. PMID 18060077.
66. King, Charles H.; Bertino, Anne-Marie (2008-01-01). “Asymmetries of poverty: why global burden of disease valuations underestimate the burden of neglected tropical diseases”. PLoS neglected tropical diseases. 2 (3): e209. doi:10.1371/journal.pntd.0000209. ISSN 1935-2735. PMC 2267491Freely accessible. PMID 18365036.

CHAPTER 8

Quantitative Parasitology

Chapter Contents

Quantifying parasites in a sample of hosts or comparing measures of infection across two or more samples can be challenging.

The parasitic infection of a sample of hosts inherently exhibits a complex pattern that cannot be adequately quantified by a single statistical measure. As the use of two or more separate indices is advisable, only two or more separate statistical tests can reliably compare infections different samples of hosts.

A few of the available statistical measures have markedly different biological interpretations, while others have more-or-less overlapping interpretations or no interpretations at all. Therefore, one should apply measures that have clear and separate biological interpretations thus do not predict each other.

INTRODUCTION

In parasitology, the quantitative study of parasitism in a host population involves the use of statistics to draw meaningful conclusions from observations of the prevalence and intensity of parasitic infection.

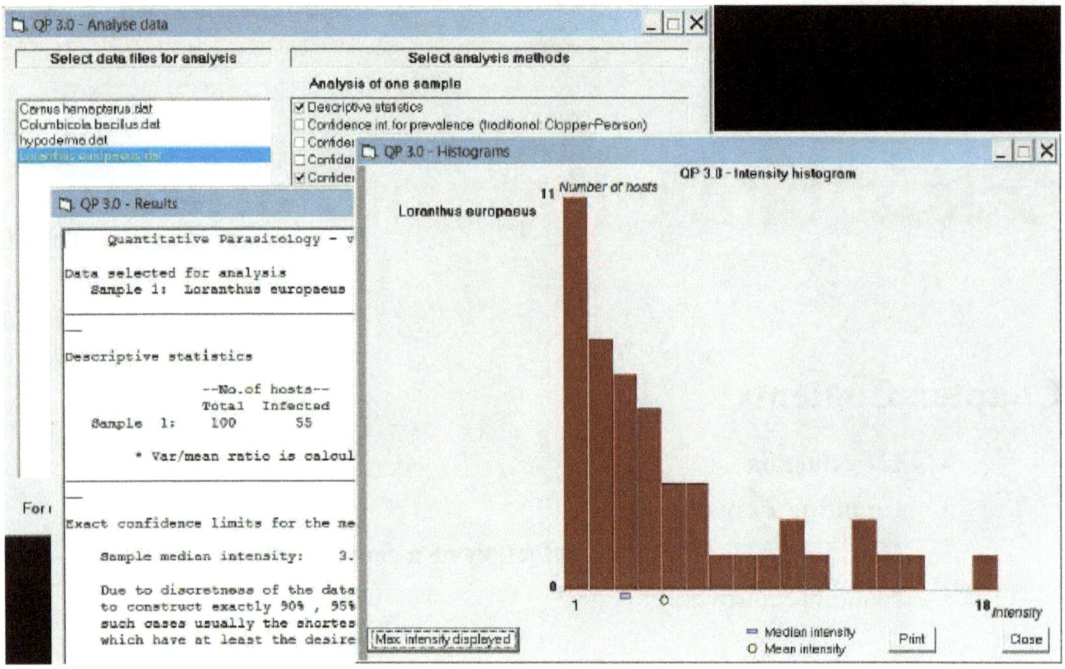

Working view of QP 3.0

COUNTING PARASITES

Quantifying parasites in a sample of hosts or comparing measures of infection across two or more samples can be challenging.

The parasitic infection of a sample of hosts inherently exhibits a complex pattern that cannot be adequately quantified by a single statistical measure. As the use of two or more separate indices is advisable, only two or more separate statistical tests can reliably compare infections different samples of hosts.

A few of the available statistical measures have markedly different biological interpretations, while others have more-or-less overlapping interpretations or no interpretations at all. Therefore, one should apply measures that have clear and separate biological interpretations thus do not predict each other.

Parasite individuals typically exhibit an aggregated (right-skewed) distribution among host individuals; most hosts harbour few if any parasites and a few hosts harbour many of them. This quantitative feature of parasitism makes the application of many traditional statistical methods inappropriate by violating assumptions about the underlying data distribution, requiring the use of more advanced computationally-intensive methods.

DESCRIBING THE PARASITIC INFECTION OF A SAMPLE OF HOSTS

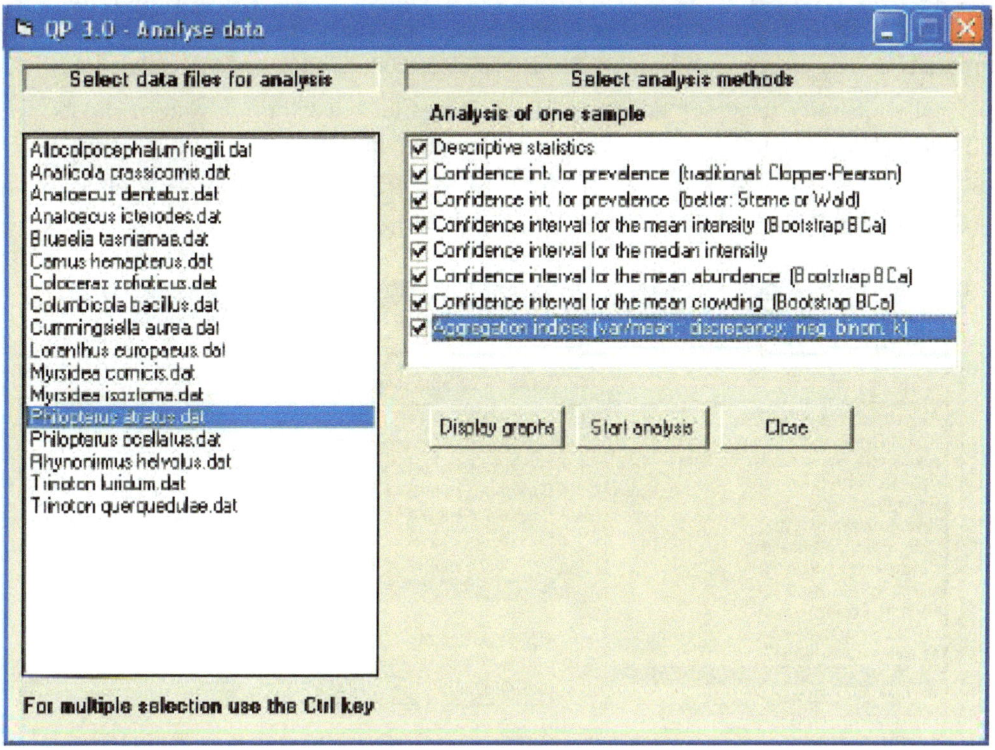

Statistical procedures to characterize the infection/infestation of a sample of hosts.

Always give the host **sample size**. In most cases, this is expressed as the number of hosts individuals examined. (Exceptionally, other units may also be used for special cases.)

Describe prevalence. This is the proportion of infected hosts among all the hosts examined. Give the confidence interval (CI) of prevalence (either as a Clopper-Pearson interval or as adjusted Wald/Sterne›s interval) to indicate the accuracy of the estimation (use of the confidence intervals belonging to the 95% probability is advisable).

Describe mean intensity. This is the mean number of parasites found in the infected hosts (the zeros of uninfected hosts are excluded). Since sample size and prevalence are known, mean intensity defines the quantity of parasites found in the sample of hosts. Given the typical aggregated (right-skewed) distribution of parasites, its actual value is highly dependent on a few extremely infected hosts. Also give CI to indicate the accuracy of the estimation. Use bias-corrected and accelerated bootstrap (BCa Bootstrap) to get this confidence interval.

Describe median intensity. This is the median number of parasites found in infected hosts (the zeros of uninfected hosts are excluded). Median intensity shows a typical level of infection among the infected hosts. Use exact CI to indicate the accuracy of the estimation. In certain cases one may prefer to use mean abundance instead of mean intensity. This is the mean number of parasites found in all hosts (involves the zero values of uninfected hosts). Give BCa Bootstrap confidence interval to indicate the accuracy of this estimation. This measure unifies two of the former ones: prevalence and mean intensity. Do not use it, unless you have a clearly specified a reason why to prefer it.

Describing mean crowding (intensity values averaged across parasite individuals) and its confidence interval is essential only for those who study density-dependent characters of parasites. BCa Bootstrap CI can be used to indicate the accuracy of the estimation.

Finally, quantify levels of skewness of the parasites' distribution among hosts. There are 3 indices widely used for this purpose, but their interpretation is quite similar. They predict each other rather well, thus it is not necessary to use all the 3 of them.

Comparing Parasite Burdens Across two or More Samples

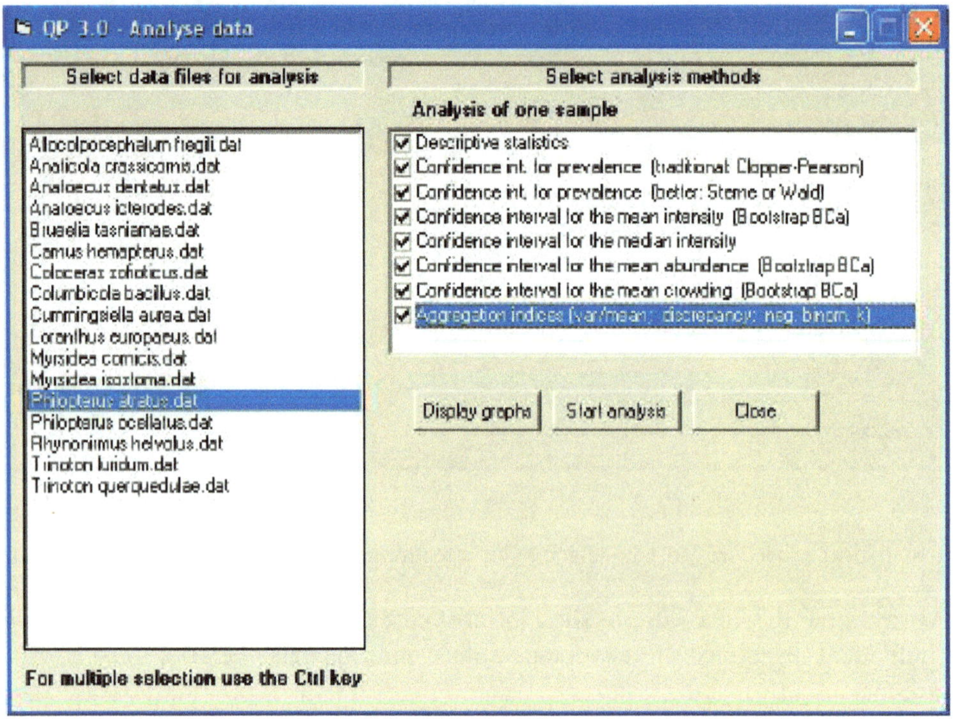

Statistical procedures to compare levels of infection/infestation across two or more samples of hosts.

Compare prevalences by Fisher's exact test. This will show whether the proportion of infected individuals differs significantly between the two (or more) samples. The time need of this test may increase dramatically when several samples are involved. Using Chi-squared test for the same purpose may be advisable in such cases.

Compare mean intensities by a Bootstrap t-test. This will show whether parasite quantities differ significantly between the infected proportions of the two samples.

Compare median intensities by Mood›s median test. This will show whether the typical level of infection differs significantly between the infected proportions of the two samples.

One can also compare the frequency distributions of intensities by a Stochastic equality test. It compares several random pairs of individual values taken from the two samples to test whether or not there is a significant tendency to get higher values from one sample than from the other.

In certain cases, one may also decide to compare mean abundances by a Bootstrap t-test. This will show whether parasite quantities differ significantly between two samples. This comparison unifies two of the former ones: the comparison of prevalences and the comparison of mean intensities.

Finally, mean crowding can be compared across samples by a simple method: provided that the two 97.5% confidence intervals do not overlap, we conclude that the two values are different at a 95% level of significance.

AVAILABLE SOFTWARE

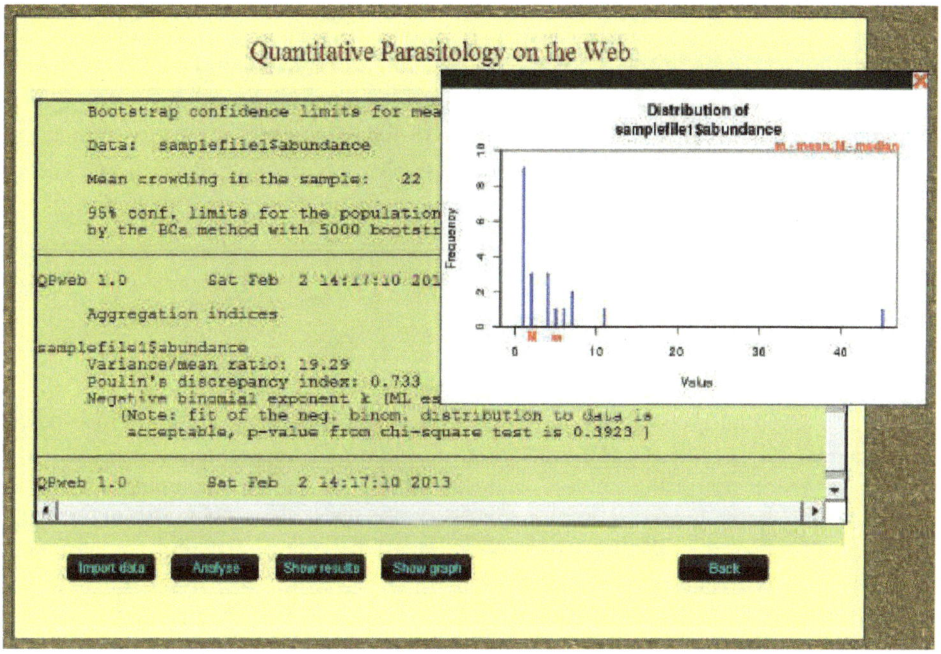

QPweb1.0: an interactive web surface to upload and analyse your data through the web

- ***Quantitative Parasitology 3.0*** is a zipped folder containing an exe file that runs under Microsoft Windows.
- ***Quantitative Parasitology on the Web 1.0*** is an interactive web surface that comes with an extended functionality. It works with Windows, Linux, Mac etc. operating systems and Explorer, Firefox, Google Chrome etc. browsers.

Morphology

Unlike other parasitic protozoa (*Giardia lamblia*, *Entamoeba histolytica* etc.), *Trichomonas vaginalis* exists in only one morphological stage, a trophozoite, and cannot encyst. The *T. vaginalis* trophozoite is oval as well as flagellated, or "pear" shaped as seen on a wet-mount. It is slightly larger than a white blood cell, measuring 9 × 7 μm. Five flagella arise near the cytostome; four of these immediately extend outside the cell together, while the fifth flagellum wraps backwards along the surface of the organism. The functionality of the fifth flagellum is not known. In addition, a conspicuous barb-like axostyle projects opposite the four-flagella bundle. The axostyle may be used for attachment to surfaces and may also cause the tissue damage seen in trichomoniasis infections.

While *T. vaginalis* does not have a cyst form, organisms can survive for up to 24 hours in urine, semen, or even water samples.

Protein Function

Trichomonas vaginalis lacks mitochondria and therefore necessary enzymes and cytochromes to conduct oxidative phosphorylation. *T. vaginalis* obtains nutrients by transport through the cell membrane and by phagocytosis. The organism is able to maintain energy requirements by the use of a small amount of enzymes to provide energy via glycolysis of glucose to glycerol and succinate in the cytoplasm, followed by further conversion of pyruvate and malate to hydrogen and acetate in an organelle called the hydrogenosome.

Virulence Factors

One of the hallmark features of *Trichomonas vaginalis* is the adherence factors that allow cervicovaginal epithelium colonization in women. The adherence that this organism illustrates is specific to vaginal epithelial cells (VECs) being pH, time and temperature dependent. A variety of virulence factors mediate this process some of which are the microtubules, microfilaments, adhesins (4), and cysteine proteinases. The adhesins are four trichomonad enzymes called AP65, AP51, AP33, and AP23 that mediate the interaction of the parasite to the receptor molecules on VECs. Cysteine proteinases may be another virulence factor because not only do these 30 kDa proteins bind to host cell surfaces but also may degrade extracellular matrix proteins like hemoglobin, fibronectin or collagen IV.

Genome Sequencing and Statistics

The *T. vaginalis* genome was found to be approximately 160 megabases in size – ten times larger than predicted from earlier gel-based chromosome sizing (The human genome is ~3.5 gigabases by comparison.) As much as two-thirds of the *T. vaginalis* sequence consists of repetitive and transposable elements, reflecting a massive, evolutionarily recent expansion of the genome. The total number of predicted protein-coding genes is ~98,000, which includes ~38,000 ‹repeat› genes (virus-like, transposon-like, retrotransposon-like, and unclassified repeats, all with high copy number and low polymorphism). Approximately 26,000 of the protein-coding genes have been classed as ‹evidence-supported› (similar either to known proteins, or to ESTs), while the remainder have no known function. These extraordinary genome statistics are likely to change downward as the genome sequence, currently very fragmented due to the difficulty of ordering repetitive DNA, is assembled into chromosomes, and as more transcription data (ESTs, microarrays) accumulate. But it appears that the gene number of the single-celled parasite *T. vaginalis* is, at minimum, on par with that of its host *H. sapiens*.

In late 2007 TrichDB.org was launched as a free, public genomic data repository and retrieval service devoted to genome-scale trichomonad data. The site currently contains all of the *T. vaginalis* sequence project data, several EST libraries, and tools for data mining and display. TrichDB is part of the NIH/NIAID-funded EupathDB functional genomics database project.

Increased Susceptibility to HIV

The damage caused by *Trichomonas vaginalis* to the vaginal epithelium increases a woman's susceptibility to an HIV infection. In addition to inflammation, the parasite also causes lysis of epithelial cells and RBCs in the area leading to more inflammation and disruption of the protective barrier usually provided by the epithelium. Having *Trichomonas vaginalis* also may increase the chances of the infected woman transmitting HIV to her sexual partner(s).

Evolution

The biology of *T. vaginalis* has implications for understanding the origin of sexual reproduction in eukaryotes. *T. vaginalis* is not known to undergo meiosis, a key stage of the eukaryotic sexual cycle. However, when Malik et al. examined *T. vaginalis* for the presence of 29 genes known to function in meiosis, they found 27 such genes, including 8 of 9 genes that are specific to meiosis in model organisms. These findings suggest that the capability for meiosis, and hence sexual reproduction, was present in recent ancestors of *T. vaginalis*. Twenty-one of the 27 meiosis genes were also found in another parasite *Giardia lamblia* (also called *Giardia intestinalis*), indicating that these meiotic genes were present in a common ancestor of *T. vaginalis* and *G. intestinalis*. Since these two species are descendants of lineages that are highly divergent among eukaryotes, Malik et al. noted that these meiotic genes were likely present in a common ancestor of all eukaryotes.

REFERENCES

1. Soper, D (2004). "Trichomoniasis: under control or undercontrolled?". American Journal of Obstetrics and Gynecology. 190 (1): 281–90. doi:10.1016/j.ajog.2003.08.023. PMID 14749674.
2. Harp, Djana F.; Chowdhury, Indrajit (2011). "Trichomoniasis: Evaluation to execution". European Journal of Obstetrics & Gynecology and Reproductive Biology. 157 (1): 3–9. doi:10.1016/j.ejogrb.2011.02.024. PMID 21440359.
3. Hook, Edward W. (1999). "Trichomonas vaginalis—No Longer a Minor STD". Sexually Transmitted Diseases. 26 (7): 388–9. doi:10.1097/00007435-199908000-00004. PMID 10458631.
4. Johnston VJ, Mabey DC (February 2008). "Global epidemiology and control of

Trichomonas vaginalis". Current Opinion in Infectious Diseases. 21 (1): 56–64. doi:10.1097/QCO.0b013e3282f3d999. PMID 18192787.

5. ^ Jump up to: a b Nanda, N; Michel, RG; Kurdgelashvili, G; Wendel, KA (2006). "Trichomoniasis and its treatment". Expert review of anti-infective therapy. 4 (1): 125–35. doi:10.1586/14787210.4.1.125. PMID 16441214.
6. Swygard H, Seña AC, Hobbs MM, Cohen MS (April 2004). "Trichomoniasis: clinical manifestations, diagnosis and management". Sex Transm Infect. 80 (2): 91–5. doi:10.1136/sti.2003.005124. PMC 1744792Freely accessible. PMID 15054166.
7. Petrin D, Delgaty K, Bhatt R, Garber G (April 1998). "Clinical and microbiological aspects of Trichomonas vaginalis". Clin. Microbiol. Rev. 11 (2): 300–17. PMC 106834Freely accessible. PMID 9564565.
8. Garber GE (January 2005). "The laboratory diagnosis of Trichomonas vaginalis". Can J Infect Dis Med Microbiol. 16 (1): 35–8. PMC 2095007Freely accessible. PMID 18159526.
9. Schwebke, J. R.; Burgess, D. (2004). "Trichomoniasis". Clinical Microbiology Reviews. 17 (4): 794–803, table of contents. doi:10.1128/CMR.17.4.794-803.2004. PMC 523559Freely accessible. PMID 15489349.
10. "Trichomoniasis". CDC Fact Sheet. Centers for Disease Control and Prevention. 2007-12-17.
11. Caini, Saverio; Gandini, Sara; Dudas, Maria; Bremer, Viviane; Severi, Ettore; Gherasim, Alin (2014). "Sexually transmitted infections and prostate cancer risk: A systematic review and meta-analysis". Cancer Epidemiology. 38 (4): 329–338. doi:10.1016/j.canep.2014.06.002. ISSN 1877-7821. PMID 24986642.
12. Avwioro O G. "Diagnosis of trichomoniasis in pap smears; How effective is it?". European Journal of Experimental Biology. Pelagia Research Library. 1 (1): 10–13.
13. Ohlemeyer, C; Hornberger, L; Lynch, D; Swierkosz, E (March 1998). "Diagnosis of Trichomonas vaginalis in adolescent females: InPouch TV® culture versus wet-mount microscopy". Journal of Adolescent Health. 22 (3): 205–8. doi:10.1016/S1054-139X(97)00214-0. PMID 9502007.
14. Sood, Seema; Mohanty, Srujana; Kapil, Arti; Tolosa, Jorge; Mittal, Suneeta (2007). "InPouch TV culture for detection of Trichomonas vaginalis" (PDF). The Indian journal of medical research. 125 (4): 567–71. PMID 17598943.
15. Huppert, Jill S.; Mortensen, Joel E.; Reed, Jennifer L.; Kahn, Jessica A.; Rich, Kimberly D.; Miller, William C.; Hobbs, Marcia M. (2007). "Rapid Antigen Testing Compares Favorably with Transcription-Mediated Amplification Assay for the Detection of Trichomonas vaginalis in Young Women". Clinical Infectious Diseases. 45 (2): 194–8. doi:10.1086/518851. PMID 17578778.
16. Schirm, Jurjen; Bos, Petra A.J.; Roozeboom-Roelfsema, Irene K.; Luijt, Dirk S.; Möller, Lieke V. (2007). "Trichomonas vaginalis detection using real-time TaqMan PCR". Journal of Microbiological Methods. 68 (2): 243–7. doi:10.1016/j.mimet.2006.08.002. PMID 17005275.

17. "Trichomonas vaginalis repeated DNA target for PCR identification". GenBank Nucleotide Database. National Center for Biotechnology Information. L23861.1.

18. Kengne P, Veas F, Vidal N, Rey JL, Cuny G (September 1994). "Trichomonas vaginalis: repeated DNA target for highly sensitive and specific polymerase chain reaction diagnosis". Cell. Mol. Biol. (Noisy-le-grand). 40 (6): 819–31. PMID 7812190.

19. "Sexually Transmitted Diseases Treatment Guidelines, 2010" (PDF). Morbidity and Mortality Weekly Report, CDC. Centers for Disease Control and Prevention. December 17, 2010.

20. Cudmore, S. L.; Delgaty, K. L.; Hayward-Mcclelland, S. F.; Petrin, D. P.; Garber, G. E. (2004). "Treatment of Infections Caused by Metronidazole-Resistant Trichomonas vaginalis". Clinical Microbiology Reviews. 17 (4): 783–93, table of contents. doi:10.1128/CMR.17.4.783-793.2004. PMC 523556Freely accessible. PMID 15489348.

21. Ryan, Kenneth James; Ray, C. George; Sherris, John C., eds. (2004). Sherris Medical Microbiology (4th ed.). McGraw Hill. ISBN 978-0-8385-8529-0.[page needed]

22. Upcroft, P.; Upcroft, J. A. (2001). "Drug Targets and Mechanisms of Resistance in the Anaerobic Protozoa". Clinical Microbiology Reviews. 14 (1): 150–64. doi:10.1128/CMR.14.1.150-164.2001. PMC 88967Freely accessible. PMID 11148007.

23. Arroyo, R.; Engbring, J.; Alderete, J. F. (1992). "Molecular basis of host epithelial cell recognition by Trichomonas vaginalis". Molecular Microbiology. 6 (7): 853–862. doi:10.1111/j.1365-2958.1992.tb01536.x. PMID 1602965.

24. Mendoza-Lopez, M. R.; Becerril-Garcia, C.; Fattel-Facenda, L. V.; Avila-Gonzalez, L.; Ruiz-Tachiquin, M. E.; Ortega-Lopez, J.; Arroyo, R. (2000). "CP30, a Cysteine Proteinase Involved in Trichomonas vaginalis Cytoadherence". Infection and Immunity. 68 (9): 4907–12. doi:10.1128/IAI.68.9.4907-4912.2000. PMC 101697Freely accessible. PMID 10948104.

25. Carlton, J. M.; Hirt, R. P.; Silva, J. C.; Delcher, A. L.; Schatz, M.; Zhao, Q.; Wortman, J. R.; Bidwell, S. L.; et al. (2007). "Draft Genome Sequence of the Sexually Transmitted Pathogen Trichomonas vaginalis". Science. 315 (5809): 207–12. doi:10.1126/science.1132894. PMC 2080659Freely accessible. PMID 17218520.

26. Lehker, M. W.; Alderete, J. F. (1999). "Resolution of Six Chromosomes of Trichomonas vaginalis and Conservation of Size and Number among Isolates". The Journal of Parasitology. 85 (5): 976–9. doi:10.2307/3285842. JSTOR 3285842. PMID 10577741.

27. Zimmer, C. (2007). "EVOLUTION: Jurassic Genome". Science. 315 (5817): 1358–9. doi:10.1126/science.315.5817.1358. PMID 17347424.

28. Aurrecoechea, Cristina; Brestelli, John; Brunk, Brian P.; Carlton, Jane M.; Dommer, Jennifer; Fischer, Steve; Gajria, Bindu; Gao, Xin; et al. (2009). "GiardiaDB and TrichDB: integrated genomic resources for the eukaryotic protist

pathogens Giardia lamblia and Trichomonas vaginalis". Nucleic Acids Research. 37 (Database issue): D526–30. doi:10.1093/nar/gkn631. PMC 2686445Freely accessible. PMID 18824479.

29. Mulla, Summaiyaa; Kosambiya, JK; Desai, Vikask; Shethwala, Nimishad (2009). "Sexually transmitted infections and reproductive tract infections in female sex workers". Indian Journal of Pathology and Microbiology. 52 (2): 198–9. doi:10.4103/0377-4929.48916. PMID 19332911.

30. Mavedzenge, Sue Napierala; Van der Pol, Barbara; Cheng, Helen; Montgomery, Elizabeth T.; Blanchard, Kelly; de Bruyn, Guy; Ramjee, Gita; Van der Straten, Ariane (2010). "Epidemiological Synergy of Trichomonas vaginalis and HIV in Zimbabwean and South African Women". Sexually Transmitted Diseases. 37 (7): 460–6. doi:10.1097/OLQ.0b013e3181cfcc4b. PMID 20562586.

31. Malik SB, Pightling AW, Stefaniak LM, Schurko AM, Logsdon JM (2008). "An expanded inventory of conserved meiotic genes provides evidence for sex in Trichomonas vaginalis". PLoS ONE. 3 (8): e2879. doi:10.1371/journal.pone.0002879. PMC 2488364 . PMID 18663385.

CHAPTER 9

Brood Parasites

Chapter Contents

- **Introduction**
- **Birds**
- **Parental-Care Parasitism**
- **Fish**
- **Insects**
- **Broodiness**

Some species of birds thrive not by carefully rearing their own young, but by pawning that task off on adults of other species. The European Cuckoo, whose distinctive call is immortalized in the sound of the "cuckoo clock," is the bird in which this habit has been most thoroughly studied. Female European Cuckoos lay their eggs only in the nests of other species of birds. A cuckoo egg usually closely mimics the eggs of the host (one of whose eggs is often removed by the cuckoo). The host may recognize the intruding egg and abandon the nest, or it may incubate and hatch the cuckoo egg. Shortly after hatching, the young European Cuckoo, using a scoop-like depression on its back, instinctively shoves over the edge of the nest any solid object that it contacts. With the disappearance of their eggs and rightful young, the foster parents are free to devote all of their care to the young cuckoo. Frequently this is an awesome task, since the cuckoo chick often grows much larger than the host adults long before it can care for itself. One of the tragicomic scenes in nature is a pair of small foster parents working like Sisyphus to keep up with the voracious appetite of an outsized young cuckoo.

INTRODUCTION

Brood parasites are organisms that rely on others to raise their young. The strategy appears among birds, insects and some fish. The brood parasite manipulates a host, either of the same or of another species, to raise its young as if it were its own.

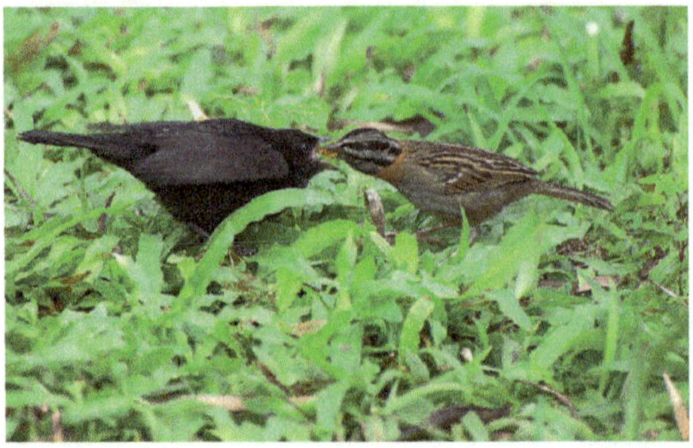

A shiny cowbird chick (left) being fed by a rufous-collared sparrow

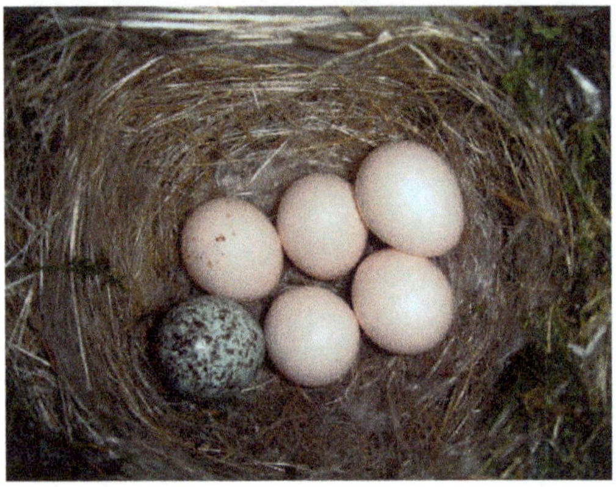

Eastern phoebe nest with one brown-headed cowbird egg (at bottom left)

Brood parasitism relieves the parasitic parents from the investment of rearing young or building nests for the young, enabling them to spend more time on other activities such as foraging and producing further offspring. Bird parasite species mitigate the risk of egg loss by distributing eggs amongst a number of different hosts. As this behaviour damages the host, it often results in an evolutionary arms race between parasite and host.

BIRDS

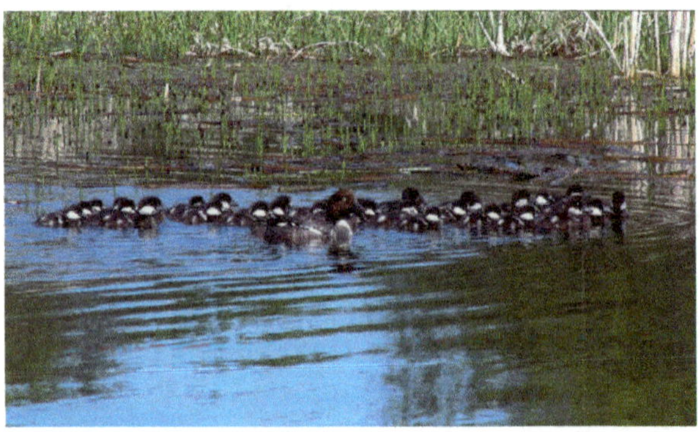

The goldeneye often lays its eggs in the nests of other females.

In many monogamous bird species, there are extra-pair matings resulting in males outside the pair bond siring offspring and used by males to escape from the parental investment in raising their offspring. This form of cuckoldry is taken a step further when females of the goldeneye (*Bucephala clangula*) often lay their eggs in the nests of other individuals. Intraspecific brood parasitism is seen in a number of duck species, where females often lay their eggs in the nests of others.

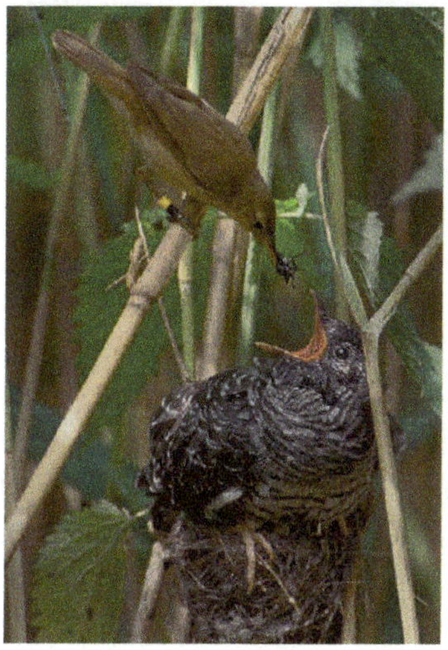

A Eurasian reed warbler raising a common cuckoo

Interspecific brood-parasites include the indigobirds, whydahs, and honeyguides in Africa, cowbirds, Old World cuckoos, black-headed ducks, and some New World cuckoos in the Americas. Seven independent origins of obligate interspecific brood parasitism in birds have been proposed. While there is still some controversy over when and how many origins of interspecific brood parasitism have occurred, recent phylogenetic analyses suggest two origins in Passeriformes (once in New World cowbirds: Icteridae, and once in African Finches: Viduidae); three origins in Old World and New World cuckoos (once in Cuculinae, Phaenicophaeinae, and in Neomorphinae-Crotophaginae); a single origin in Old World honeyguides (Indicatoridae); and in a single species of waterfowl, the black-headed duck (*Heteronetta atricapilla*).

Most avian brood parasites are specialists which parasitize only a single host species or a small group of closely related host species, but four out of the five parasitic cowbirds are generalists,(with the exception of the screaming cowbird) which parasitize a wide variety of hosts; the brown-headed cowbird has 221 known hosts. They usually lay only one egg per nest, although in some cases, particularly the cowbirds, several females may use the same host nest.

The common cuckoo presents an interesting case in which the species as a whole parasitizes a wide variety of hosts, including the reed warbler and dunnock, but individual females specialize in a single species. Genes regulating egg coloration appear to be passed down exclusively along the maternal line, allowing females to lay mimetic eggs in the nest of the species they specialize in. Females generally parasitize nests of the species which raised them. Male common cuckoos fertilize females of all lines, which maintains sufficient gene flow among the different maternal lines to prevent speciation.

The mechanisms of host selection by female cuckoos are somewhat unclear, though several hypotheses have been suggested in attempt to explain the choice. These include genetic inheritance of host preference, host imprinting on young birds, returning to place of birth and subsequently choosing a host randomly ("natal philopatry"), choice based on preferred nest site (nest-site hypothesis), and choice based on preferred habitat (habitat-selection hypothesis). Of these hypotheses the nest-site selection and habitat selection have been most supported by experimental analysis.

Adaptations for Parasitism

Among specialist avian brood parasites, mimetic eggs are a nearly universal adaptation. There is even some evidence that the generalist brown-headed cowbird may have evolved an egg coloration mimicking a number of their hosts.

Most avian brood parasites remove a host egg when they lay one of their own in a nest. Depending upon the species, this can happen either in the same visit to the host nest or in a separate visit before or after the parasitism. This both prevents the host species from realizing their nest has been parasitized and reduces competition for the parasitic nestling once it hatches. Most avian brood parasites have very short egg incubation periods and rapid nestling growth. This gives the parasitic nestling a head start on growth over its nestmates, allowing it to outcompete them. In many brood parasites, such as cuckoos and honeyguides, this short egg incubation period is due to internal incubation periods up to 24 hours longer in cuckoos than hosts. Some non-parasitic cuckoos also have longer internal incubation periods, suggesting that this longer internal incubation period was not an adaptation following brood parasitism, but predisposed birds to become brood parasites. Where the host nestlings are significantly smaller than the parasite nestling, the host nestlings often starve to death. Some brood parasites eliminate all their nestmates shortly after hatching, either by ejecting them from the nest or killing them with sharp mandible hooks which fall off after a few days.

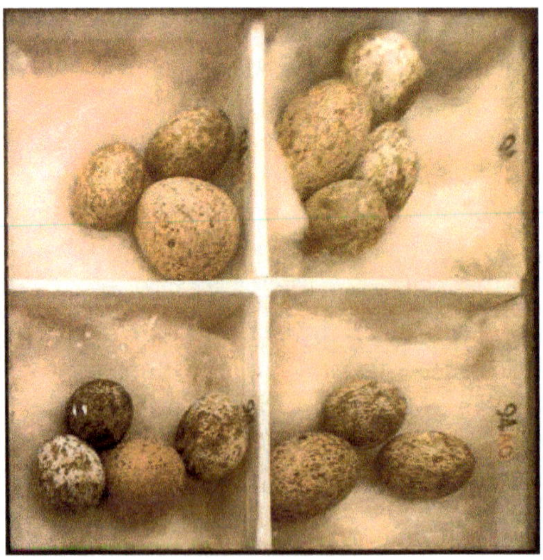

Four clutches of reed warbler eggs, each containing one (larger) cuckoo egg

Mafia Hypothesis

There is a question as to why the majority of the hosts of brood parasites care for the nestlings of their parasites. Not only do these brood parasites usually differ significantly in size and appearance, but it is also highly probable that they reduce the reproductive success of their hosts. The "mafia hypothesis" evolved through studies in an attempt to answer this question. This hypothesis revolves around host manipulations induced by behaviors of the brood parasite. Upon the detection and rejection of a brood parasite›s egg, the host›s nest is depredated upon, its nest destroyed and nestlings injured or killed. This threatening response indirectly enhances selective pressures favoring aggressive parasite behavior that may result in positive feedback between mafia-like parasites and compliant host behaviors.

There are two avian species that have been speculated to portray this mafia-like behavior: the brown-headed cowbird of North America, *Molothrus ater*, and the great spotted cuckoo of Europe, *Clamator glandarius*. The great spotted cuckoo lays the majority of its eggs in the nests of the European magpie, *Pica pica*. It has been observed that the great spotted cuckoo repeatedly visits the nests that it has parasitised, a precondition for the mafia hypothesis. An experiment was run by Soler *et al.* from April to July 1990 – 1992 in the high-altitude plateau Hoya de Guadix, Spain. They observed the effects of the removal of cuckoo eggs on the reproductive success of the magpie and measured the magpie›s reaction; the egg was considered accepted if it remained in the nest, ejected if gone in between visits, or abandoned if the eggs were present but cold. If any nest contents were gone between consecutive visits, the nests were considered to have been depredated. The magpie›s reproductive success was measured by number of nestlings that survived to their last visit, which was just before the nestling had been predicted to fledge from the nest. The results from these experiments show that after the removal of the parasitic eggs from the great spotted cuckoo, these nests are predated at much higher rates than those where the eggs were not removed. Through the use of plasticine eggs that model those of the magpie, it was confirmed that the nest destruction was caused by the great spotted cuckoo. This destruction benefits the cuckoo, for the possibility of re-nesting by the magpie allows another chance for the cuckoo egg to be accepted.

Another similar experiment was done in 1996–2002 by Hoover *et al.* on the relationship between the parasitic brown-headed cowbird and a host, the prothonotary warbler, *Protonotaria citrea*. In their experiment, researchers manipulated the cowbird egg removal and cowbird access to the predator proof nests of the warbler. They found that 56% of egg ejected nests were depredated upon in comparison to 6% of non-ejected nests when cowbirds were not prevented from getting to the hosts' nest. Of the nests that were rebuilt by hosts that had previously been predated upon, 85% of those were destroyed. The number of young produced by the hosts that ejected eggs dropped 60% compared to those that accepted the cowbird eggs.

Nest-site hypothesis

In this hypothesis, female cuckoos select a group of host species with similar nest sites and egg characteristics to her own. This population of potential hosts is monitored and a nest is chosen from within this group.

Research of nest collections has illustrated a significant level of similarity between cuckoo eggs and typical eggs of the host species. A low percentage of parasitized nests were shown to contain cuckoo eggs not corresponding to the specific host egg morph.

In these mismatched nests a high percent of the cuckoo eggs were shown to correlate to the egg morph of another host species with similar nesting sites. This has been pointed to as evidence for nest- site selection.

A criticism of the hypothesis is that it provides no mechanism by which nests are chosen, or which cues might be used to recognize such a site.

PARENTAL-CARE PARASITISM

Parental-care parasitism emphasizes the relationship between the host and the parasite in brood parasitism. Parental-care parasitism occurs when individuals raise offspring of other unrelated individuals. The host are the parents of offspring and the parasites are individuals who take advantage of either the nest or eggs within the family construct. Such dynamics occur when the parasites attempt to reduce their parental investment so they can invest the extra energy into other endeavors.

Cost of the Hosts

Given the detrimental effects avian brood parasites can have on their hosts' reproductive success, host species have come up with various defenses against this unique threat. Given that the cost of egg removal concurrent with parasitism is unrecoverable, the best defense for hosts is avoiding parasitism in the first place. This can take several forms, including selecting nest sites which are difficult to parasitize, starting incubation early so they are sitting on the nests when parasites visit them early in the morning, and aggressive territorial defense. Birds nesting in aggregations can also benefit from group defense.

The hosts Reject Offspring

The host may be the one that ultimately ends up raising offspring after they return from foraging. Once parasitism has occurred, the next most optimal defense is to eject the parasitic egg. According to parental investment theory, the host can possibly adopt some defense to protect their own eggs if they distinguish which eggs are not theirs. Recognition of parasitic eggs is based on identifying pattern differences or changes in the number of eggs. This can be done by grasp ejection if the host has a large enough beak, or otherwise by puncture ejection. Ejection behavior has some costs however, especially when host species have to deal with mimetic eggs. Hosts inevitably mistake one of their own eggs for a parasite egg on occasion and eject it. In any case, hosts sometimes damage their own eggs while trying to eject a parasite egg.

Among hosts not exhibiting parasitic egg ejection, some abandon parasitized nests and start over again. However, at high enough parasitism frequencies, this becomes maladaptive as the new nest will most likely also be parasitized. Some host species modify their nests to exclude the parasitic egg, either by weaving over the egg or in some cases rebuilding a new nest over the existing one. For instance, American coots may kick the parasites' eggs out, or build a new nest beside the brood nests where the parasites' babies starve to death.

Cost of the Parasites

While parental-care parasitism significantly increased the breeding number of the parasite, only about half of the parasite eggs survived.Parasitism for the individual (the brood parasite) also has significant drawbacks. As an example, the parasitic offspring of the bearded tits, *Panurus biarmicus*, compared to the offspring in non-parasitic nests, tend to develop much more slowly and often don't reach full maturity. Parasitic females however can adopt either floater traits or nesting traits. Floater females are entirely dependent on others to raise their eggs because they do not have their own nests. Hence, they reproduce significantly less because the hosts reject their 'intruder' eggs or they may just miss the egg-laying period of the bird they are trying to pass their eggs to. Nesting females who have their own nests may also be parasitic due to temporary situations like sudden loss of nests, or they lay surplus eggs, which overload their parental care ability.

The Hosts Raise Offspring

Sometimes hosts are completely unaware that they are caring for a bird that is not their own. This most commonly occurs because the host cannot differentiate the parasitic eggs from their own. It may also occur when hosts temporarily leave the nest after laying the eggs. The parasites lay their own eggs into these nests so their nestlings share the food provided by the host. It may occur in other situations. For example, female eiders would prefer to lay eggs in the nests with one or two existing eggs of others because the first egg is the most vulnerable to predators. The presence of others' eggs reduces the probability that a predator will attack her egg when a female eider leaves the nest after laying the first egg.

Sometimes, the parasitic offspring kills the host nest-mates during competition for resources. As an example, the parasite offspring of the cowbird chick kill the host nest-mates if food intake for each of them is low, but do not do so if the food intake is adequate, as a result of their interactions with co-inhabitants of the nest.

FISH

Mouthbrooding Parasites

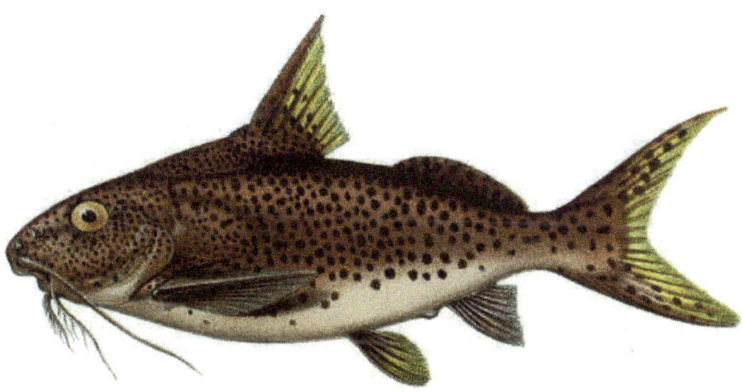

Synodontis multipunctatus

A mochokid catfish of Lake Tanganyika, *Synodontis multipunctatus*, is a brood parasite of several mouthbrooding cichlid fish. The catfish eggs are incubated in the host's mouth, and—in the manner of cuckoos—hatch before the host's own eggs. The young catfish eat the host fry inside the host's mouth, effectively taking up virtually the whole of the host's parental investment.

Nest Parasites

A cyprinid minnow, *Pungtungia herzi* is a brood parasite of the Serranid freshwater perch *Siniperca kawamebari*, which live in the south of the Japanese islands of Honshu, Kyushu and Shikoku, and in South Korea. Host males guard territories against intruders during the breeding season, creating a patch of reeds as a spawning site or "nest". Females (one or more per site) visit the site to lay eggs, which the male then defends. The parasite›s eggs are smaller and stickier than the host›s. 65.5% of host sites were parasitised in a study area.

INSECTS

Kleptoparasites

There are many different types of cuckoo bees, all of which lay their eggs in the nest cells of other bees, but they are normally referred to as kleptoparasites (Greek: klepto-, to steal), rather than as brood parasites, because the immature stages are almost never fed directly by the adult hosts. Instead, they simply take food gathered by their hosts. Examples of cuckoo bees are *Coelioxys rufitarsis*, *Melecta separata*, *Bombus bohemicus, Nomada* and *Epeoloides*.

Kleptoparasitism in insects is not restricted to bees; several lineages of wasp including most of the Chrysididae, the cuckoo wasps, are kleptoparasites. The cuckoo wasps lay their eggs in the nests of other wasps, such as those of the potters and mud daubers.

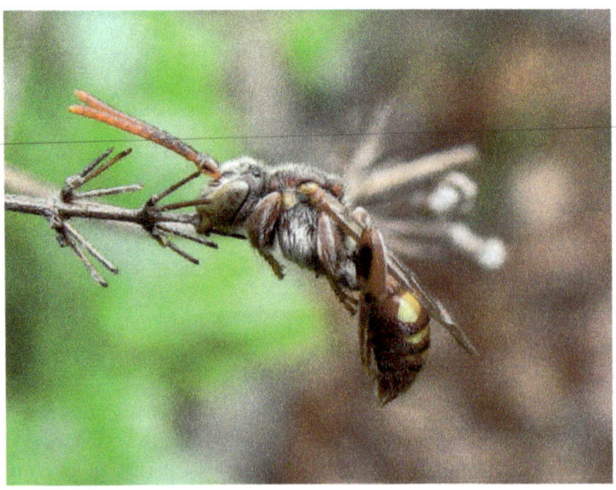

A cuckoo bee from the genus *Nomada*

Brood Parasites

Among the few exceptions, which are indeed fed by adult hosts, are cuckoo bumblebees in the subgenus *Psithyrus*. Their queens kill and replace the existing queen of a colony of the host species then use the host workers to feed their brood.

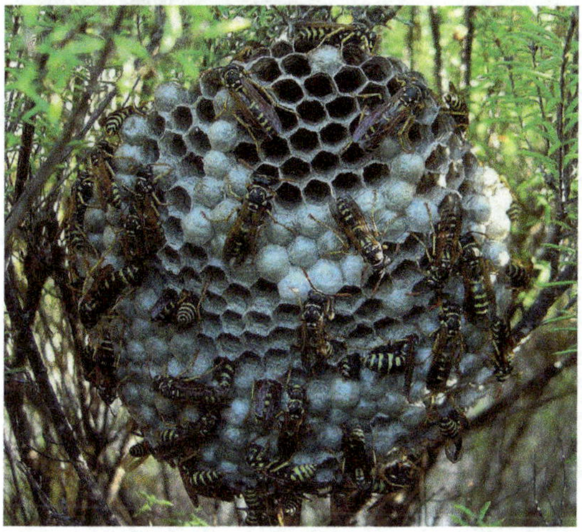

Nest of *Polistes dominula*, host species to the cuckoo wasp *Polistes sulcifer*

An example of a true brood-parasitic wasp is *Polistes sulcifer*. This species of paper wasp has lost the ability to build their own nests, and relies on its host species, *Polistes dominula*, to raise its brood, with the adult hosts feeding the parasite larvae directly, unlike typical kleptoparasitic insects.

In the bee species of *Euglossa cordata*, dominant reproductive females will display brood parasitism by replacing her daughter's eggs with her own eggs, diverting her resources from producing grand-offspring to producing more of her own offspring. In addition, to increase her longevity and fecundity, a mother will also eat her daughter's eggs to gain more nutrients.

Host insects are sometimes tricked into bringing offspring of another species into their own nests, as is the case with the parasitic butterfly, *Phengaris rebeli*, and the host ant *Myrmica schencki*. The butterfly larvae release chemicals that confuse the host ant into believing that the *P. rebeli* larvae are actually ant larvae. Thus, the *M. schencki* ants bring back the *P. rebeli* larvae to their nests and feed them, much like the chicks of cuckoos and other brood-parasitic birds.

BROODINESS

Broodiness is the action or behavioral tendency to sit on a clutch of eggs to incubate them, often requiring the non-expression of many other behaviors including feeding and drinking. Being **broody** has been defined as "Being in a state of readiness to brood eggs that is characterized by cessation of laying and by marked changes in behavior and physiology". Broody birds often pluck feathers from their chest and abdomen, using them to cover the eggs. As a consequence of this, they develop one or several patches of bare skin on the ventral surface. These reddish, well-vascularized areas of skin are usually called brood patches, and improve heat transfer to the eggs. Broodiness is usually associated with female birds, although males of some bird species become broody and some non-avian animals also show broodiness.

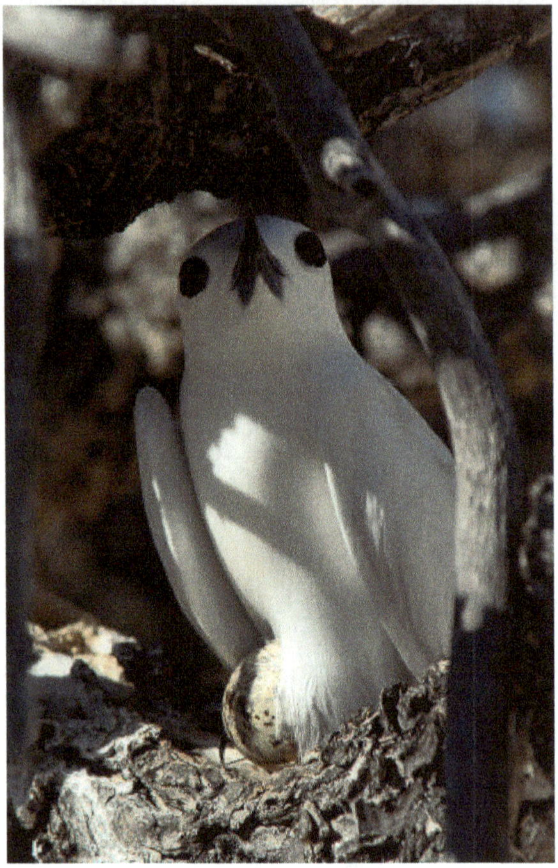

A brooding White tern (*Gygis alba*).

In Wild Birds

In wild birds, egg incubation is a normal and essential phase in the process of reproduction, and in many families of birds, e.g. pigeons, the eggs are incubated by both male and female parents.

Broodiness in males

In all the species of phalaropes the males become broody rather than the female. The females leave the nest after finishing laying to let the males incubate the eggs and take care of the young. Male emus (*Dromaius novaehollandiae*) become broody after their mates start laying, and begin to incubate the eggs before the laying period is complete.

Non-broodiness

A small number of atypical birds such as *Passeriformes* of the genus *Molothrus* do not become broody but lay their eggs in the nests of other species for incubation, known as brood parasitism. The Australian Brushturkey *(Alectura lathami)* also does not become broody, rather, it covers the eggs with a large mound of vegetable matter which decomposes keeping the eggs warm until hatching. The Crab-plover, (*Dromas ardeola*), which live on the coasts and islands of the Indian Ocean, let their eggs incubate primarily by the heat of the sun and will leave their nests unattended, occasionally for days at a time.

In Domestic Poultry

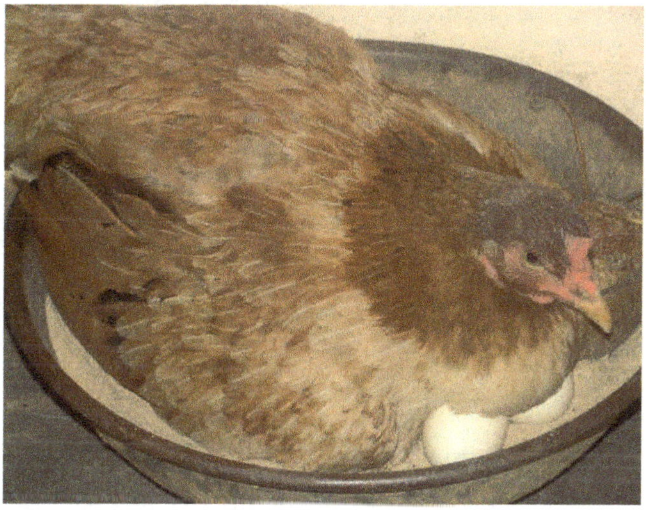

A brooding domestic hen.

Broody hens can be recognized by their behaviour. They sit firmly over the eggs, and when people approach or try to remove the eggs, threaten the person by erecting their feathers, emitting a characteristic sound like *clo-clo-clo* and will peck aggressively. When broody, hens often temporarily cease eating or reduce their feed consumption.

Letting eggs accumulate in a relatively dark place near the floor often stimulates hens to become broody. Placing artificial eggs into nests also stimulates broodiness. Keeping hens in dark places with warm temperatures and in view of vocalising orphan chicks can induce broodiness, even in breeds that normally do not go broody.

Some environmental conditions stimulate broodiness. In heavy breeds of chickens, warm weather tends to bring about broodiness. Removing eggs each day, out of the sight of the hens, helps avoid broodiness not only in domestic poultry but also in some wild species in captivity. This continued egg laying means more eggs are laid than would occur under natural conditions. Poultry farming in battery cages also helps to avoid broodiness.

In Commercial egg-laying

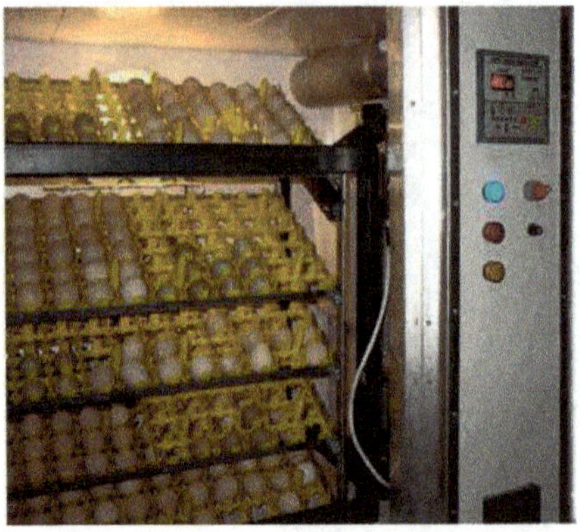

An egg incubator.

Because hens stop laying when they become broody, commercial poultry breeders perceive broodiness not as a normal physiological process, but as a drawback to egg and poultry meat production. With domestication, it has become more profitable to incubate eggs artificially, while keeping hens in full egg production. To help achieve this, there has been intense artificial selection for non-broodiness in commercial egg laying chickens Gallus gallus domesticus and parent stock of poultry. As a result of this artificial selection, broodiness has been greatly reduced to very low levels in present breeds of commercial fowl, both among egg-laying and meat-producing breeds.

Physiological Basis

Broodiness is due to the secretion of prolactine hormone by the front lobe of the hypophysis. Prolactine injection in hens provokes egg laying to stop within a few days, vitellum reabsorbtion, ovary regression (hens only have a left ovary) and finally broodiness. However, attempts to stop broodiness by the administration of several hormones have failed because this state, once evoked, requires time to revert.

Prolactine injections inhibit the production of gonadotropin hormone, a hormone that stimulates ovarian follicles which is produced in the frontal lobe of hypophysis.

Castrated males can go broody with baby chicks, showing that broodiness is not limited to females, however, castrated males do not incubate eggs.

Contrary to common opinion, the temperature of broody hens barely differs from that of laying hens. Broody hens pluck feathers from their chest, using them to cover the eggs. As a consequence of this, they develop one or several patches of bare skin on the ventral surface. These reddish, well-vascularized areas of skin are usually called brood patches. which improve heat transfer to the eggs.

Genetic Basis

Broodiness is more common in some chicken breeds than others, indicating that it is an inherited characteristic. Breeds such as Cochin, Cornish and Silkie exhibit a tendency to broodiness, including brooding eggs from other species such as quails, pheasants, turkeys and geese. In some breeds such as the White Leghorn, broodiness is extremely rare.

Some studies on crosses of chicken breeds point to the hypothesis of complementary genes acting on broodiness. Other results point to the hypothesis of sex-linked genes, or, inheritance through the maternal chromosome. Although these studies have been made on different breeds of chickens, their results are not contradictory. There is common agreement that artificial selection for egg production succeeded in reducing the incidence of broody hens in chicken populations.

Chicken Breeds that Commonly Exhibit Broodiness

- Cochin
- Manx Rumpy
- Plymouth Rock
- Silkie
- Saipan Jungle Fowl
- Orpington
- Kraienköppe
- Belgian Bearded d'Anvers
- Icelandic chicken
- Java (chicken)
- Philippine Native Chicken
- Belgian Bearded d'Uccle
- Iowa Blue
- Nankin
- Delaware
- Booted Bantam
- New Hampshire
- Pekin
- Dutch Bantam
- Indian Game (Cornish)

Chicken Breeds that rarely Exhibit Broodiness

- Leghorn
- Polish
- Norwegian Jærhøne
- Brabanter
- Orloff
- Sultan

- Scots Grey
- Sussex
- Sebright
- Menorca
- Wyandotte
- Egyptian Fayoumi

Broodiness in Non-Avian Animals

There is some evidence that non-avian dinosaurs also practiced brooding. A specimen of the Mongolian oviraptorid *Citipati osmolskae* was discovered in a chicken-like brooding position in 1993, which may indicate that they had begun using an insulating layer of feathers to keep the eggs warm.

Several deinonychosaur and oviraptorosaur specimens have also been found preserved on top of their nests, likely brooding in a bird-like manner.

Lungless salamanders in the family *Plethodontidae* lay a small number of eggs in a cluster among damp leaf litter. The female salamander often broods the eggs and in the genus *Ensatinas*, she has been observed to coil around them and press her throat area against them, effectively massaging them with a mucous secretion. The black mountain salamander mother broods her eggs, guarding them from predation as the larvae feed on the yolks of their eggs. They eventually break their way out of the egg capsules and disperse. Some species of Gymnophiona (caecilians, with long, cylindrical, limbless bodies) brood their eggs.

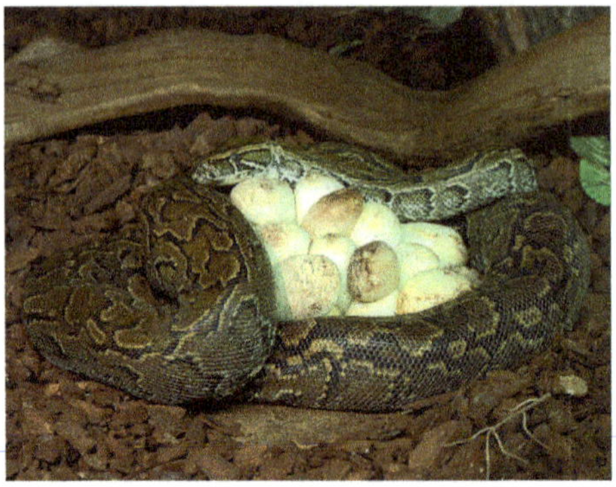

A brooding female python.

Most pythons coil around their egg-clutches and remain with them until they hatch. A female python will not leave the eggs, except to occasionally bask in the sun or drink water. She will even "shiver" to generate heat to incubate the eggs.

Some cichlid fish lay their eggs in the open, on rocks, leaves, or logs. Male and female parents usually engage in differing brooding roles. Most commonly, the male patrols the pair's territory and repels intruders, while females fan water over the eggs, removing the infertile and leading the fry while foraging. However, both sexes are able to perform the full range of parenting behaviours.

Mouthbrooding

Mouthbrooding, also known as oral incubation, refers to the care given by some groups of animals to fertilized eggs or their offspring by holding them in the mouth of the parent for extended periods of time. Although it has been observed in a variety of animals, most mouthbrooders are fish. The parent performing this behavior invariably feeds less often and afterwards will be underweight, requiring a period of feeding and restoring the depleted energy reserves.

Others

Marsupial frogs are so-called because they possess a dorsal brood pouch. In some species the eggs are fertilized on the female's lower back, and are inserted in her pouch with the aid of the male's toes. The eggs remain in contact with the female's vascular tissue, which provides them oxygen.

Some animals have a common name that includes the word ‹brood› or its derivatives, although it is arguable whether the animals show ‹broodiness› per se. For example, the female gastric-brooding frog (*Rheobatrachus sp.*) from Australia, now probably extinct, swallows her fertilized eggs, which then develop inside her stomach. She ceases to feed and stops secreting stomach acid and the tadpoles rely on the yolks of the eggs for nourishment. After six or seven weeks the mother opens her mouth wide and regurgitates the tadpoles which hop away from her mouth. The Brooding sea anemone (*Epiactis prolifera*) is a colonial hermaphrodite that fertilizes and incubates its eggs internally. The motile larvae, after swimming out of the mouth, migrate down to the disk and become fixed there until they become little anemones, ready to move and feed independently.

In Darwin's Frog (*Rhinoderma darwinii*), the female lays about 30 eggs and then the male guards them for about two weeks, until they hatch. The male then takes all the survivors and carries around the developing young in his vocal pouch. When the tiny tadpoles have developed they hop out and swim away. In this animal, the parents hold the hatched young rather than eggs in their mouths, so is arguably not showing 'broodiness'.

REFERENCES

1. David Attenborough (1998) [1998]. The Life of Birds. New Jersey: Princeton University Press. p. 246. ISBN 0-691-01633-X.
2. Payne, R. B. 1997. Avian brood parasitism. In D. H. Clayton and J. Moore (eds.), Host-parasite evolution: General principles and avian models, 338–369. Oxford University Press, Oxford.
3. Rothstein, S.I (1990). "A model system for coevolution: avian brood parasitism". Annual Review of Ecology and Systematics. **21**: 481–508. doi:10.1146/annurev.ecolsys.21.1.481.
4. Stephen M. Yezerinac, Patrick J. Weatherhead 1997. Extra-Pair Mating, Male Plumage Coloration and Sexual Selection in yellow warblers (Dendroica petechia). Proc. R. Soc. London B. 264(1381):527–532

5. Andersson, M.; Eriksson, M.O.G. (1982). "Nest parasitism in goldeneyes Bucephala clangula: some evolutionary aspects". American Naturalist. **120**: 1–16. doi:10.1086/283965.

6. Aragon, S.; Møller, A. P.; Soler, J. J.; Soler, M. (1999). "Molecular phylogeny of cuckoos supports a polyphyletic origin of brood parasitism". Journal of Evolutionary Biology. **12**: 495–506. doi:10.1046/j.1420-9101.1999.00052.x.

7. Sorenson, M.D; Payne, R.B. (2001). "A single ancient origin of brood parasitism in African finches: implications for host-parasite coevolution". Evolution. **55**: 2550–2567. doi:10.1554/0014-3820(2001)055[2550:asaoob]2.0.co;2.

8. Sorenson, M.D.; Payne, R.B. (2002). "Molecular genetic perspectives on avian brood parasitism". Integrative and Comparative Biology. **42**: 388–400. doi:10.1093/icb/42.2.388. PMID 21708732.

9. Vogl, W.; Taborsky, M.; Taborsky, B.; Teuschl, Y.; Honza, M. (2002). "Cuckoo females preferentially use specific habitats when searching for hot nests". Animal Behaviour. **64**: 843–850. doi:10.1006/anbe.2003.1967.

10. Teuschl, Y; Taborsky, B; Taborsky, M (1998). "How do cuckoos find their hosts? The role of habitat imprinting". Animal Behaviour. **56**: 1425–1433. doi:10.1006/anbe.1998.0931.

11. Brian Peer, Scott Robinson, and James Herkert in The Auk 117(4):892–901

12. Birkhead, T. R.; Hemmings, N.; Spottiswoode, C. N.; Mikulica, O.; Moskát, C.; Ban, M.; Schulze-Hagen, K. (2011). "Internal incubation and early hatching in brood parasitic birds". Proceedings of the Royal Society Series B. **278**: 1019–1024. doi:10.1098/rspb.2010.1504.

13. Soler, M.; Soler, J. J.; Martinez, J. G.; Moller, A. P. (1995). "Magpie host manipulation by great spotted cuckoos: Evidence for an avian mafia?". *Evolution.* **49**: 770–775. doi:10.2307/2410329.

14. Hoover, J.P.; Robinson, S.K. (2007). "Retaliatory mafia behavior by a parasitic cowbird favors host acceptance of parasitic eggs". Proceedings of the National Academy of Sciences of the United States of America. **104**: 4479–4483. doi:10.1073/pnas.0609710104.

15. ^ Jump up to:[a] [b] Moksnes, A; Roskaft, E (1995). "Egg-morphs and host preference in the common cuckoo (Cuculus canorus): an analysis of cuckoo and host eggs form European museums and collections". J. Zool. **236**: 625–648. doi:10.1111/j.1469-7998.1995.tb02736.x.

16. Vogl, W; Taborsky, M; Taborsky, B; Teuschl, Y; Honza, M (2002). "Cuckoo females preferentially use specific habitats when searching for hot nests". Animal Behaviour. **64**: 843–850. doi:10.1006/anbe.2003.1967.

17. Roldán, M.; Soler, M. (2011). "Parental-care parasitism: How do unrelated offspring attain acceptance by foster parents?". *Behavioral Ecology.* **22** *(4): 679–691. doi:10.1093/* beheco/arr041.

18. Lyon, Bruce E (2003). "Egg recognition and counting reduce costs of avian conspecific brood parasitism". Nature. **422**: 495–499. doi:10.1038/nature01505.

19. ^ Jump up to:[a] [b] Lyon, B. E. (1993). "Conspecific brood parasitism as a flexible female reproductive tactic in American coots". Animal Behaviour. **46** *(5): 911–928. doi:10.1006/anbe.1993.1273.*

20. Hoi, H.; Darolová, A.; Krištofík, J. (2010). "Conspecific brood parasitism and anti-parasite strategies in relation to breeding density in female bearded tits". Behaviour. **147** *(12): 1533–1549.* doi:10.1163/000579510X511060.

21. Robertson, G. J. (1998). "Egg adoption can explain joint egg-laying in common eiders". Behavioral Ecology and Sociobiology. **43** *(4-5): 289–296.* doi:10.1007/s002650050493.

22. Gloag, R.; Tuero, D. T.; Fiorini, V. D.; Reboreda, J. C.; Kacelnik, A. (2012). "The economics of nestmate killing in avian brood parasites: A provisions trade-off". Behavioral Ecology. **23** *(1): 132–140. doi:10.1093/*beheco/arr166.

23. Sato, Tetsu (4 September 1986). "A brood parasitic catfish of mouthbrooding cichlid fish in Lake Tanganyika". Nature. **323**: 58–59. doi:10.1038/323058a0. PMID 3748180.

24. Baba, Reiko; Nagata, Yoshikazu; Yamagishi, Satoshi (October 1990). "Brood parasitism and egg robbing among three freshwater fish". Animal Behaviour. **40**: 776–778. doi:10.1016/s0003-3472(05)80707-9.

25. Pawelek, Jaime; Coville, Rollin. "Cuckoo Bees". UC Berkeley. Retrieved 24 February 2015.

26. Kawakita, Atsushi; Sota, Teiji; Ito, Masao; Ascher, John S.; Tanaka, Hiroyuki; Kato, Makoto; Roubik, David W. (May 2004). "Phylogeny, historical biogeography, and character evolution in bumble bees (Bombus: Apidae) based on simultaneous analysis of three nuclear gene sequences". Molecular Phylogenetics and Evolution. **31** *(2): 799–804. doi:10.1016/j.ympev.2003.12.003.*

27. Dapporto L, Cervo R, Sledge MF, Turillazzi S (2004). "Rank integration in dominance hierarchies of host colonies by the paper wasp social parasite Polistes sulcifer (Hymenoptera, Vespidae)". Journal of Insect Physiology **50** :217–223

28. Ortolani, I.; Cervo, R. (2009). "Coevolution of daily activity timing in a host-parasite system". Biological Journal of the Linnean Society. **96** *(2): 399–405. doi:10.1111/j.1095-8312.2008.01139.x.*

29. Akino, T; JJ Knapp; JA Thomas; GW Elmes (1999). "Chemical mimicry and host specificity in the butterfly Maculinea rebeli, a social parasite of Myrmica ant colonies". Proceedings of the Royal Society B. **266** *(1427): 1419–1426. doi:10.1098/rspb.1999.0796.*

CHAPTER 10

Obligate Parasite

Chapter Contents

Parasites are organisms that depend on other living beings for their survival. They need a host to get nutrition and grow. They are ectoparasites and endo parasites. The endoparasites can further be classified into intracellular(these live in the host's cells) and intercellular parasites(these live in the spaces in the host's body). The parasites have specialized parts that can absorb nutrition from the cells of the host to thrive and grow. Social parasites , epiparasites are another kind of parasites. Obligate parasites cannot live outside the hosts body. They die once they leave the hosts body as they are completely dependent on the host for their nutrition and completion of their life cycle.

INTRODUCTION

An **obligate parasite** or **holoparasite**, is a parasitic organism that cannot complete its life-cycle without exploiting a suitable host. If an obligate parasite cannot obtain a host it will fail to reproduce. This is opposed to a facultative parasite, which can act as a parasite but does not rely on its host to continue its life-cycle. Obligate parasites have evolved a variety of parasitic strategies to exploit their hosts.

It is advantageous for the parasite to preserve the health of their host when this is compatible with their nutritional and reproductive requirements, except when the death of the host is necessary for transmission.

SPECIES

Obligate parasitism is exhibited in a range of organisms, with examples in viruses, bacteria, fungi, plants, and animals. They are unable to complete their development without passing through at least one parasitic stage which is necessary to their life-cycle.

Whether one regards viruses as living organisms or not, they cannot reproduce except by means of resources within living cells, and accordingly, it is convenient and customary to regard them as obligate intracellular parasites.

Among the Vespidae family, Vespula austriaca is an example of an obligate parasite; its common host is Vespula acadica. In the genus Bombus, B. bohemicus is an obligate parasite of B. locurum, B. cryptarum, and B. terrestris.

HOST-PARASITE INTERACTION

Life-Cycle

Parasitic life-cycles involve the exploitation of at least one host. Parasites that infect a single species are said to have **direct** life-cycles. For example, the hookworm species *Necator americanus*. Parasites that infect more than one host are said to have a **complex** or **indirect** life-cycle. For example, the Malaria plasmodium.

Intermediate or final Host

An **intermediate** or **secondary** host is exploited by the parasite only for a short transition period. A **final** or **primary** host is exploited by the parasite and is the only location in which the parasite is able to reach maturity and if possible, reproduce sexually. For example, *Ribeiroia ondatrae* uses Ramshorn snail as its first intermediate host, amphibians and fish as second intermediate hosts and birds as definitive hosts.

Parasitic Permanence

Obligate parasites may not necessarily spend all of their time behaving as parasites. When a parasite is **permanent**, a number of generations occur in or on the host of an infested individual. Head lice are an example of this. **Temporary** parasites are organisms whose parasitic mode of life is limited to a few or even one stage of development. An example of this is the larval stage of harvest mites, while the adult stage is non-parasitic.

Location on Host

The parasite may live outside of the host **ectoparasite** for example, a tick. Alternatively, the parasite may live within the host **endoparasite** for example, the fluke. A special alternative whereby the obligate parasite does not live directly in or on the host, but rather acts at a distance. For example, a cuckoo which hatches and is raised by non-relatives, is known as a brood parasite.

Invasion Strategies

In order to establish infestation in a susceptible host, obligate parasites must evade defences before, during and after entry into the host. Due to the wide range of obligate parasite types, it is impossible to identify a general invasion strategy. Intracellular parasites use various strategies to invade cells and subvert cellular signalling pathways. Most bacteria and viruses undergo passive uptake, where they rely on the host cell for uptake. However, apicomplexans engage in active entry. One obligate wasp parasite, *Polistes atrimandibularis*, infiltrates their hosts' colony by modifying their chemical signature to match that of the hosts'. This tricks the host wasps into thinking the parasite is one of their own.

Evasion of Host Defences

A number of obligate intracellular parasites have evolved mechanisms for evading their hosts cellular defences, including the ability to survive in distinct cellular compartments. One of the mechanisms that hosts employ in their attempt to reduce the replication and spread of pathogens is apoptosis (programmed cell death). Some obligate parasites have developed ways to suppress this phenomena, for example *Toxoplasma gondii* although the mechanism is not yet fully understood.

Manipulation of Host Behaviour

Changes in a host's behaviour following infection with obligate parasites are extremely common. Unusual behaviour observed in infected individuals is noted, and if its complexity suggests that this behaviour will benefit the transmission of the parasite, then this is said to be an example of adaptive manipulation. However, there is a difficulty in demonstrating changes in behaviour are the result of a selective process favouring transmission of the parasite. It has been suggested that these changes may merely be a side-effect of infection. Most behaviour changes have not been demonstrated to lead to fitness gains in either the host or the parasite. An example of this behaviour is the attraction of rats to cat urine after infection with *Toxoplasma gondii*.

Extended Phenotype

In some cases the behaviour we observe in an organism is not due to the expression of their genes, but rather to the genes of parasites infecting them. This behaviour is an extended phenotype.

Evolution of Host Behaviour Manipulation

Three main evolutionary routes have been suggested for the appearance of host behaviour manipulation by parasites. The first is a *parasite driven* scenario Of manipulation, while the second and third are *host driven* scenarios of manipulation.

- Manipulation *sensu stricto* (extended phenotype- abhorrent behaviour displayed by parasitised hosts results from the expression of the parasites genes) this capacity could have been the product of natural selection in an ancestral parasite with the trait.

- The mafia-like strategy- retaliation for non-compliance (eg.great spotted cuckoo and magpie) magpies that eject the cuckoos eggs from their nest suffer a much greater rate of cuckoo predation.
- The exploitation of compensatory responses induce host compensatory responses since these may at least partially match with the transmission routes of parasites. E.g. the sexually transmitted ectoparasite *Chrysomelobia labidomerae*, parasitizing the leaf beetle host *Labidomera clivicollis~* infected males exhibit increased sexual behaviour and as a result enhance inter- and intra- sexual contacts (copulation and competition) which provide more opportunities for parasite transmission.

It has been suggested that extended phenotype behaviours are not adaptive, but are Exaptative. While they may have a benefit for the parasitic organism, they did not arise with the intention of this benefit.

PARASITIC MIMICRY IN BROOD PARASITES

The cowbird and cuckoo require the nests and parental care of other passerines in order for their young to fledge. These are known as brood parasites. The parasitic bird species mimics egg patterns and colours of the host species, which reduces egg rejection. The chicks of some species are able to manipulate host behaviour by making rapid calls that mimic the sound made by up to four of the host chicks. Mimicry of the host species also occurs in the paper wasp species *Polistes semenowi* and *Polistes sulcifer* and the bumblebee species *Bombus bohemicus*, with the parasite changing its proportions of cuticular hydrocarbons, species- and colony-specific identifying chemicals, to match that of the usurped host species.

It is proposed that this mimicry has evolved through two processes: either as coevolutionary responses to host defences against brood parasites or modifying pre-existing host provisioning strategies. Competition between the parasite and host young for parental resources might lead to exaggeration of the aspects of the signal that most effectively exploit host parents. The parasitic young are likely to experience stronger selection for exaggerated signals than host young, because they are unrelated to the other chicks in the nest and therefore under selection to behave more selfishly.

EVOLUTION OF OBLIGATE PARASITISM

Current theory in evolutionary biology indicates that host-parasite relationships may evolve towards equilibrial states of severe disease. This differs from the conventional belief that commensalism is the ideal equilibrium for both the host and parasite.

Intracellular Parasite

Intracellular parasites are parasitic microorganisms - microparasites that are capable of growing and reproducing inside the cells of a host.

Facultative

Facultative intracellular parasites are capable of living and reproducing either inside or outside cells.

Bacterial examples include:

- *Bartonella henselae*
- *Francisella tularensis*
- *Listeria monocytogenes*
- *Salmonella typhi*
- *Brucella*
- *Legionella*
- *Mycobacterium*
- *Nocardia*
- *Rhodococcus equi*
- *Yersinia*
- *Neisseria meningitidis*

Fungal examples include:

- *Histoplasma capsulatum.*
- *Cryptococcus neoformans*

Obligate intracellular parasites cannot reproduce outside their host cell, meaning that the parasite's reproduction is entirely reliant on intracellular resources.

Obligate intracellular parasites of humans include:

- Viruses
- Certain bacteria, including:
    - *Chlamydia*, and closely related species.
    - *Rickettsia*
    - *Coxiella*
    - Certain species of *Mycobacterium* such as *Mycobacterium leprae*
- Certain protozoa, including:
    - Apicomplexans (*Plasmodium* spp., *Toxoplasma gondii* and *Cryptosporidium parvum*)
    - Trypanosomatids (*Leishmania* spp. and *Trypanosoma cruzi*)
- Certain fungi
    - Pneumocystis jirovecii

The mitochondria in eukaryotic cells may also have originally been such parasites, but ended up forming a mutualistic relationship (endosymbiotic theory).

Study of obligate pathogens is difficult because they cannot usually be reproduced outside the host. However, in 2009 scientists reported a technique allowing the Q-fever pathogen *Coxiella burnetii* to grow in an axenic culture and suggested the technique may be useful for study of other pathogens.

Nutrition

The majority of intracellular parasites must keep host cells alive as long as possible while they are reproducing and growing. In order to grow they need nutrients that might be scarce in their free form in the cell. To study the mechanism that intracellular parasites use to obtain nutrients *Legionella pneumophila*, a facultative intracellular parasite, has been used as a model. It is known that *Legionella pneumophila* obtains nutrients by promoting host proteasomal degradation. Self-degradation of host proteins into amino acids provides the parasite with its primary carbon and energy source.

Susceptibility

People with T cell deficiencies are particularly susceptible to intracellular pathogens.

REFERENCES

1. *Jantsch, J.; Chikkaballi, D.; Hensel, M. (2011). «Cellular aspects of immunity to intracellular Salmonella enterica». Immunological Reviews.* ***240*** *(1): 185–195. doi:10.1111/j.1600-065X.2010.00981.x. PMID 21349094.*
2. *Kelly, B. G.; Wall, D. M.; Boland, C. A.; Meijer, W. G. (2002). «Isocitrate lyase of the facultative intracellular pathogen Rhodococcus equi». Microbiology (Reading, England).* ***148*** *(Pt 3): 793–798. PMID 11882714.*
3. *Spinosa MR, Progida C, Talà A, Cogli L, Alifano P, Bucci C (July 2007). «The Neisseria meningitidis capsule is important for intracellular survival in human cells». Infect. Immun.* ***75*** *(7): 3594–603. doi:10.1128/IAI.01945-06. PMC 1932921. PMID 17470547.*
4. *Sebghati TS, Engle JT, Goldman WE (November 2000). «Intracellular parasitism by Histoplasma capsulatum: fungal virulence and calcium dependence». Science.* ***290*** *(5495): 1368–72. doi:10.1126/science.290.5495.1368. PMID 11082066.*
5. *Alvarez, M.; Burns, T.; Luo, Y.; Pirofski, L. A.; Casadevall, A. (2009). «The outcome of Cryptococcus neoformans intracellular pathogenesis in human monocytes». BMC Microbiology.* ***9****: 51. doi:10.1186/1471-2180-9-51. PMC 2670303. PMID 19265539.*
6. *Amann R, Springer N, Schönhuber W, et al. (January 1997). «Obligate intracellular bacterial parasites of acanthamoebae related to Chlamydia spp». Applied and Environmental Microbiology.* ***63*** *(1): 115–21. PMC 168308. PMID 8979345.*
7. *Deng, M.; Lancto, C. A.; Abrahamsen, M. S. (2004). «Cryptosporidium parvum regulation of human epithelial cell gene expression». International Journal for Parasitology.* ***34*** *(1): 73–82. doi:10.1016/j.ijpara.2003.10.001. PMID 14711592.*
8. Page 28 in: Title: Rook›s textbook of dermatology, Volume 4, Rook›s Textbook of Dermatology, Tony Burns (FRCP.) Authors: Arthur Rook, Tony Burns (FRCP.) Edition: 8 Publisher: John Wiley and Sons, 2010 ISBN 1-4051-6169-8, ISBN 978-1-4051-6169-5
9. *Lynn Sagan (1967). «On the origin of mitosing cells». J Theor Biol.* ***14*** *(3): 255–274. doi:10.1016/0022-5193(67)90079-3. PMID 11541392.*

10. *Omsland, Anders; Cockrell, Diane C.; Howe, Dale; Fischer, Elizabeth R.; Virtaneva, Kimmo; Sturdevant, Daniel E.; Porcella, Stephen F.; Heinzen, Robert A. (Mar 17, 2009). «Host cell-free growth of the Q fever bacterium Coxiella burnetii». Proceedings of the National Academy of Sciences USA.* ***106*** *(11): 4430–4. doi:10.1073/pnas.0812074106. PMC 2657411. PMID 19246385.*

11. Heuner K; Swanson M (editors). (2008). Legionella: Molecular Microbiology. Caister Academic Press.

12. Page 432, Chapter 22, in: *Jones, Jane; Bannister, Barbara A.; Gillespie, Stephen H. (2006). Infection: Microbiology and Management. Wiley-Blackwell. ISBN 1-4051-2665-5.*

13. Combes, C. (1997) Fitness of Parasites: Pathology and Selection International Journal for Parasitology 27 (1): 1-10.

14. Balashov, Yu.S. (2011) Parasitism and Ecological Parasitology. Entomological Review 91 (9): 1216-1223.

15. Schmidt, J.O; Reed, H.C; Akre, R.D (1984). "Venoms of a Parasitic and Two Nonparasitic Species of Yellowjackets (Hymenoptera: Vespidae)". Journal of the Kansas Entomological Society. JSTOR 25084514.

16. Kreuter, Kirsten; Elfi Bunk (November 23, 2011). "How the social parasitic bumblebee Bombus bohemicus sneaks into power of reproduction". Behavioral Ecology and Sociobiology 66 (3): 475–486. doi:10.1007/s00265-011-1294-z. Retrieved 21 September 2015.

17. May, R.M. & Anderson, R.M (1979) Population biology of infectious diseases. Nature 280: 455-461.

18. Goodman, B. A. & Johnson, PTJ. (2011) Disease and extended phenotype: Parasites control host performance and survival through induced changes in body plan. Plos One 6(5):1-10.

19. Hall, B. F.; Joiner, K. A. (1991). "Strategies of obligate intracellular parasites for evading host defences". Immunology Today. 12 (3): A22–7. doi:10.1016/S0167-5699(05)80007-6. PMID 2069674.

20. Sibley, L. D. (2004) Parasite invasion strategies. Science 304(5668): 284-253.

21. Cervo, Rita (December 2006). "Polistes Wasps and Their Social Parasites: An Overview" (PDF). Ann. Zool. Fennici.

22. Hackstadt, T. (1998) The diverse habitats of obligate intracellular parasites. Current Opinion in Microbiology 1: 82-87.

23. Laliberté, J. & Carruthers, V.B. (2008) Host cell manipulation by the human pathogen toxoplasma gondii. Cellular and Molecular Life Sciences 65: 1900-1915.

24. Poulin, R. (1995) "Adaptive" changes in the behaviour of parasitized animals: A critical review. International Journal for Parasitology 5 (12): 1371-1383.

25. ^ Jump up to: a b Hughes, D. (2013) Pathways to understanding the extended phenotype of parasites in their hosts. The Journal of Experimental Biology 216: 142-147.

26. Combes, C. (1991) Ethological aspects of parasite transmission. The American

Naturalist 138 (4): 866-880.

27. McNair D. M. & Timmons E. H. 1977. Effects of Aspiculuris tetraptera and Syphacia obvelata on exploratory behaviour of an inbred mouse strain. Laboratory Animal Science 27:38-42.
28. Pullin, R. (1995) "Adaptive" changes in the behaviour of parasitized animals: A critical review. International Journal for Parasitology 25 (12): 1371-1383.
29. Berdoy, M.F., Webster, J. P & MacDonald, D. W. (2000) Fatal Attraction in rats infected with Toxoplasma gondii. Proceedings of the Royal Society B 267:1591-1594.
30. Adamo, S. A. (2012) The strings of the puppet master: How parasites change host behaviour in Hughes, D.P., Brodeur, J. & Thomas, F. (Eds.), Host Manipulation by Parasites (pp.36-51).Oxford, UK: Oxford University Press.
31. Abbot, P. & Dll, L. M. (2001). Sexually transmitted parasites and sexual selection in the milkweed leaf beetle, Labidomera clivicollis. Oikos 92: 91-100
32. Gould, S. J. & Vrba, E.S. (1982) Exaptation: a missing term in the science form. Paleobiology. 8:4-15.
33. May, R. M., & Robinson, S.K. (1984) Population dynamics of avian brood parasitism. The American Naturalist 126(4):475-494.
34. Kilner, R. M., & Davies, N. B. (1999). How selfish is a cuckoo chick? Animal Behaviour 58:797-808.
35. Sledge, M.F., Dani, F.R., Cervo, R., Dapporto, L., Turillazzi, S. (2001). "Recognition of social parasites as nestmates: adoption of colony-specific host cuticular odours by the paper wasp parasite Polistes sulcifer". Proceedings of the Royal Society of London B 268: 2253–2260.
36. Cervo, R. (2006). Polistes wasps and their social parasites: an overview. Ann. Zool. Fennici, 43, 531-549.
37. Langmore, N. E. & Spottiswoode, C. N. (2012) Visual Trickery in avian brood parasites in Hughes, D.P., Brodeur, J. & Thomas, F. (Eds.), Host Manipulation by Parasites (pp.36-51).Oxford, UK: Oxford University Press.
38. Hauber, M. E. & Kilner, R. M. (2007) Coevolution, communication and host-chick mimicry in parasitic finches: who mimics whom? Behavioural Ecology and Sociobiology 61: 497-503.
39. Lichtensten, G. (2001). Low success of shiny cowbird chicks parasitizing rufous-bellied thrushes: chick-chick competition or parental discrimination? Animal Behaviour 61:401-413.
40. Ewald, P.W. (1983). Host-parasite relations, vectors, and the evolution of disease severity. Annual Review of Ecology and Systematics 14:465-485.

Index